Atlas of Radiologic-Cytopathologic Correlations

Armanda Tatsas, MD
Assistant Professor of Pathology
The Johns Hopkins Hospital
Baltimore, Maryland

Syed Z. Ali, MD
Professor of Pathology and Radiology
The Johns Hopkins Hospital
Baltimore, Maryland

Justin A. Bishop, MD
Assistant Professor of Pathology
The Johns Hopkins Hospital
Baltimore, Maryland

Salina Tsai, MD
Instructor of Radiology
The Johns Hopkins Hospital
Baltimore, Maryland

Sheila Sheth, MD
Associate Professor of Radiology
The Johns Hopkins Hospital
Baltimore, Maryland

Anil V. Parwani, MD, PhD
Associate Professor of Pathology
Director, Pathology Informatics
University of Pittsburgh Medical Center-Shadyside Hospital
Pittsburgh, Pennsylvania

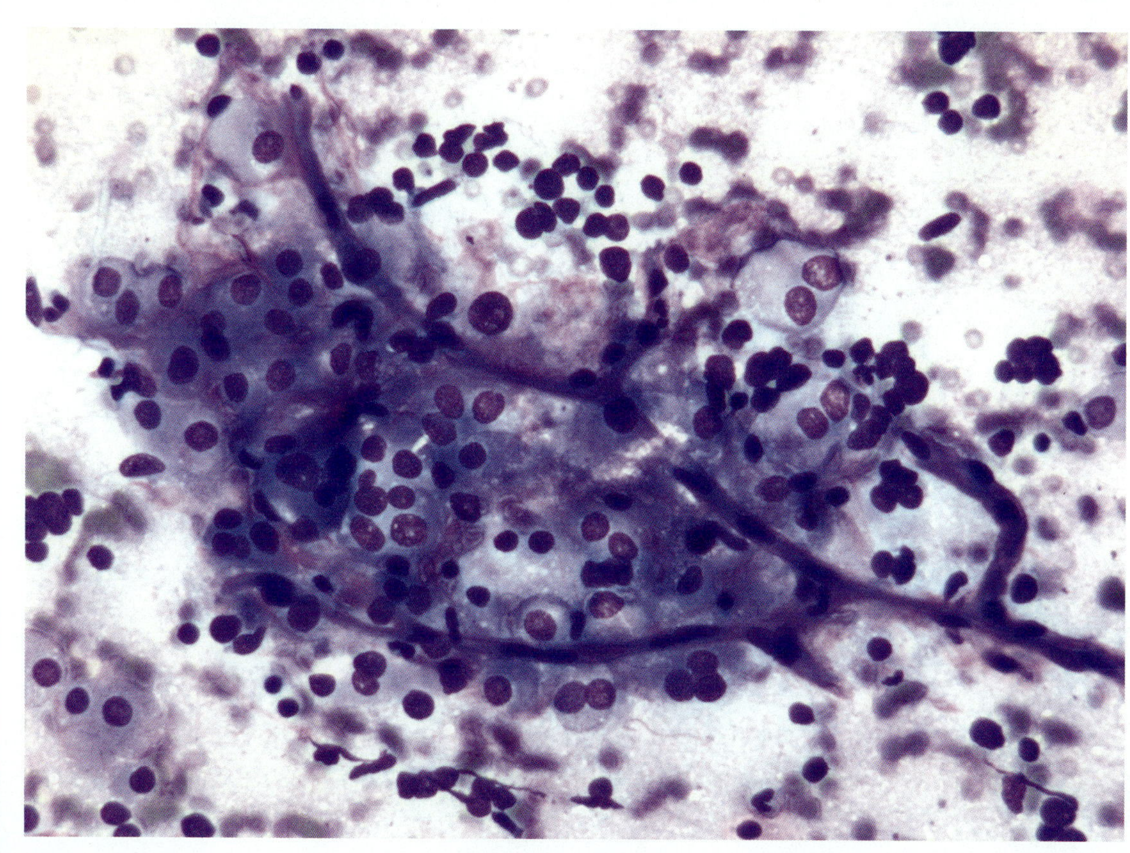

Atlas of Radiologic-Cytopathologic Correlations

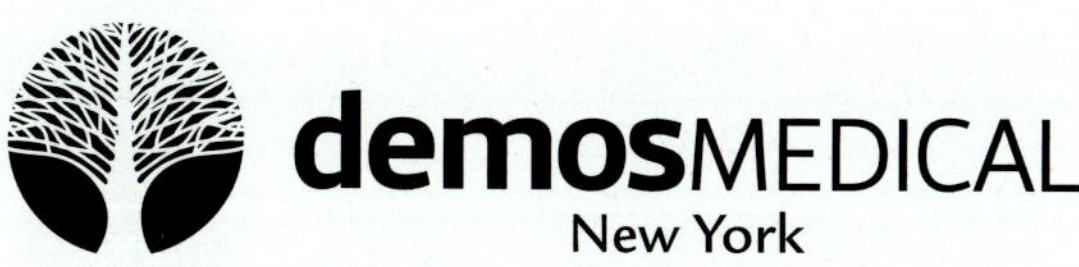
demosMEDICAL
New York

Visit our website at www.demosmedpub.com

ISBN: 9781936287697
e-book ISBN: 9781617051265

Acquisitions Editor: Rich Winters
Compositor: Techset

Medicine is an ever-changing science. Research and clinical experience are continually expanding our knowledge, in particular our understanding of proper treatment and drug therapy. The authors, editors, and publisher have made every effort to ensure that all information in this book is in accordance with the state of knowledge at the time of production of the book. Nevertheless, the authors, editors, and publisher are not responsible for errors or omissions or for any consequences from application of the information in this book and make no warranty, express or implied, with respect to the contents of the publication. Every reader should examine carefully the package inserts accompanying each drug and should carefully check whether the dosage schedules mentioned therein or the contraindications stated by the manufacturer differ from the statements made in this book. Such examination is particularly important with drugs that are either rarely used or have been newly released on the market.

Library of Congress Cataloging-in-Publication Data
CIP data is available from the Library of Congress.

Printed in the United States of America by Bang Printing.
12 13 14 15 / 5 4 3 2 1

Contents

Preface

Cytopathology, one of the most clinically oriented fields within the discipline of Pathology, relies heavily on a multidisciplinary approach since it uses small tissue samples procured through minimally invasive techniques in order to arrive at a diagnosis. As such, cytopathologists frequently depend on the clinical and radiographic impression to align with the cytomorphologic findings in order to arrive at an accurate diagnosis, needed for timely patient management. Furthermore, correlation of a cytopathologic interpretation with a follow-up surgical specimen when available is essential to reinforcing features seen in these small cytologic samples. Therefore, close collaboration of cytopathologists with radiologists and surgical pathologists is pivotal to accurate interpretation leading to optimal patient care.

For this reason, we at The Johns Hopkins Hospital arranged a unique "Radiology-Pathology Correlation Conference" jointly between the Departments of Pathology and Radiology, held since 1997. The educational impact of the conference has been huge and enormously rewarding for both departments involved. In each conference, diagnostically challenging cytology cases performed via fine-needle aspiration are presented followed by an extensive academic and clinical discussion using high-resolution digitized images of the corresponding radiology, cytopathology, and, if available, surgical pathology. Herein we share many of the most challenging, interesting, and illustrative cases we have collected from the conference over the years, encompassing a wide variety of organ systems and body sites.

We hope that this volume will serve as a reference to a wide range of providers who have an interest in understanding the radiographic correlates to cytopathologic diagnoses and that it will promote understanding of how critical radiologic-cytopathologic correlation is for an accurate interpretation of a pathologic process. We also hope that the detailed descriptions of numerous entities will aid in diagnosis of some of the most challenging cases seen in cytopathology.

Armanda Tatsas
Syed Z. Ali
Justin A. Bishop
Salina Tsai
Sheila Sheth
Anil V. Parwani

Baltimore, Maryland

Head and Neck

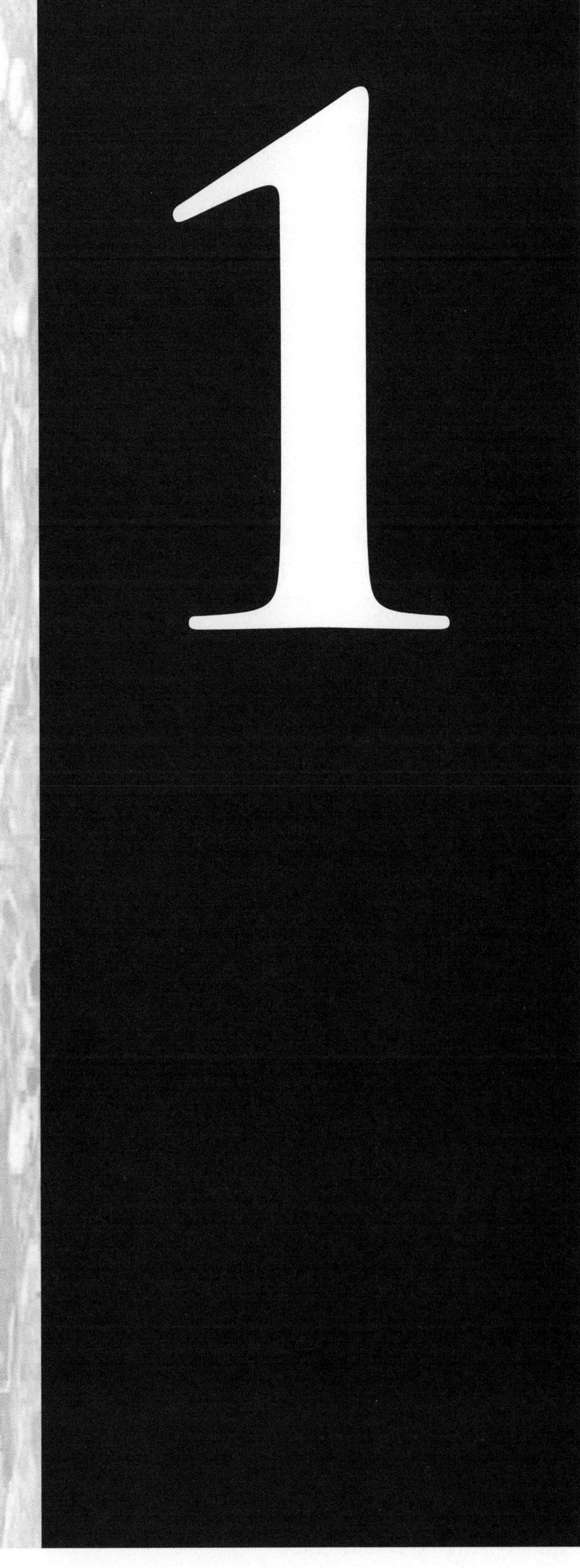

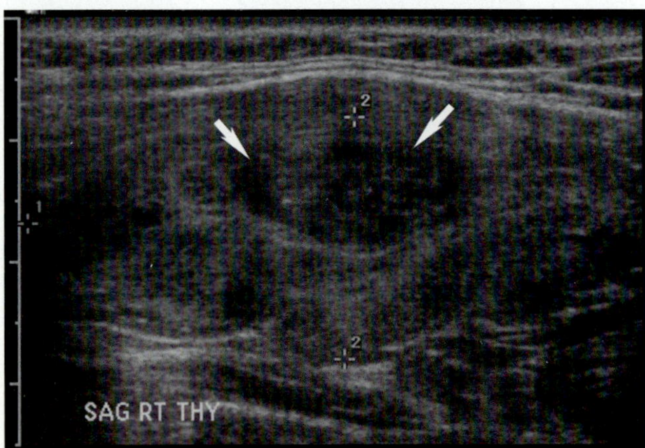

Figure 1.1 — Thyroid, Papillary Carcinoma. Sonographic image demonstrates a diffusely heterogeneous thyroid containing areas of ill-defined hypoechogenicity compatible with Hashimoto thyroiditis. There is also a dominant hypoechoic nodule in the right lobe of the thyroid (arrows).

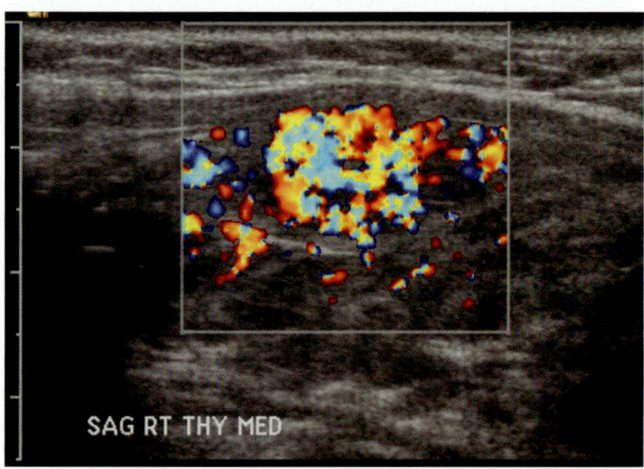

Figure 1.2 — Thyroid, Papillary Carcinoma. This nodule demonstrates marked internal vascularity with color Doppler which can be seen with papillary thyroid carcinoma.

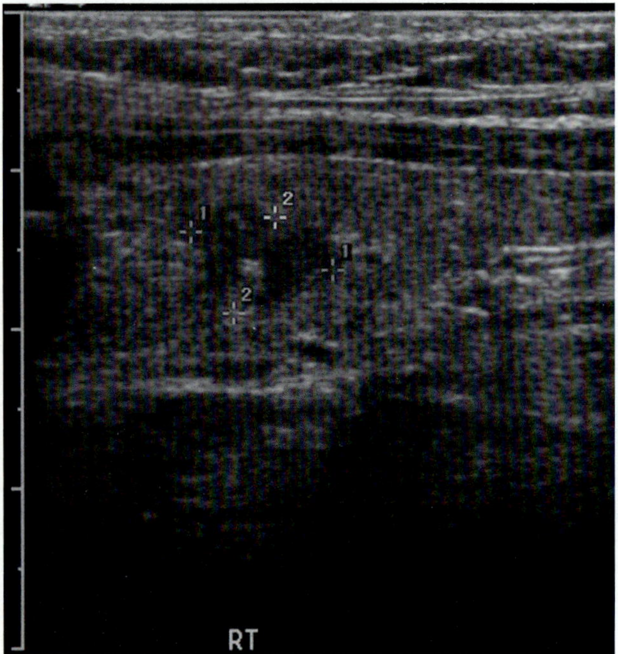

Figure 1.3 — Thyroid, Papillary Carcinoma. Sonographic image in a different patient shows an irregular, hypoechoic right thyroid nodule. Hypoechoic appearance, irregular borders, and the presence of microcalcifications in the mass are suggestive of papillary thyroid carcinoma.

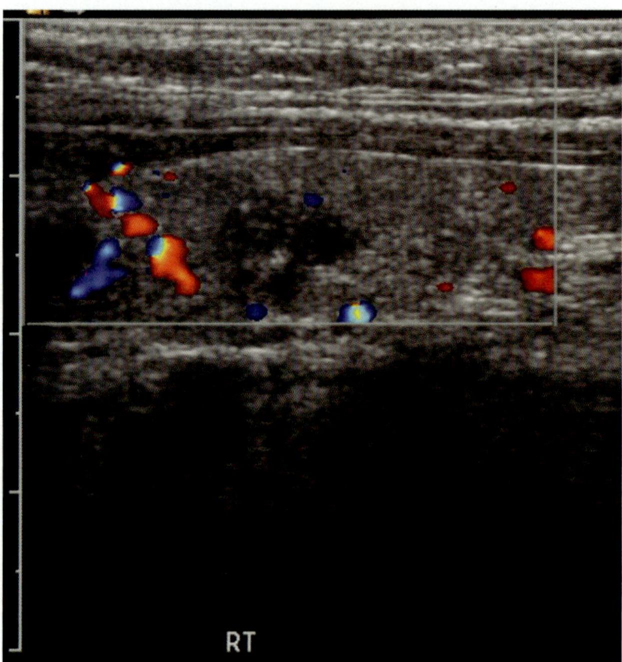

Figure 1.4 — Thyroid, Papillary Carcinoma. There is only minimal vascularity in this nodule with color Doppler. Although papillary thyroid carcinoma can be markedly vascular, the gray scale appearance is highly suspicious for papillary thyroid carcinoma.

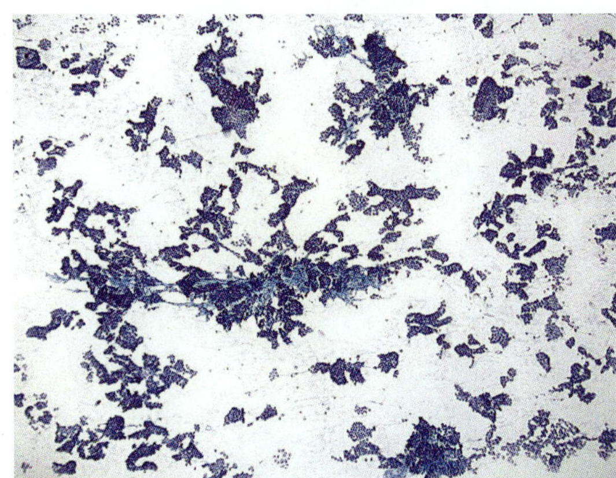

Figure 1.5 — Thyroid, Papillary Carcinoma. Aspirates from papillary thyroid carcinoma are typically hypercellular, consisting of numerous monolayer sheets of malignant epithelial cells. Fragments with papillary architecture and true fibrovascular cores may be encountered, but are not required for the cytologic diagnosis. (Papanicolaou stain, low power)

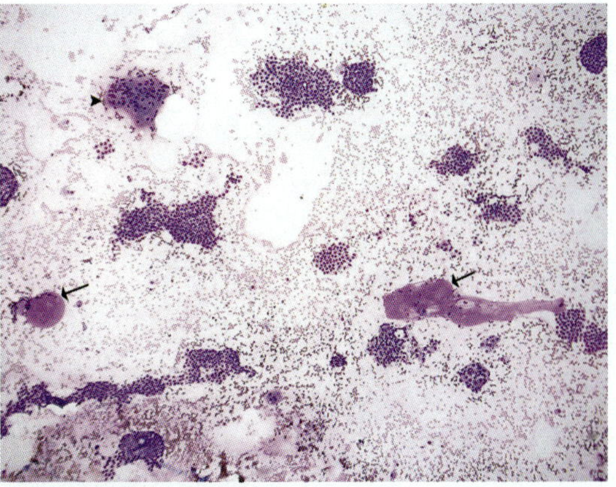

Figure 1.6 — Thyroid, Papillary Carcinoma. Numerous small flat sheets of malignant follicular cells are present. Thick, dense so-called "bubble-gum" colloid (arrows) is characteristic of papillary thyroid carcinoma. Multinucleated giant cells (arrowhead) are often encountered, but are not a specific finding for this tumor. (Diff Quik stain, low power)

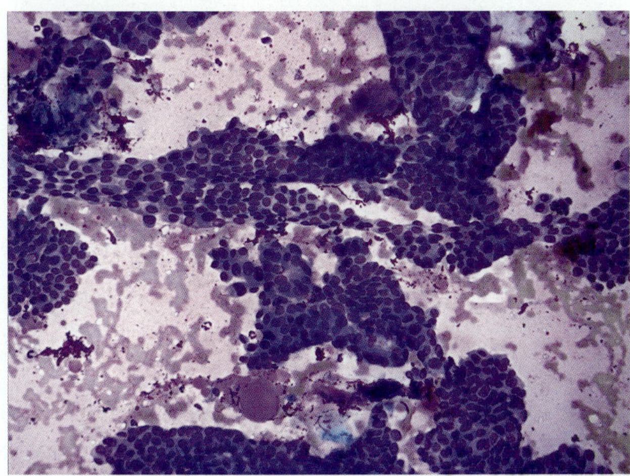

Figure 1.7 — Thyroid, Papillary Carcinoma. A densely cellular aspirate smear shows flat monolayer sheets composed of tumor cells with enlarged, oval-shaped nuclei. A small amount of dense colloid is present. (Diff Quik stain, medium power)

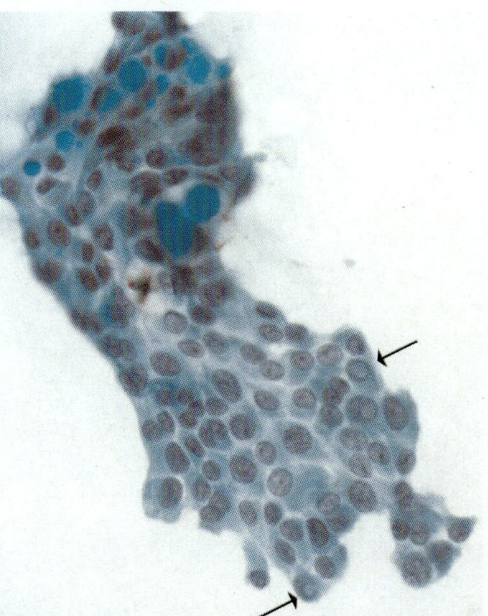

Figure 1.8 — Thyroid, Papillary Carcinoma. Characteristic nuclear features of papillary thyroid carcinoma are typically best demonstrated on Papanicolaou stained material. A flat sheet of malignant cells with ample cytoplasm and oval-shaped nuclei with pale, powdery chromatin is shown. Sharply defined intranuclear pseudoinclusions (arrows), representing cytoplasmic invagination into the nucleus, are evident along with longitudinal nuclear grooves. (Papanicolaou stain, high power)

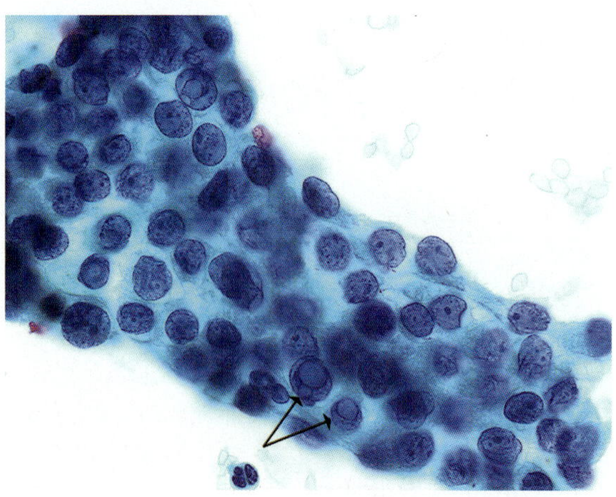

Figure 1.9 — Thyroid, Papillary Carcinoma. Oval-shaped nuclei show irregular nuclear contours and pale chromatin with very small, peripherally-placed "marginal" nucleoli. Intranuclear pseudoinclusions (arrows) match the color of the cytoplasm and are round with sharply defined edges. Intranuclear pseudoinclusions are not entirely specific for papillary thyroid carcinoma, as they may be seen in medullary thyroid carcinoma, hyalinizing trabecular adenoma, and rarely in non-neoplastic settings (e.g., Hashimoto thyroiditis). (Papanicolaou stain, high power)

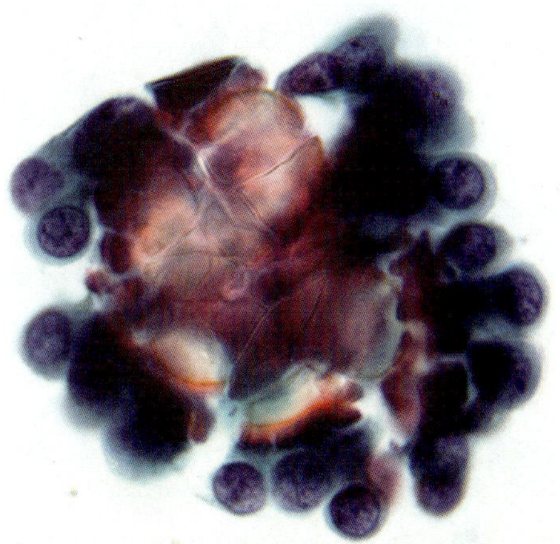

Figure 1.10 — Thyroid, Papillary Carcinoma. A psammoma body (PB) is present surrounded by malignant epithelial cells of papillary thyroid carcinoma. PBs are round calcifications that demonstrate laminated appearance and often appear radially cracked when present on aspirate smears. PBs are not specific for papillary thyroid carcinoma, but their presence should prompt careful examination of the remaining aspirate material and consideration of papillary thyroid carcinoma. (Papanicolaou stain, high power)

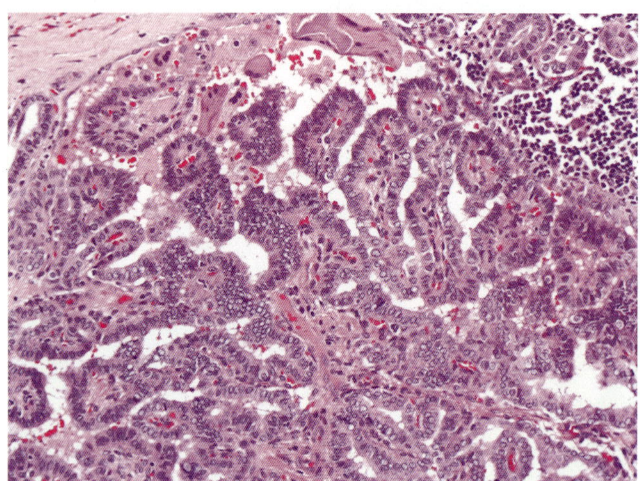

Figure 1.11 — Thyroid, Papillary Carcinoma (Histology). The tumor consists of papillae with fibrovascular cores lined by elongated nuclei that are disordered and overlapping. Note the characteristic ground-glass appearance of nuclei with nuclear grooves. Mitoses are not a usual finding in papillary thyroid carcinoma. (Hematoxylin and eosin stain, high power)

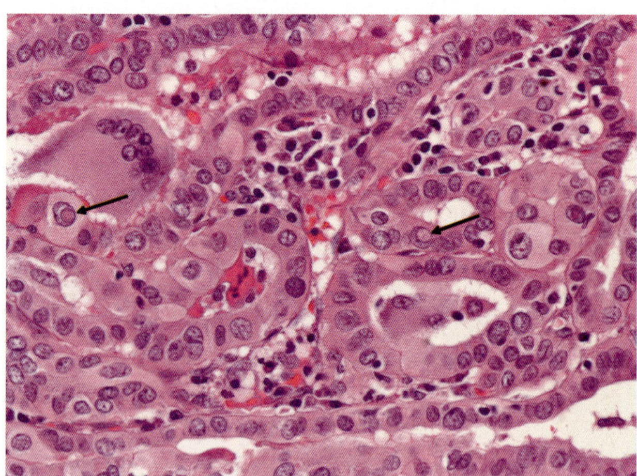

Figure 1.12 — Thyroid, Papillary Carcinoma (Histology). This case shows features of the tall cell variant of papillary carcinoma, with many tumor cells displaying a height greater than two times their width with abundant eosinophilic cytoplasm. Overlapping vesicular nuclei with characteristic nuclear clearing or an "Orphan Annie eye" appearance are evident. Nuclear grooves and pseudoinclusions (arrows) are present. An intrafollicular multinucleated giant cell is seen in the top left portion of the image. (Hematoxylin and eosin stain, high power)

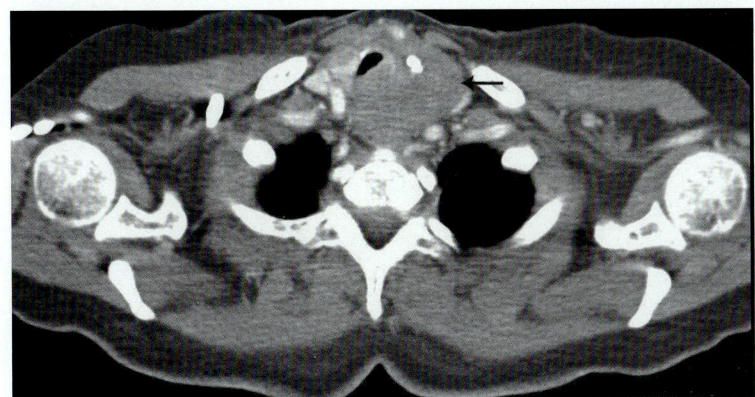

Figure 1.13 — Thyroid, Undifferentiated (Anaplastic) Carcinoma. Axial contrast-enhanced CT image of the neck shows a mass in the left lobe of the thyroid (arrow) containing a focal coarse calcification. The mass deviates the trachea to the right. There is loss of the fat plane between the mass and the trachea and esophagus, suggestive of tumor invasion.

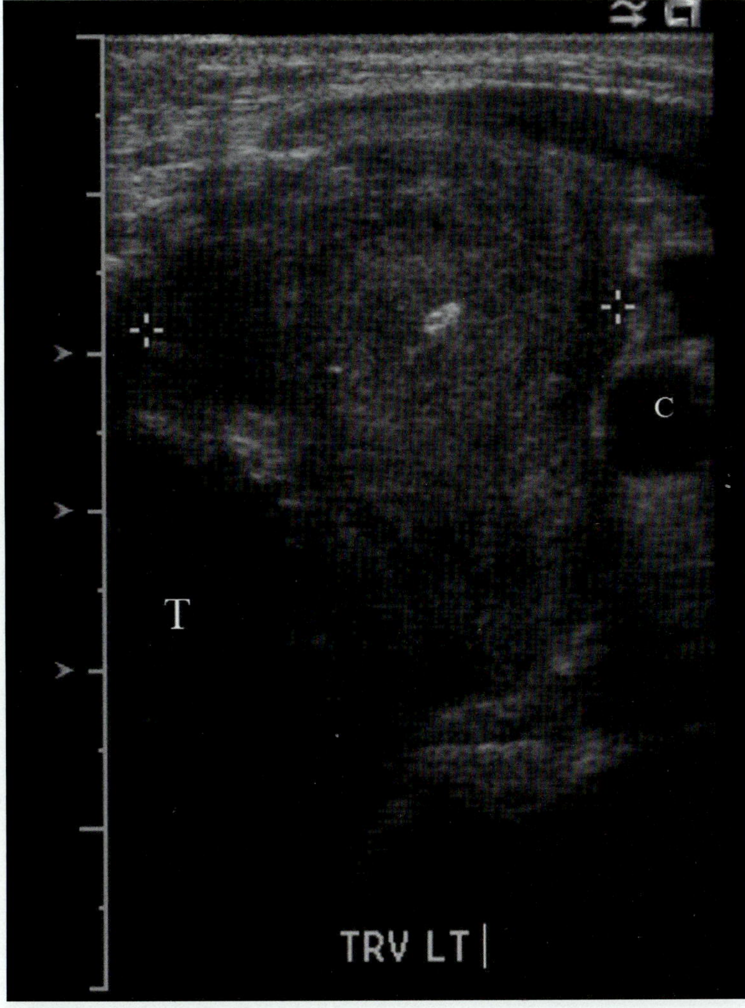

Figure 1.14 — Thyroid, Undifferentiated (Anaplastic) Carcinoma. Transverse sonographic image of the left lobe of the thyroid confirms a heterogeneous mass in the left lobe of the thyroid (T= trachea, C = common carotid artery). Aggressive local invasion is common with anaplastic thyroid carcinoma and lymphoma.

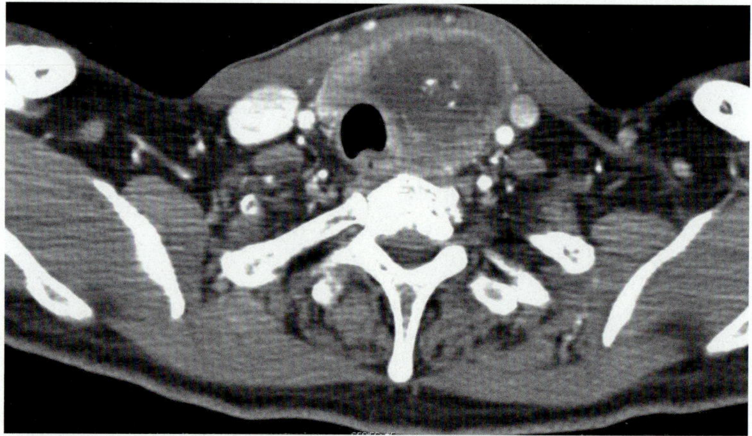

Figure 1.15 — Thyroid, Undifferentiated (Anaplastic) Carcinoma. Axial contrast-enhanced CT image of the neck in a different patient shows a large heterogeneous mass in the left lobe of the thyroid with central necrosis and scattered coarse calcifications. The mass deviates the trachea to the right.

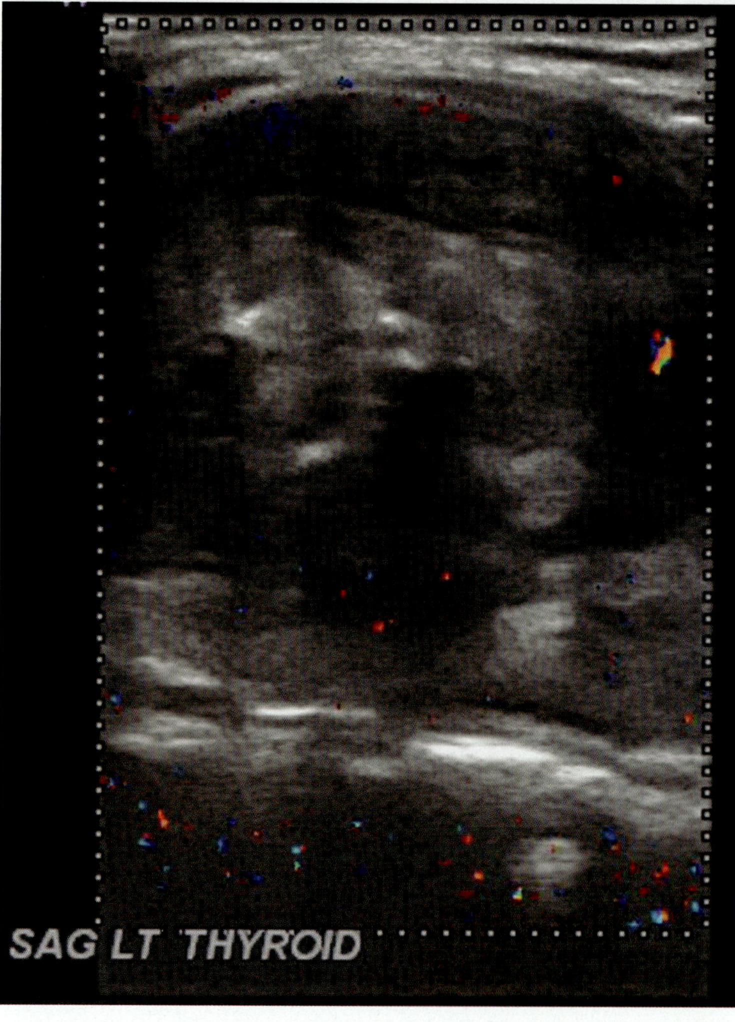

Figure 1.16 — Thyroid, Undifferentiated (Anaplastic) Carcinoma. Sonographic image confirms a large, heterogeneous left thyroid nodule containing coarse calcifications. Anaplastic thyroid carcinomas are rare, representing less than 5% of thyroid cancers.

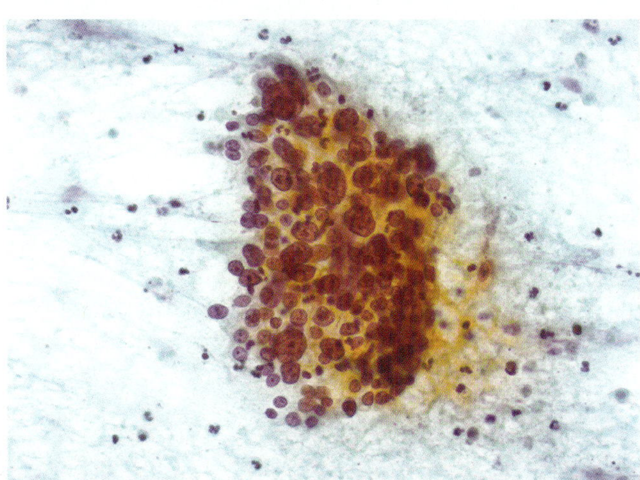

Figure 1.17 — Thyroid, Undifferentiated (Anaplastic) Carcinoma. A cellular fragment demonstrating a disrupted, haphazard architecture is evident. Malignant epithelial cells with marked anisonucleosis are admixed with neutrophils. The background is granular or "grungy" due to necrosis, which is characteristic of anaplastic thyroid carcinoma. (Papanicolaou stain, medium power)

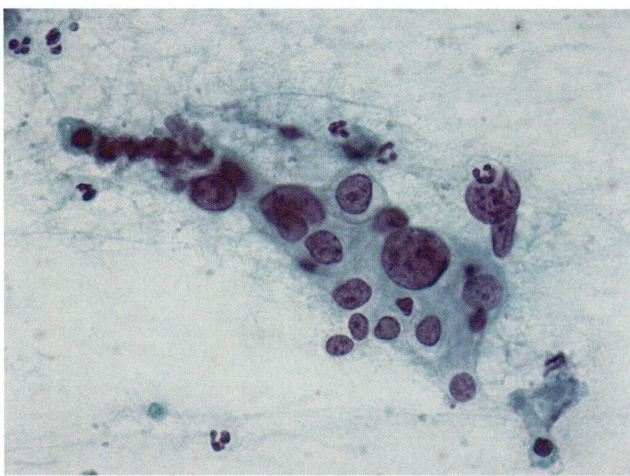

Figure 1.18 — Thyroid, Undifferentiated (Anaplastic) Carcinoma. Markedly pleomorphic cells show nuclear enlargement, hyperchromasia and variably sized nucleoli. Scattered neutrophils embedded in the epithelial fragment are characteristic of anaplastic thyroid carcinoma. A classical clinical history of patient age over 60 years and a rapidly enlarging large thyroid mass supports the diagnosis of anaplastic thyroid carcinoma. (Papanicolaou stain, medium power)

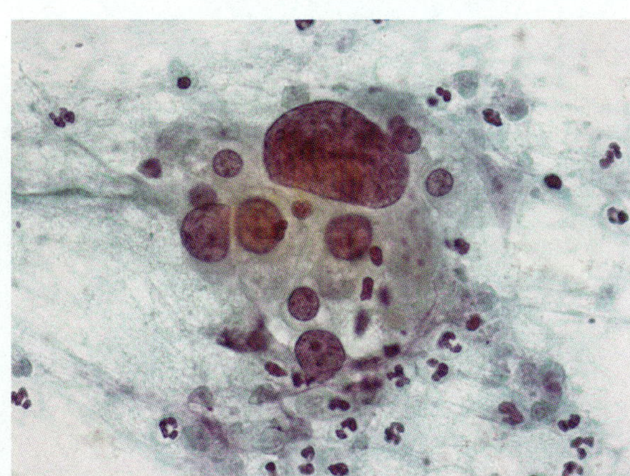

Figure 1.19 — Thyroid, Undifferentiated (Anaplastic) Carcinoma. A small fragment of malignant epithelial cells shows marked anisonucleosis beyond what is expected from any other primary thyroid malignancy. Neutrophils are prominent in and around the epithelial fragment. Occasionally acute inflammation is so prominent that scant malignant epithelial cells may be overlooked and the aspirate mistaken for an abscess or other inflammatory process. (Papanicolaou stain, high power)

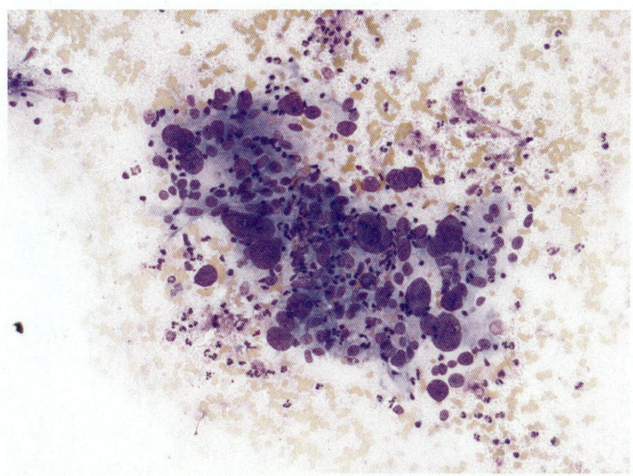

Figure 1.20 — Thyroid, Undifferentiated (Anaplastic) Carcinoma. The neoplastic cells comprising this fragment show both spindled and epithelioid morphology. The cells are cohesive, but show no architectural organization. Anaplastic thyroid carcinomas most likely arise from a pre-existing papillary, follicular or Hürthle-cell carcinoma, thus elements of a better differentiated thyroid malignancy may be present in aspirate smears (not shown). (Diff Quik stain, medium power)

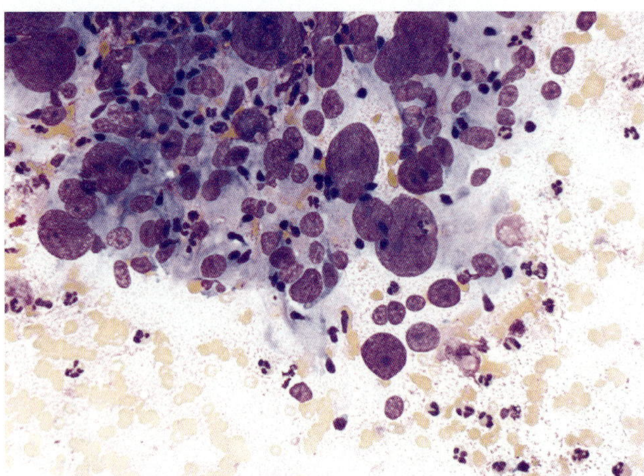

Figure 1.21 — Thyroid, Undifferentiated (Anaplastic) Carcinoma. Nuclei show nuclear hyperchromasia, marked anisonucleosis and prominent nucleoli. Prior to rendering a diagnosis of anaplastic thyroid carcinoma, a metastatic carcinoma, or a sarcoma (primary or metastatic) should be considered. If sufficient sample is obtained for cell block, immunostains may be useful, but anaplastic thyroid carcinomas often lose immunoreactivity for the thyroid-specific markers TTF-1 and thyroglobulin. PAX-8 immunoreactivity, on the other hand, is often retained and can be useful in confirming a thyroid follicular origin. (Diff Quik stain, high power)

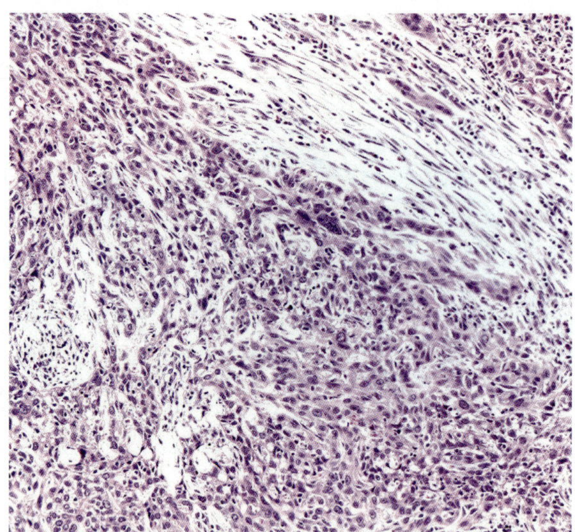

Figure 1.22 — Thyroid, Undifferentiated (Anaplastic) Carcinoma (Histology). Histologically, the three main variants of anaplastic thyroid carcinoma are squamoid, spindle cell, and pleomorphic-giant cell. The current case demonstrates the squamoid variant. (Hematoxylin and eosin stain, low power)

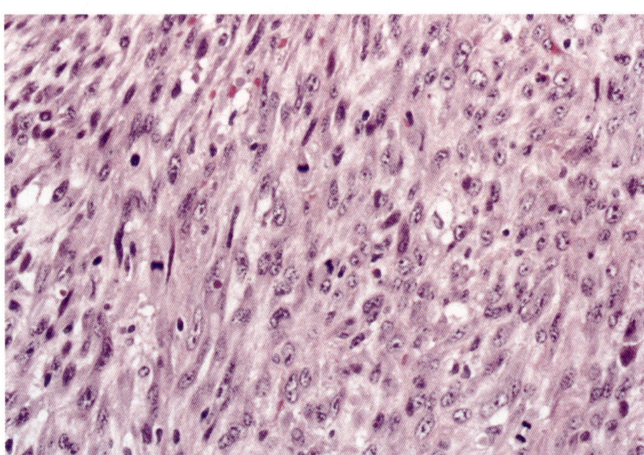

Figure 1.23 — Thyroid, Undifferentiated (Anaplastic) Carcinoma (Histology). A spindled appearance of anaplastic carcinoma is demonstrated. Note the high mitotic activity and pleomorphic nuclei. The carcinoma does not show thyroid follicular differentiation at the light microscopic level, and a true soft tissue sarcoma could be considered in the differential diagnosis. (Hematoxylin and eosin stain, high power)

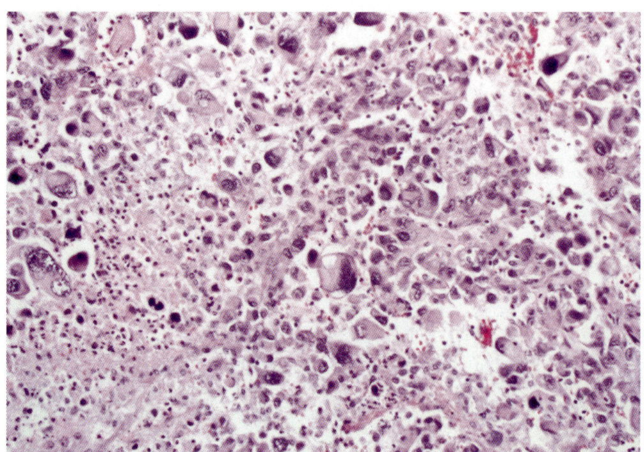

Figure 1.24 — Thyroid, Undifferentiated (Anaplastic) Carcinoma (Histology). This anaplastic thyroid carcinoma, pleomorphic/giant cell type, shows large, bizarre nuclei. Necrosis and an abundance of neutrophils are also evident. Mitotic activity is very high in these tumors. Although these tumors are undifferentiated at the light microscopic level, they are often (but not always) positive for low-molecular-weight cytokeratins and PAX-8. (Hematoxylin and eosin stain, high power)

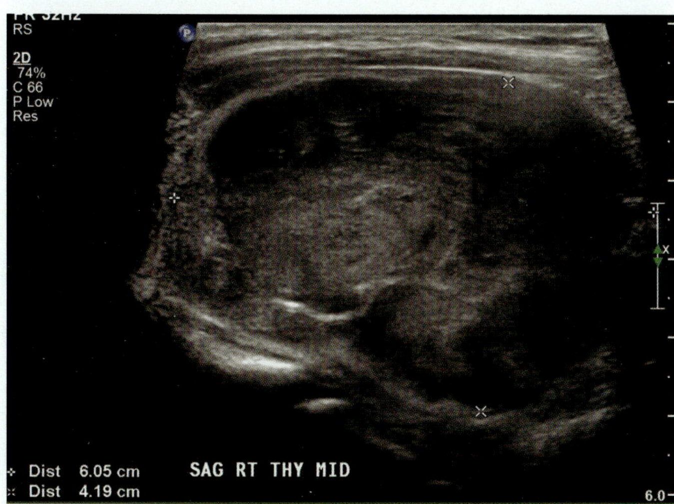

Figure 1.25 — Thyroid, Hürthle Cell Neoplasm. Sonographic image shows a large heterogeneous nodule in the right lobe of the thyroid.

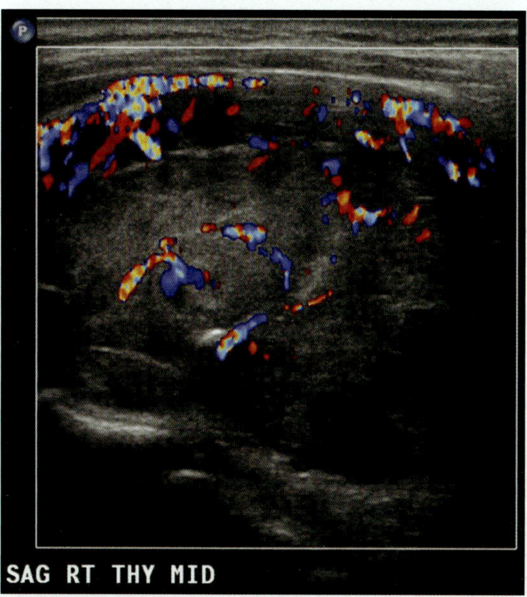

Figure 1.26 — Thyroid, Hürthle Cell Neoplasm. Marked internal vascularity is seen with color Doppler. This nodule did not contain calcifications. The appearance is nonspecific, however Hürthle cell carcinomas can be large, heterogeneous, and lack calcifications as seen in this case.

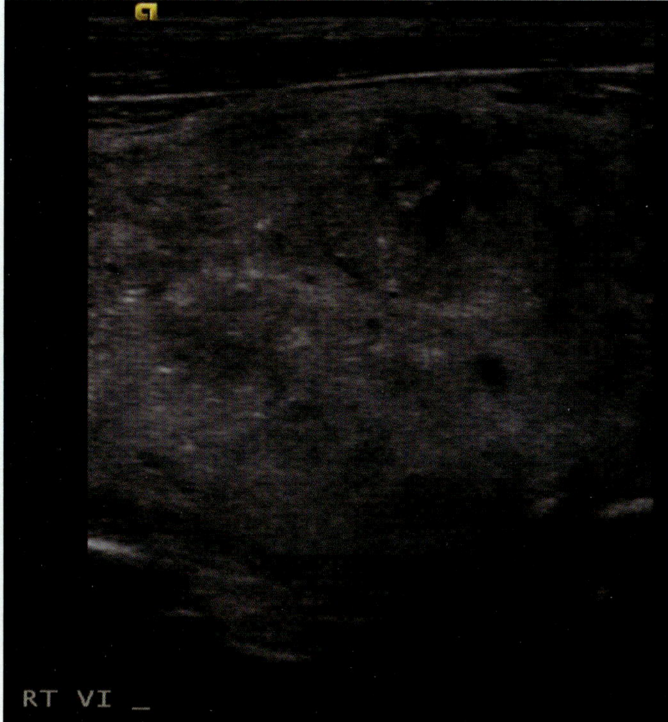

Figure 1.27 — Thyroid, Hürthle Cell Neoplasm. Sonographic image in a different patient demonstrates a large heterogeneous mass in the right lobe of the thyroid.

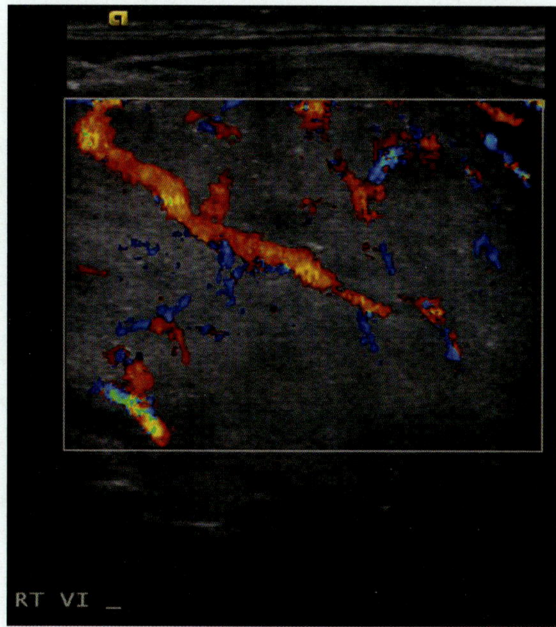

Figure 1.28 — Thyroid, Hürthle Cell Neoplasm. The mass shows marked internal vascularity with color Doppler.

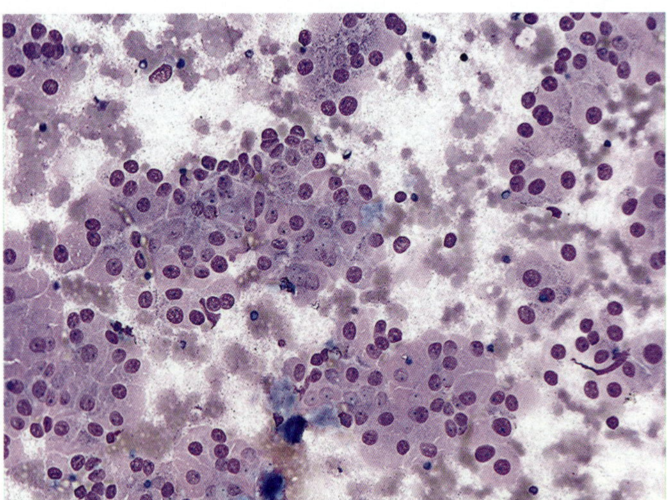

Figure 1.29 — Thyroid, Hürthle Cell Neoplasm. Hürthle-type cells (oncocytes) represent a metaplastic change of follicular epithelium and are characterized by abundant granular cytoplasm with round, centrally-placed nuclei with prominent nucleoli. Hürthle cells may be encountered in benign adenomatoid nodules, in the setting of lymphocytic (Hashimoto) thyroiditis, or in a pure Hürthle cell neoplasm (adenoma or carcinoma). Aspirates from Hürthle cell neoplasms are typically highly cellular, as seen here, and show scant to absent colloid. (Diff Quik stain, medium power)

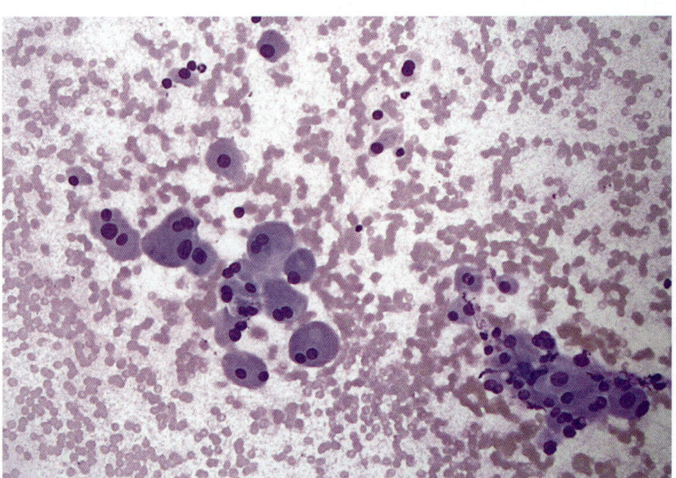

Figure 1.30 — Thyroid, Hürthle Cell Neoplasm. The cells in Hürthle cell neoplasms are frequently dispersed singly or in small clusters and may show bi- or multi-nucleation. Anisonucleosis is characteristic of Hürthle cells in general, and does not indicate a neoplastic process. The distinction between Hürthle cell adenoma and carcinoma cannot be made on cytologic preparations as the diagnosis of carcinoma relies on histologic criteria including capsular and vascular invasion. (Diff Quik stain, high power)

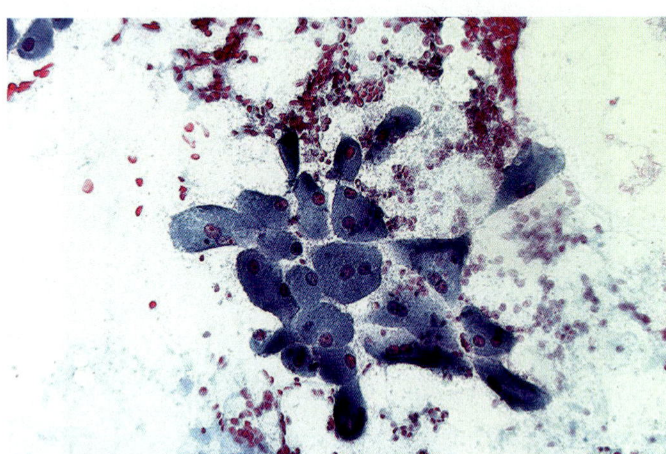

Figure 1.31 — Thyroid, Hürthle Cell Neoplasm. The abundant granular cytoplasm of Hürthle cells is evident on Papanicolaou stained preparations. These neoplastic cells show frequent binucleation. The dyshesive appearance of neoplastic Hürthle cells is likened to "fried eggs in a pan," as seen here. (Papanicolaou stain, high power)

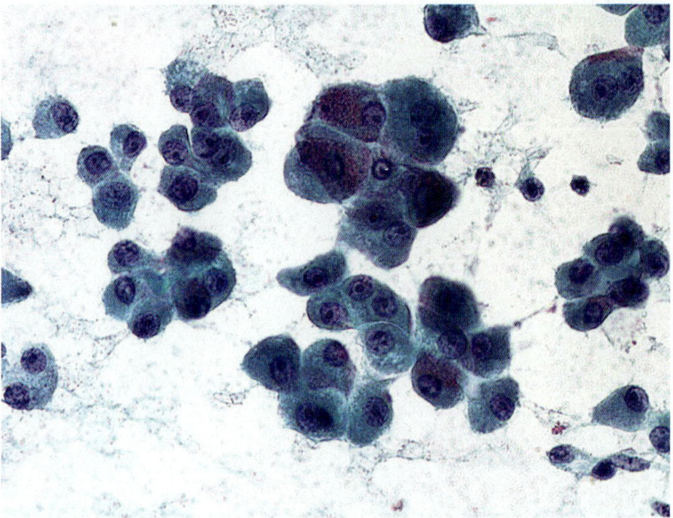

Figure 1.32 — Thyroid, Hürthle Cell Neoplasm. Neoplastic Hürthle cells are present singly and in loose clusters. Abundant granular cytoplasm and round nuclei with prominent nucleoli characteristic of Hürthle cells are evident at high power. Note lack of any background lymphocytes. (Papanicolaou stain, high power)

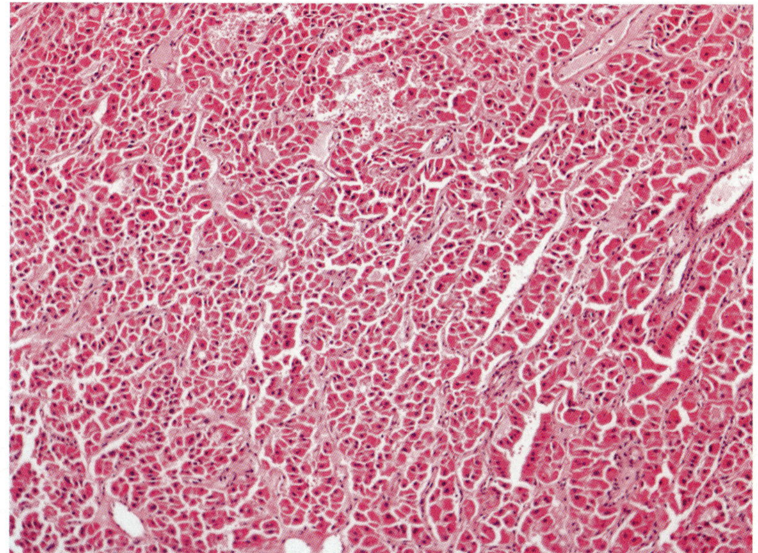

Figure 1.33 — Thyroid, Hürthle Cell Carcinoma (Histology). The cells in Hürthle cell neoplasms have an abundance of mitochondria resulting in a characteristic pink and granular cytoplasm. The nucleus is centrally located and round. (Hematoxylin and eosin stain, medium power)

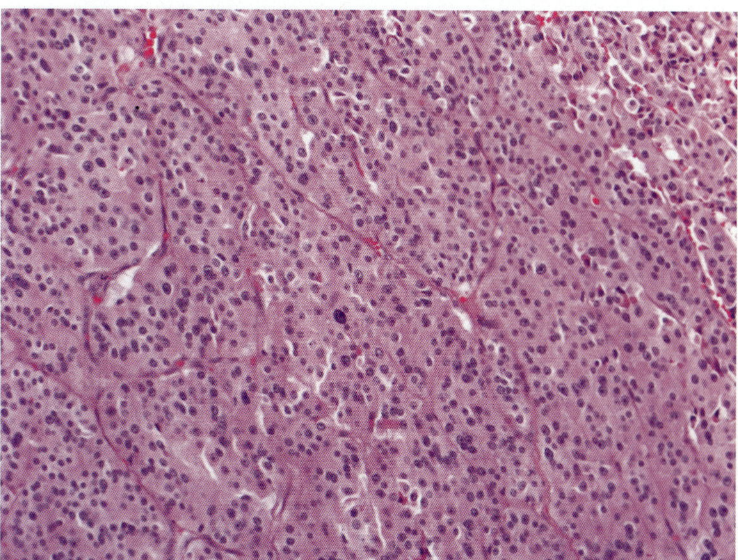

Figure 1.34 — Thyroid, Hürthle Cell Carcinoma (Histology). Hürthle cells with abundant granular cytoplasm and a central, round nucleus with a prominent nucleolus are shown. There is some pleomorphism, with degenerative, "endocrine-type" atypia seen at the center of the image. This atypia is of no prognostic significance, and the diagnosis of Hürthle cell carcinoma depends on identifying invasive tumor growth. (Hematoxylin and eosin stain, high power)

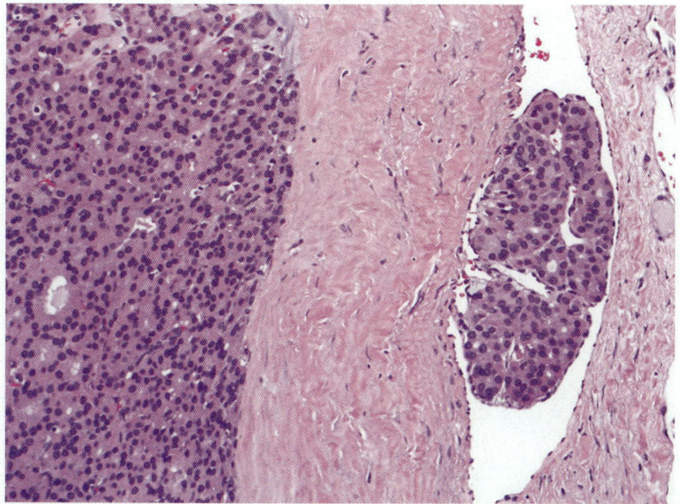

Figure 1.35 — Thyroid, Hürthle Cell Carcinoma (Histology). The diagnosis of Hürthle cell carcinoma rests on the demonstration of vascular invasion, capsular invasion, and/or distant metastasis. Depicted is a focus of vascular invasion in a medium-caliber blood vessel in the tumor capsule; the tumor has been endothelialized, and is focally adherent to the wall of the vessel. (Hematoxylin and eosin stain, high power)

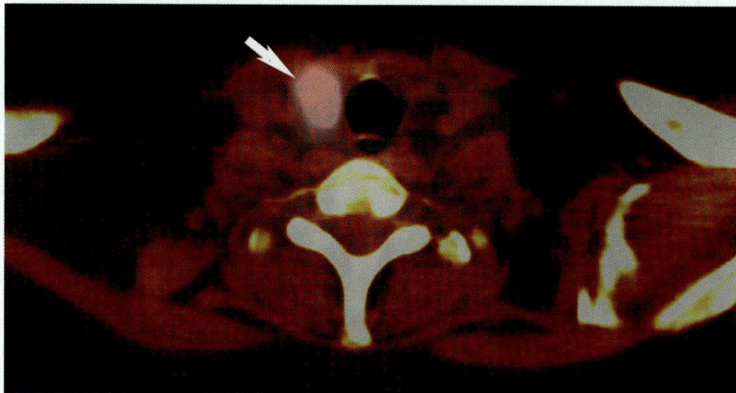

Figure 1.36 — Thyroid, Metastatic Merkel Cell Carcinoma. Axial fused PET/CT shows a FDG-avid right thyroid nodule in a patient with a history of Merkel cell carcinoma which was not present on a PET/CT four months prior. Although metastases to the thyroid gland are uncommon, this diagnosis should be consider if a solid thyroid nodule develops in a patient with a known extrathyroidal primary malignancy.

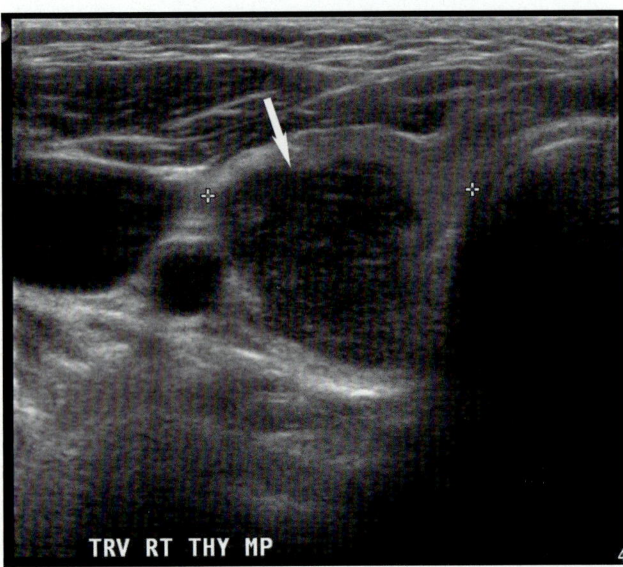

Figure 1.37 — Thyroid, Metastatic Merkel Cell Carcinoma. Sonographic image confirms a well-defined, hypoechoic right thyroid nodule (arrow).

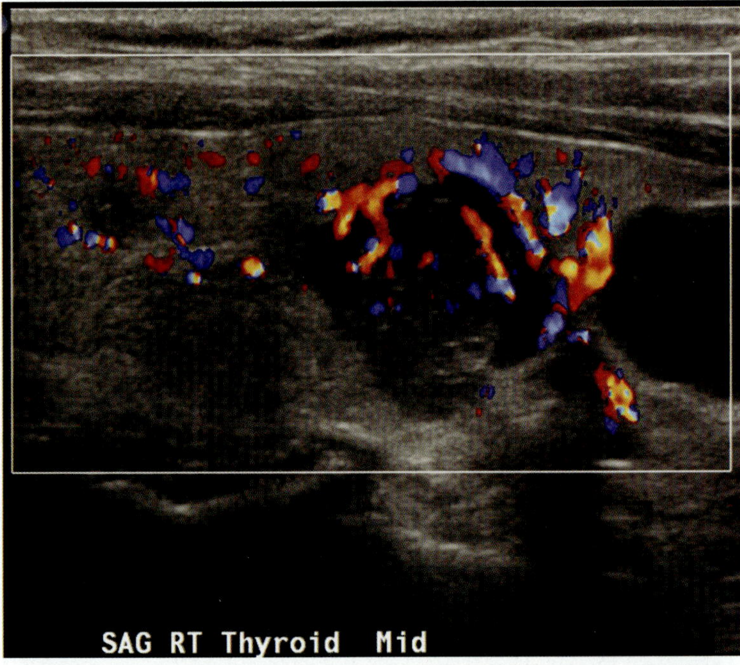

Figure 1.38 — Thyroid, Metastatic Merkel Cell Carcinoma. The nodule shows marked internal vascularity with color Doppler.

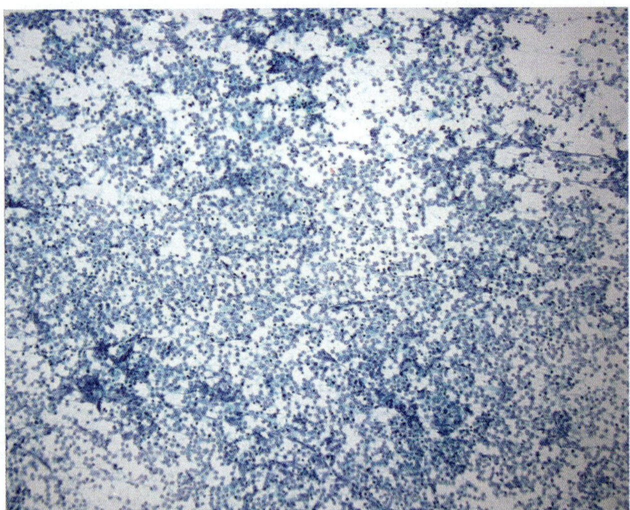

Figure 1.39 — Thyroid, Metastatic Merkel Cell Carcinoma. Merkel cell carcinoma is a rare, aggressive neuroendocrine carcinoma of the skin typically seen in older patients. Lymph node and distant metastases are common. At low power, a markedly hypercellular aspirate is appreciated. In the absence of a clinical history, a hematopoietic neoplasm should be considered at the time of on-site evaluation and additional sample obtained for immunophenotyping (flow cytometry) studies. (Papanicolaou stain, low power)

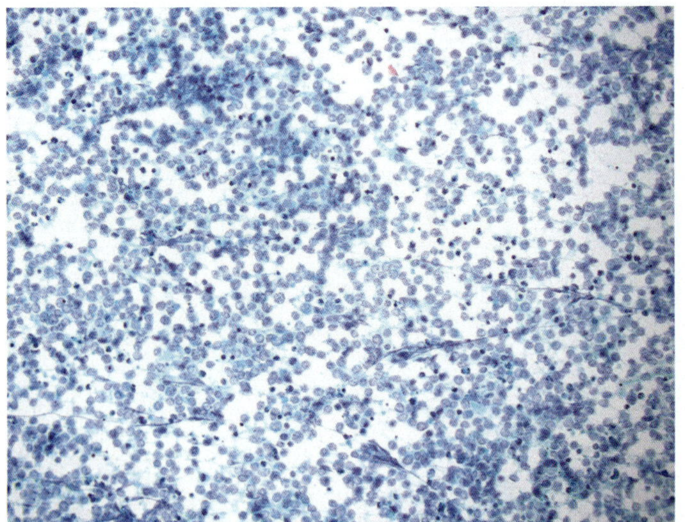

Figure 1.40 — Thyroid, Metastatic Merkel Cell Carcinoma. A monotonous population of neoplastic cells showing scant cytoplasm and round nuclei with fine chromatin is evident. Apoptotic bodies are numerous. Metastatic small cell carcinoma, particularly from a lung primary, should also be considered in the differential diagnosis. (Papanicolaou stain, medium power)

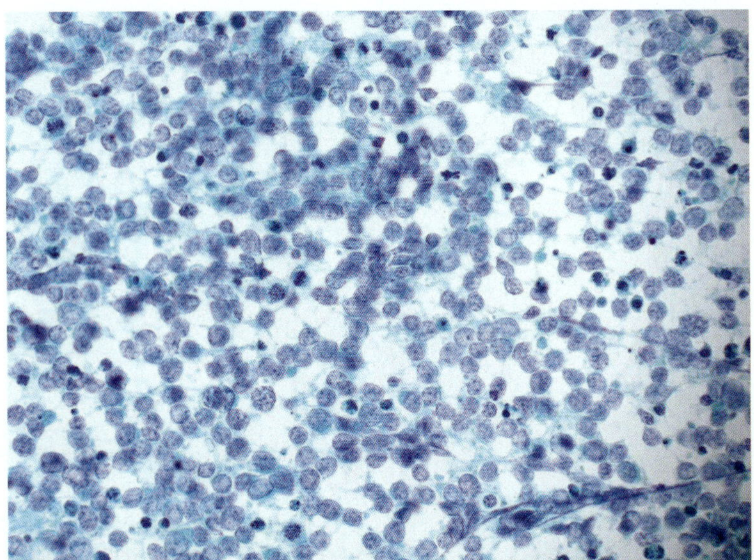

Figure 1.41 — Thyroid, Metastatic Merkel Cell Carcinoma. Malignant Merkel cells show scant cytoplasm, round nuclei with finely dispersed chromatin and occasional nucleoli. Mitoses and apoptotic bodies are present. Distinction from a malignant lymphoid population or from small cell carcinoma is difficult on routine smears. (Papanicolaou stain, high power)

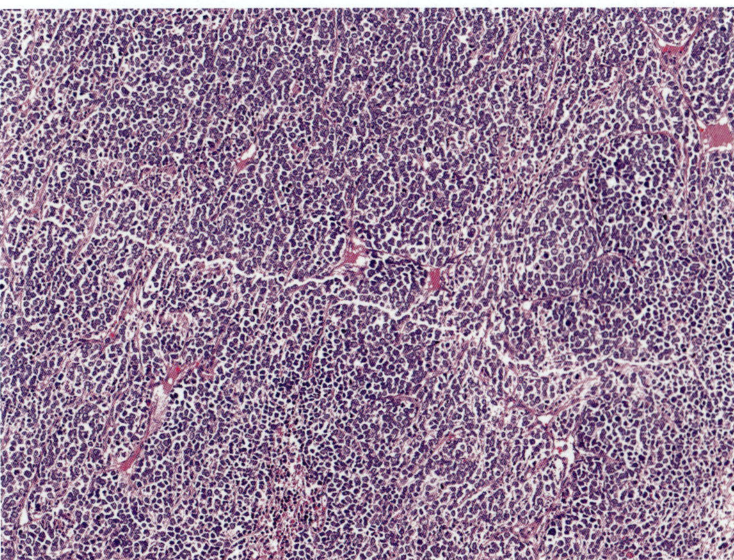

Figure 1.42 — Thyroid, Metastatic Merkel Cell Carcinoma (Histology). Merkel cell carcinoma is composed of undifferentiated small round blue cells. The tumor cells have scant rim of cytoplasm and hyperchromatic nuclei. The nuclei have a "salt and pepper" chromatin pattern with inconspicuous nucleoli. There is extensive apoptosis and mitotic activity. (Hematoxylin and eosin stain, medium power).

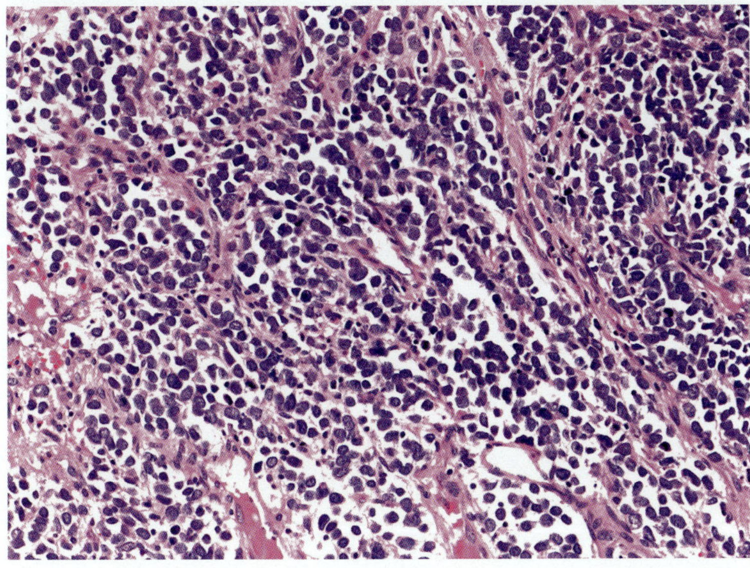

Figure 1.43 — Thyroid, Metastatic Merkel Cell Carcinoma (Histology). Metastatic neoplastic cells are growing in solid sheets of small blue cells with hyperchromatic nuclei. The chromatin pattern is fine and cells have scant cytoplasm. Mitoses were frequent and many apoptotic bodies are seen. Merkel cell carcinoma expresses neuroendocrine markers such as synaptophysin and chromogranin as well as cytokeratin markers; characteristically, Merkel cell carcinoma is positive for CK20 (in a dot-shaped cytoplasmic reactivity) and neurofilament and negative for TTF-1. (Hematoxylin and eosin stain, high power)

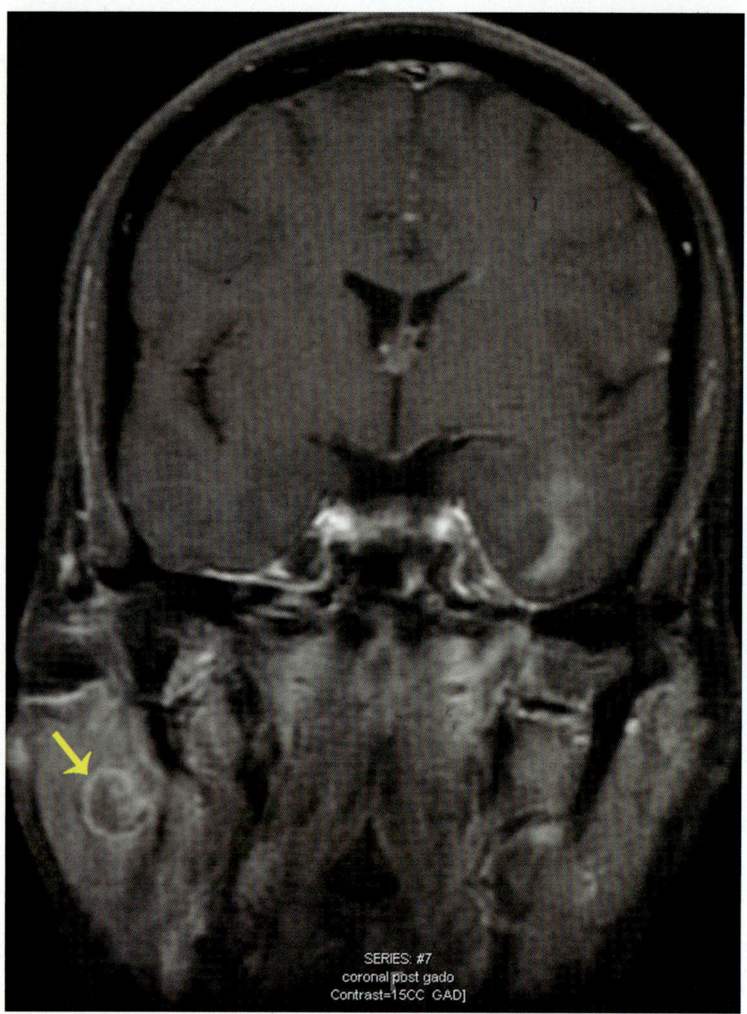

Figure 1.44 — Parotid Gland, Benign Mixed Tumor (Pleomorphic Adenoma). Coronal T1 fat saturated post-contrast MR image shows a well-defined mass in the right parotid gland with peripheral enhancement (arrow).

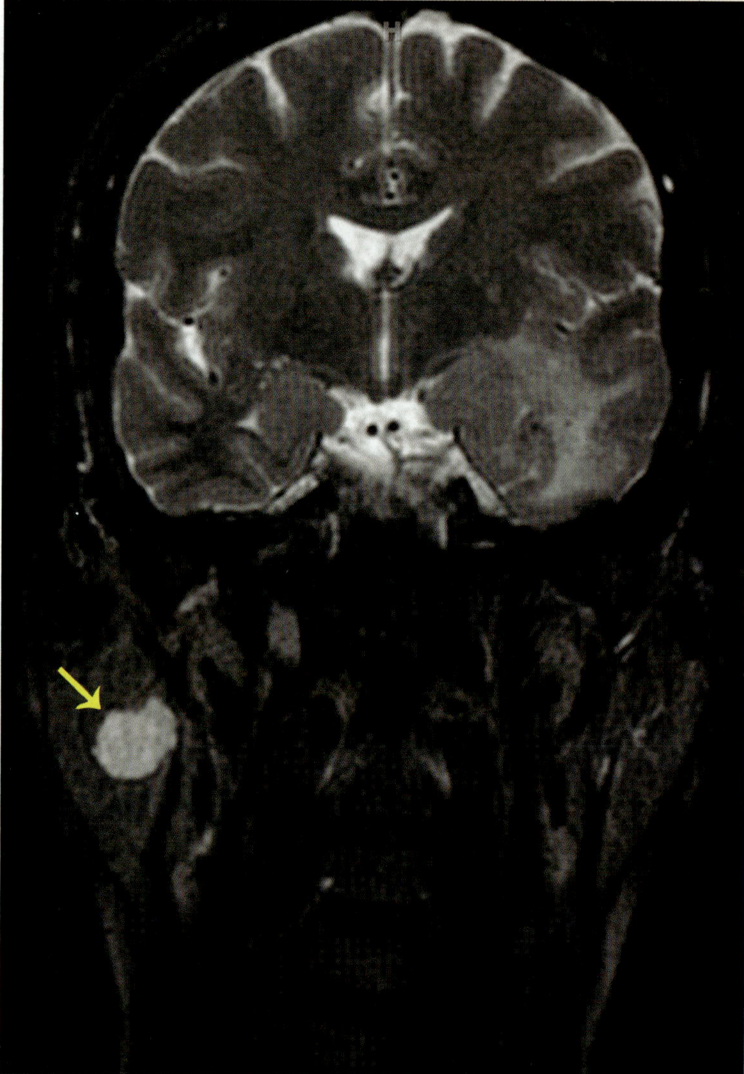

Figure 1.45 — Parotid Gland, Benign Mixed Tumor (Pleomorphic Adenoma). Coronal T2-weighted MR image confirms a well-defined mass in the right parotid gland (arrow) which is T2 hyperintense.

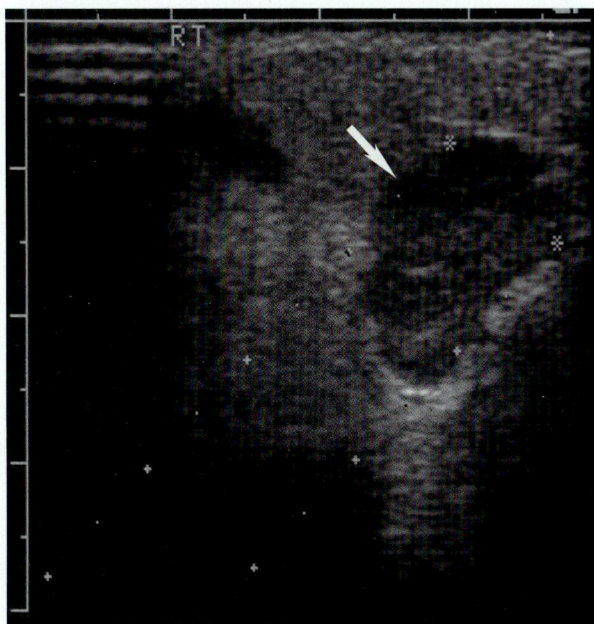

Figure 1.46 — Parotid Gland, Benign Mixed Tumor (Pleomorphic Adenoma). Sonographic image shows the right parotid mass is hypoechoic (arrow). Pleomorphic adenomas are the most common benign parotid tumor, and have a slight female predominance.

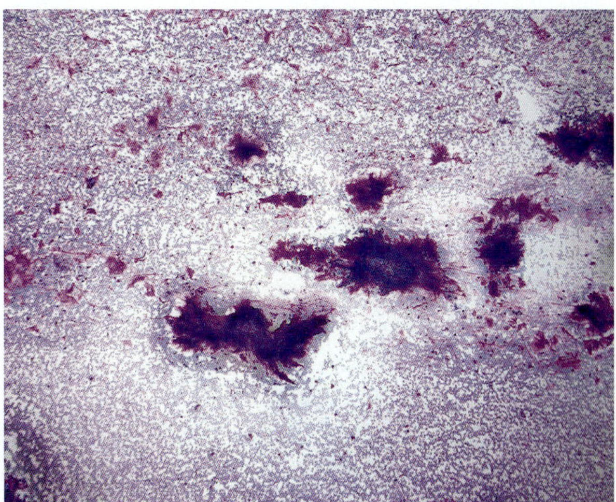

Figure 1.47 — Parotid Gland, Benign Mixed Tumor (Pleomorphic Adenoma). Pleomorphic adenoma is the most common of all salivary gland tumors, and the parotid is the most common site. The most striking cytologic feature is the brightly magenta colored (metachromatic) fibrillary stroma seen here on Diff Quik stain. The stroma appears pale and much less prominent on Papanicolaou stain. The diagnosis can be suspected even at the time of aspiration by gross examination of the shiny tenacious material that is expressed out from the needle. (Diff Quik stain, low power)

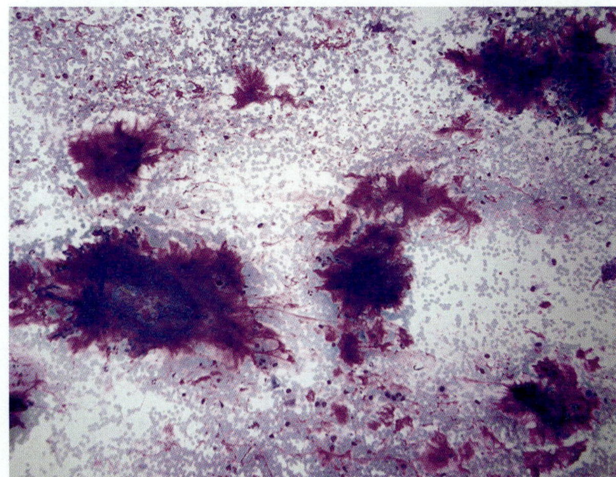

Figure 1.48 — Parotid Gland, Benign Mixed Tumor (Pleomorphic Adenoma). A combination of epithelial and myoepithelial cells are seen along with abundant metachromatic stroma. The stroma appears fibrillary, and should be distinguished from the globoid magenta material seen in adenoid cystic carcinoma of the salivary gland. (Diff Quik stain, medium power)

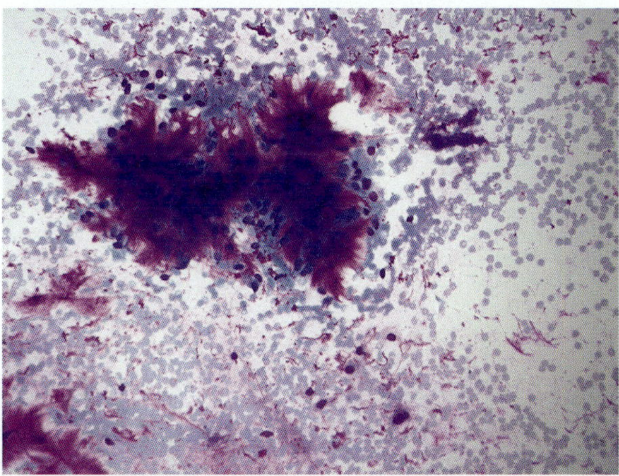

Figure 1.49 — Parotid Gland, Benign Mixed Tumor (Pleomorphic Adenoma). Myoepithelial cells are typically uniform, plump spindle to epithelioid cells which are embedded in the myxoid stroma. They may occasionally show intranuclear inclusions. Other mesenchymal elements may be present, including chondroid and osteoid matrix (not shown). (Diff Quik stain, high power)

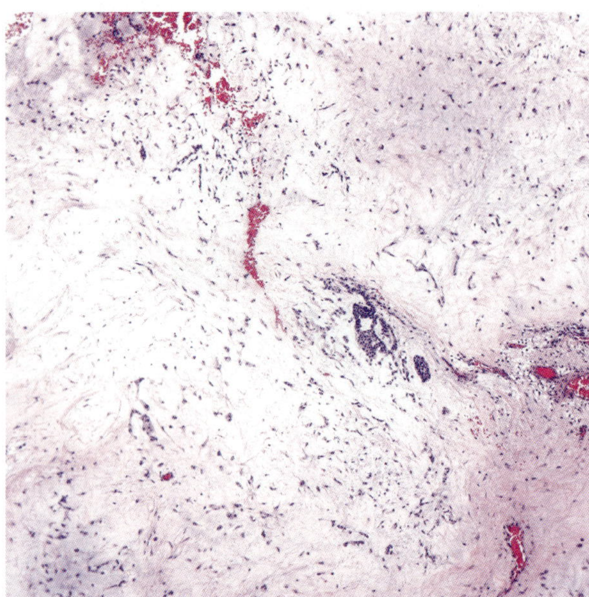

Figure 1.50 — Parotid Gland, Benign Mixed Tumor (Pleomorphic Adenoma) (Histology). Pleomorphic adenomas are composed of both epithelial and stromal components. This section has a predominance of chondromyxoid stroma with scant epithelial component. (Hematoxylin and eosin stain, low power).

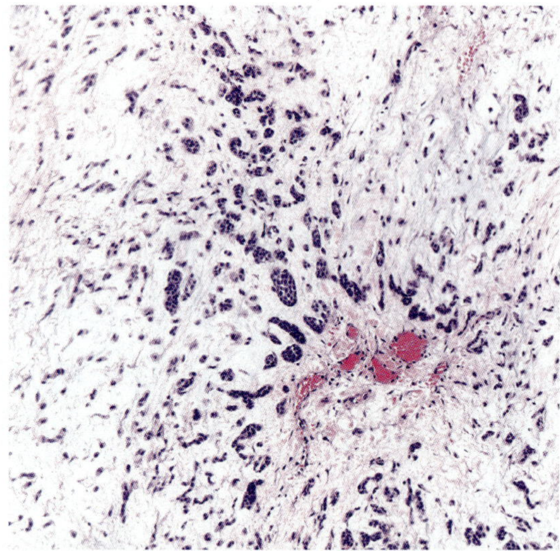

Figure 1.51 — Parotid Gland, Benign Mixed Tumor (Pleomorphic Adenoma) (Histology). The epithelial component is composed of strands and cords of bland epithelial cells that form ductal structures embedded in the myxoid stroma. In this section, there is an abundance of the epithelial component. Note several epithelial fragments are radiating around the central blood vessels. (Hematoxylin and eosin stain, medium power).

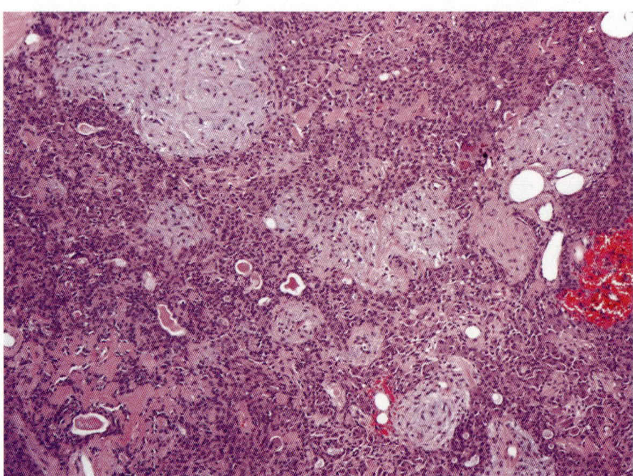

Figure 1.52 — Parotid Gland, Benign Mixed Tumor (Pleomorphic Adenoma). Several features of pleomorphic adenoma are depicted. There is a predominance of myoepithelial cells with scattered ducts (center). Hyaline stroma (bottom left) is often seen in tumors, like pleomorphic adenoma, that contain myoepithelial cells. Finally, interspersed throughout the epithelium are islands of blue-gray chondromyxoid stroma. (Hematoxylin and eosin stain, medium power).

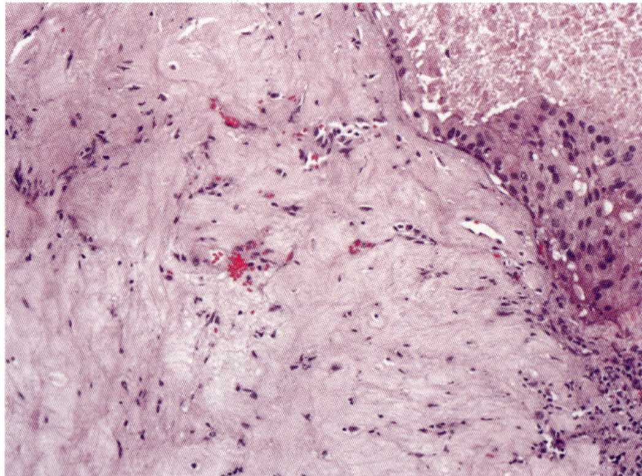

Figure 1.53 — Parotid Gland, Carcinoma Ex-Mixed Tumor (Histology). In a background of chondromyxoid stroma with embedded bland myoepithelial cells, there were foci of epithelium with overt malignant features including marked pleomorphism and mitotic activity. The juxtaposition of carcinoma and foci of pleomorphic adenoma define carcinoma ex-mixed tumor. The prognosis of these tumors depends on the type and grade of the carcinoma (in this case, a high grade salivary duct carcinoma) and, especially, the degree of invasion beyond the tumor capsule. (Hematoxylin and eosin stain, high power)

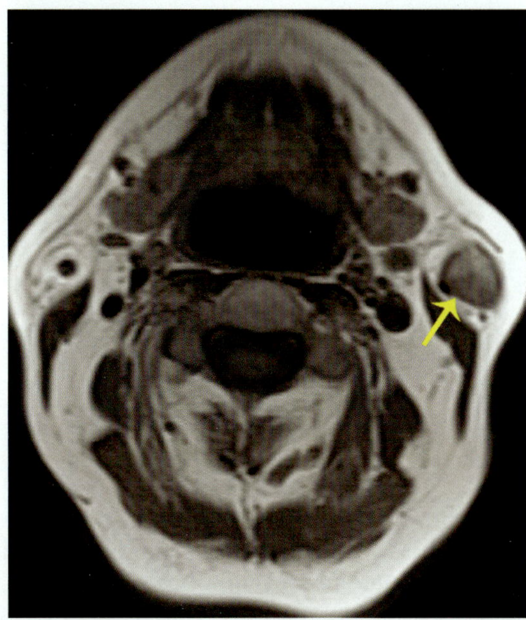

Figure 1.54 — Parotid Gland, Warthin Tumor. Axial T1-weighted MR image demonstrates a well-defined, heterogeneous predominantly hypointense mass in the inferior aspect of the left parotid gland (arrow).

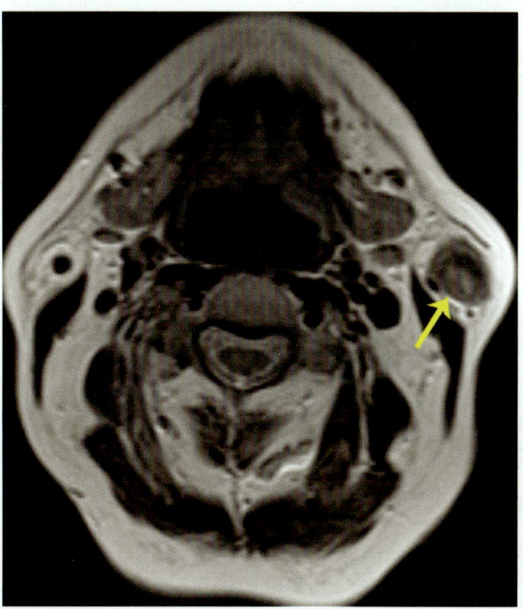

Figure 1.55 — Parotid Gland, Warthin Tumor. Axial T2-weighted MR image shows heterogeneous T2 signal intensity within the mass (arrow).

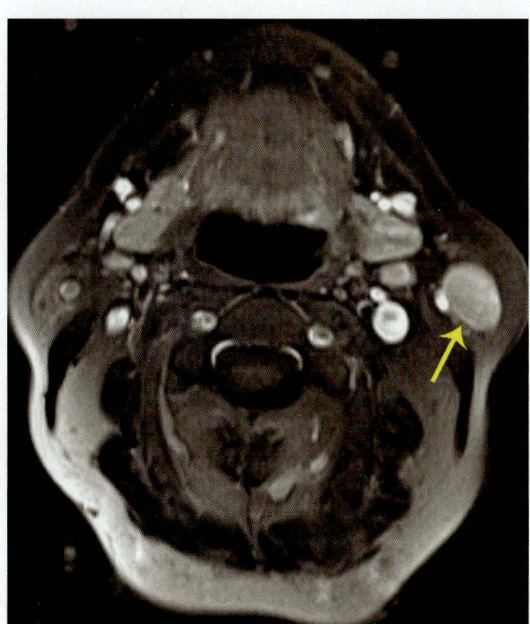

Figure 1.56 — Parotid Gland, Warthin Tumor. Axial T1 fat saturated post-contrast MR image shows mild diffuse enhancement in the mass (arrow).

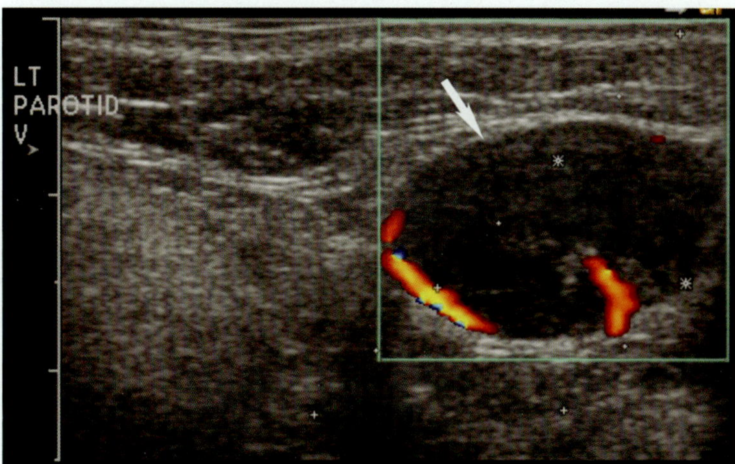

Figure 1.57 — Parotid Gland, Warthin Tumor. Sonographic image confirms a well-defined hypoechoic nodule with internal vascularity in the left parotid gland (arrow). Warthin tumors more commonly occur in older men and are associated with smoking.

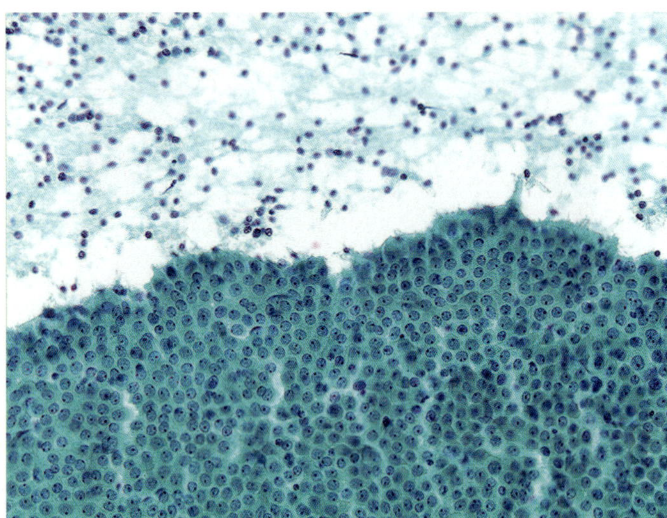

Figure 1.58 — Parotid Gland, Warthin Tumor. Warthin tumor (papillary cystadenoma lymphomatosum) is the second most common benign tumor of salivary glands, and is most often encountered in the parotid gland. The tumor consists of two components: oncocytes and lymphocytes, as seen here. (Papanicolaou stain, medium power)

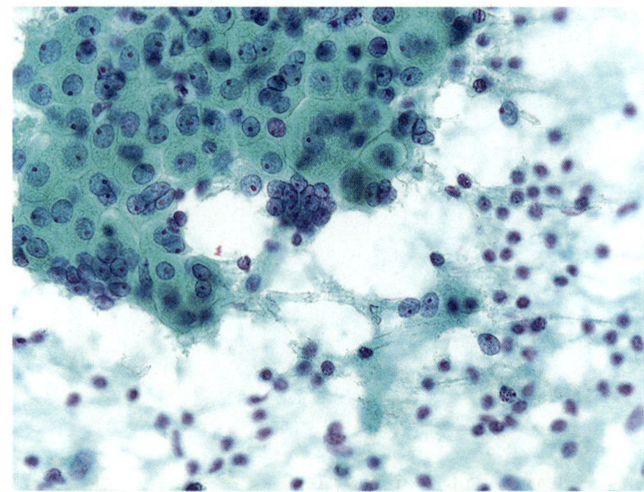

Figure 1.59 — Parotid Gland, Warthin Tumor. Oncocytes are typically present in sheets or small groups and show abundant granular cytoplasm, round nuclei and prominent nucleoli. Lymphocytes are typically numerous and scattered in the background, but can be scant, raising the differential diagnosis of oncocytoma. (Papanicolaou stain, high power)

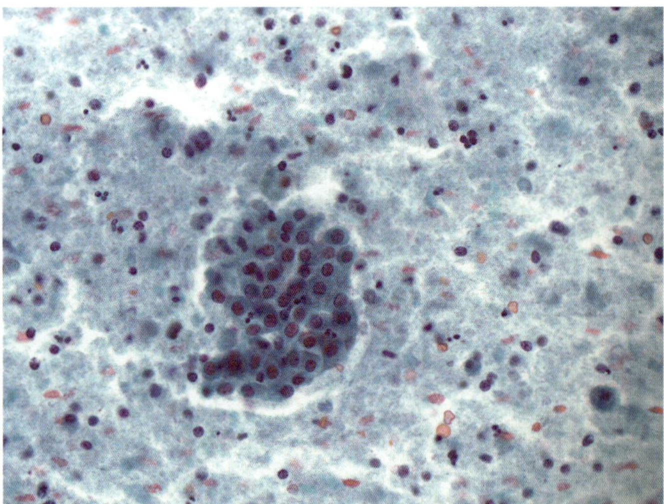

Figure 1.60 — Parotid Gland, Warthin Tumor. A small fragment of oncocytes is present demonstrating abundant cytoplasm and round nuclei. The background is composed of granular debris which is often seen in Warthin tumors. This background debris corresponds to the cyst fluid associated with this lesion that is grossly likened to motor oil. (Papanicolaou stain, high power)

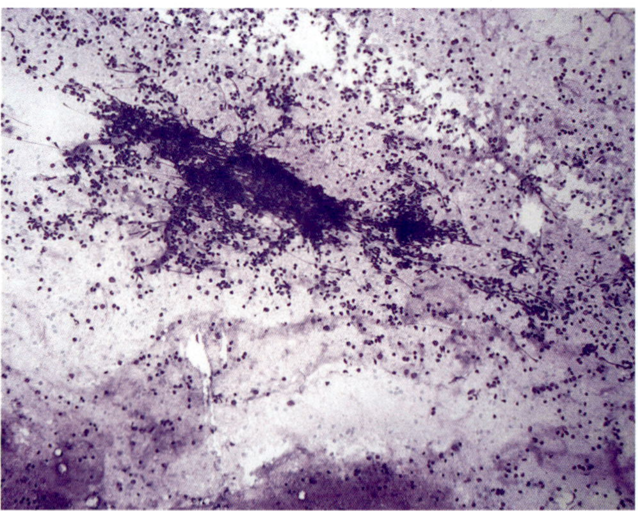

Figure 1.61 — Parotid Gland, Warthin Tumor. The lymphoid component consisting primarily of small lymphocytes admixed with scattered larger reactive lymphoid cells may be prominent, raising the possibility of chronic sialadenitis or a hematopoietic neoplasm. Careful examination of the aspirate smears for oncocytic epithelium is warranted to clarify the diagnosis. (Diff Quik stain, medium power)

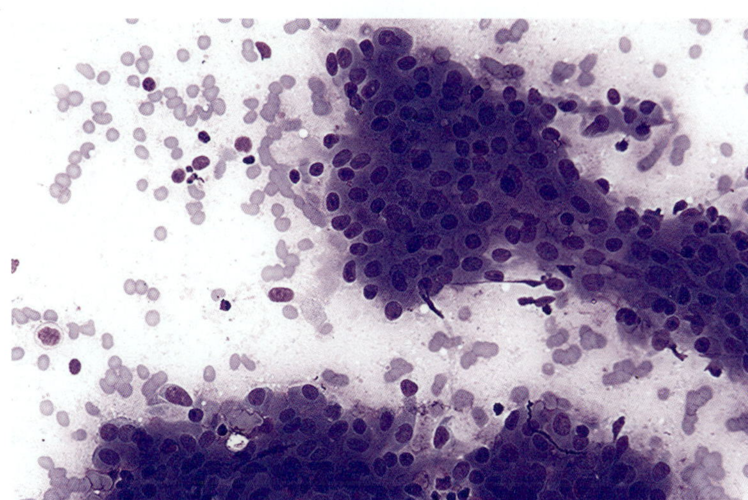

Figure 1.62 — Parotid Gland, Warthin Tumor. Oncocytes are present in small fragments. Few lymphocytes are seen dispersed throughout the epithelium and in the background. The main differential diagnosis in this case is an oncocytoma. (Diff Quik stain, high power)

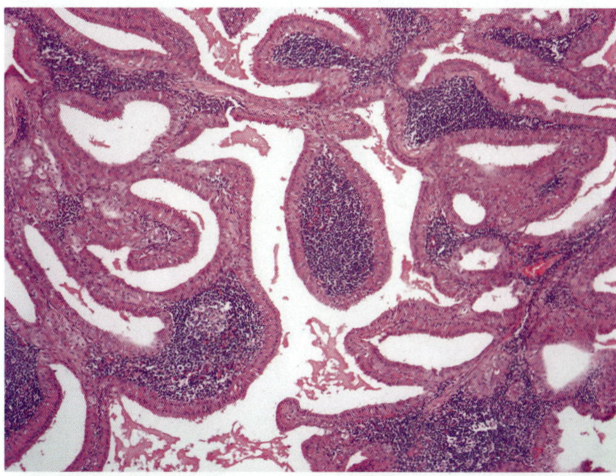

Figure 1.63 — Parotid Gland, Warthin Tumor (Histology). The neoplasm is composed of multiple irregular cystic spaces lined by two layers of cells with a papillary configuration. The surrounding stroma is predominantly lymphoid with prominent germinal centers. Scant cystic fluid is also evident in the luminal spaces. (Hematoxylin and eosin stain, medium power)

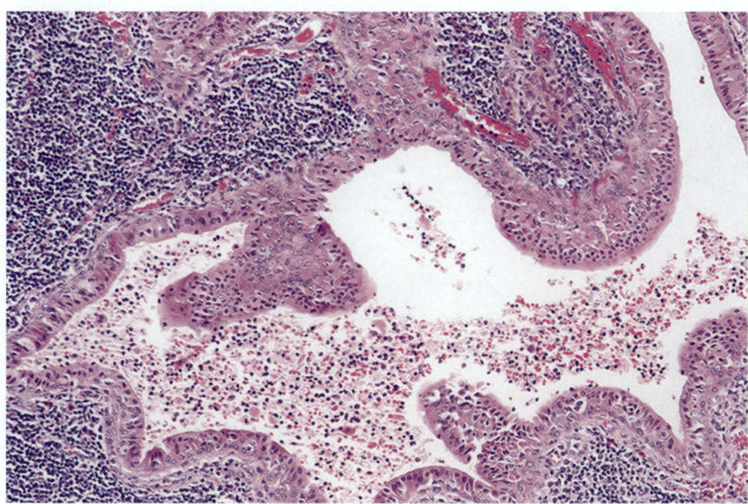

Figure 1.64 — Parotid Gland, Warthin Tumor. Characteristic dual layered tall columnar cells with prominent granular cytoplasm line the cystic spaces. Note the papillary configuration and the dense lymphoid cells in the stroma. (Hematoxylin and eosin stain, high power)

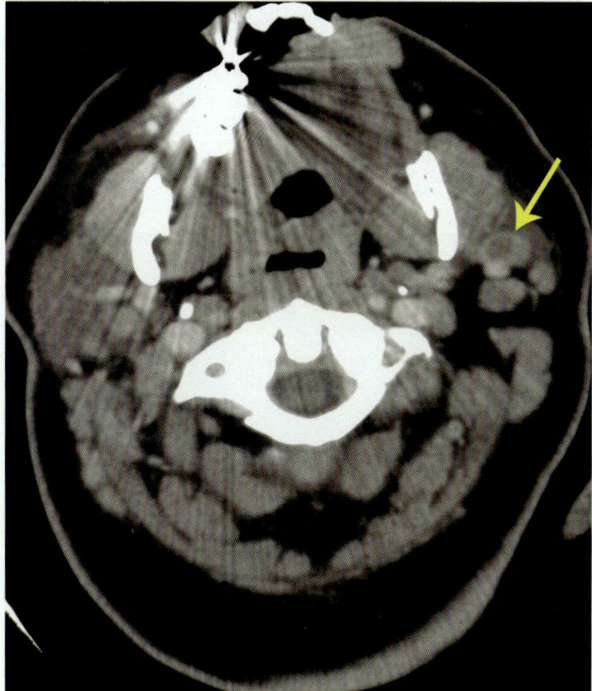

Figure 1.65 — Parotid Gland, Lymphoepithelial Cyst. Axial contrast-enhanced CT image of the neck in a HIV positive patient demonstrates several soft tissue nodules in the parotid glands. One of the nodules contains a necrotic center (arrow).

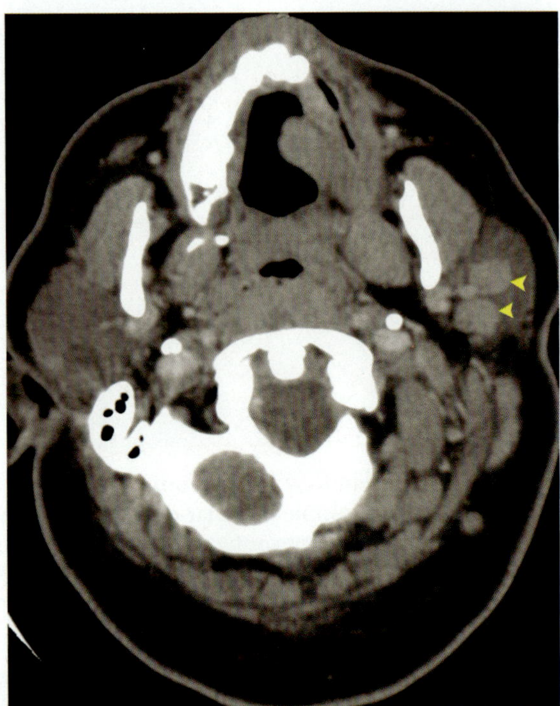

Figure 1.66 — Parotid Gland, Lymphoepithelial Cyst. Axial contrast-enhanced CT image of the neck slightly more inferiorly in the same patient demonstrates several additional soft tissue nodules in the left parotid gland (arrowheads). Lymphoepithelial cysts can be solid and cystic and are usually multiple.

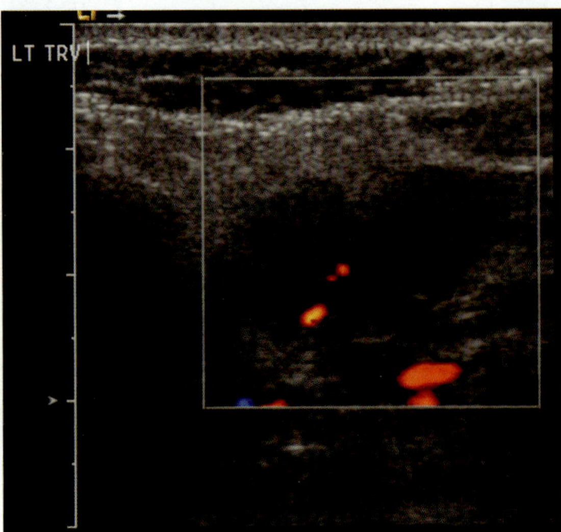

Figure 1.68 — Parotid Gland, Lymphoepithelial Cyst. The nodules show minimal internal vascularity with color Doppler.

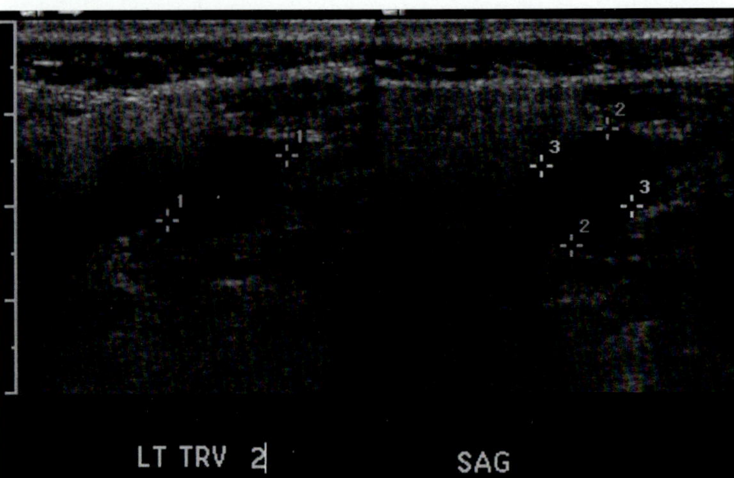

Figure 1.67 — Parotid Gland, Lymphoepithelial Cyst. Sonographic image confirms hypoechoic nodules in the left parotid gland (calipers).

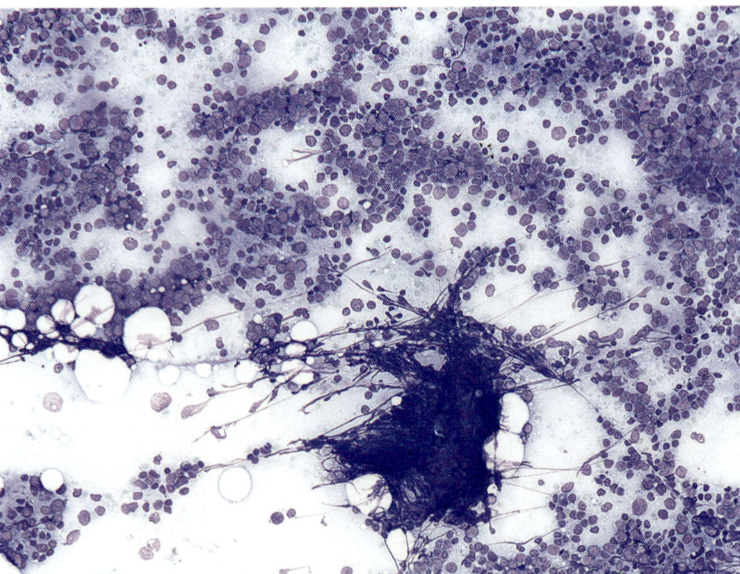

Figure 1.69 — Parotid Gland, Lymphoepithelial Cyst. Simple, sporadic lymphoepithelial cysts (LEC) are typically solitary, whereas HIV-associated LEC (as in this case) are often multiple and bilateral. A cellular aspirate consisting of a mixed population of lymphocytes is shown here. An epithelial component is less often seen. Also present is a crushed lymphoid tangle. LEC often tend to recur and patient may give history of previous aspirations performed on the same mass. (Diff Quik stain, medium power)

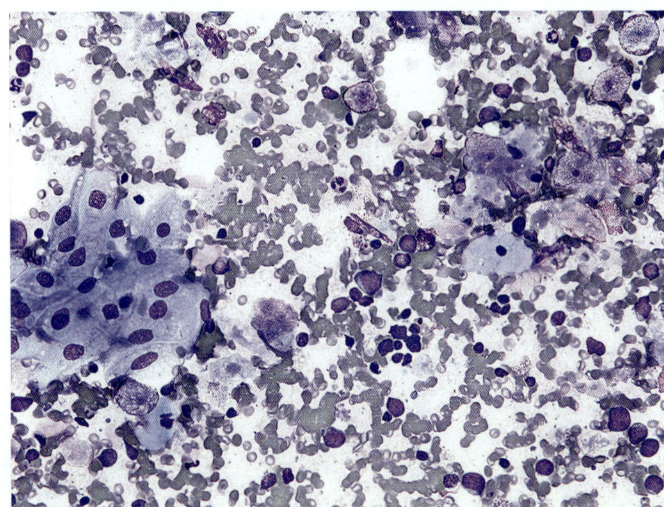

Figure 1.70 — Parotid Gland, Lymphoepithelial Cyst. Small fragments of benign squamous epithelium with scattered single squamous cells are seen in a background of small to intermediate-sized lymphocytes and histiocytes. Some keratin debris may be present and raise the possibility of branchial cleft cyst or, less likely, a squamous cell carcinoma, but nuclear atypia should not be encountered in a LEC. (Diff Quik stain, high power)

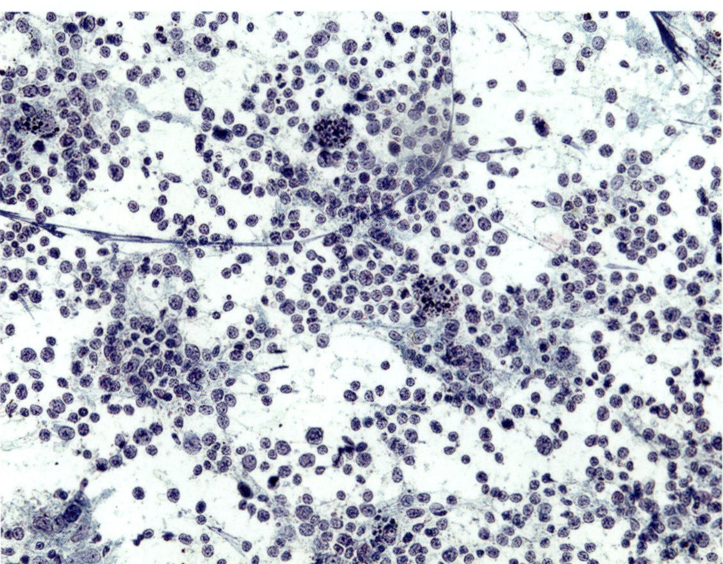

Figure 1.71 — Parotid Gland, Lymphoepithelial Cyst. Numerous small lymphocytes are present with scattered tingible-body macrophages filled with cellular debris. This portion of the aspirate represents aspiration of a germinal center. In the absence of the epithelial component, the aspirate may be interpreted as a lymph node. (Papanicolaou stain, high power)

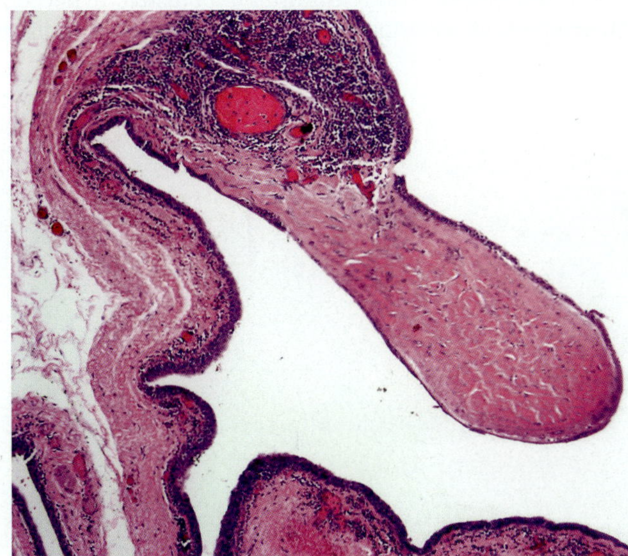

Figure 1.72 — Parotid Gland, Lymphoepithelial Cyst (Histology). Lymphoepithelial cysts are lined by either squamous or glandular epithelium that is often attenuated and undulating, as seen here. These cysts are surrounded by dense lymphoid tissue. (Hematoxylin and eosin stain, medium power)

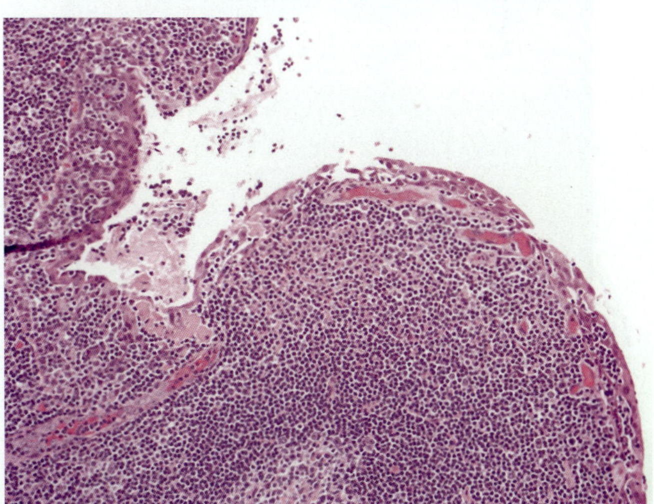

Figure 1.73 — Parotid Gland, Lymphoepithelial Cyst (Histology). Lymphoepithelial cysts are usually lined by flattened squamous (shown here) or columnar epithelium. There is no nuclear atypia. Note the characteristic dense lymphoid tissue beneath the epithelial lining as well as the intraepithelial lymphocytes. (Hematoxylin and eosin stain, high power)

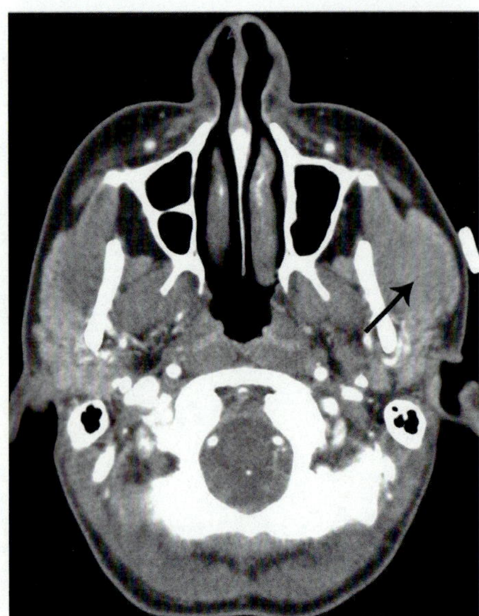

Figure 1.74 — Parotid Gland, Extranodal Marginal Zone Lymphoma of Mucosa-Associated Lymphoid Tissue (MALT Lymphoma). Axial contrast-enhanced CT image of the neck shows an infiltrative soft tissue mass in the left parotid gland (arrow). Note the asymmetry compared to the right parotid gland.

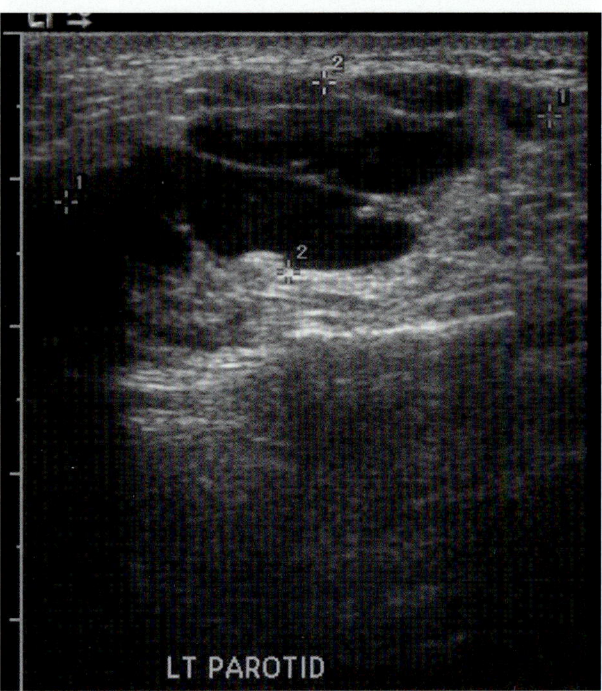

Figure 1.75 — Parotid Gland, Extranodal Marginal Zone Lymphoma of Mucosa-Associated Lymphoid Tissue (MALT Lymphoma). Sonographic image confirms a lobulated, hypoechoic mass with several thin septations in the left parotid gland (calipers).

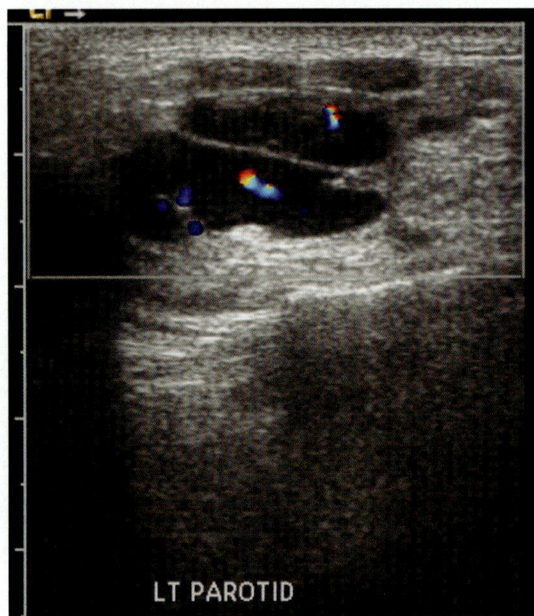

Figure 1.76 — Parotid Gland, Extranodal Marginal Zone Lymphoma of Mucosa-Associated Lymphoid Tissue (MALT Lymphoma). Internal flow is seen in this mass with color Doppler. MALT lymphomas often arise in a background of Sjögren syndrome, thus a clinical history may be useful in establishing the diagnosis.

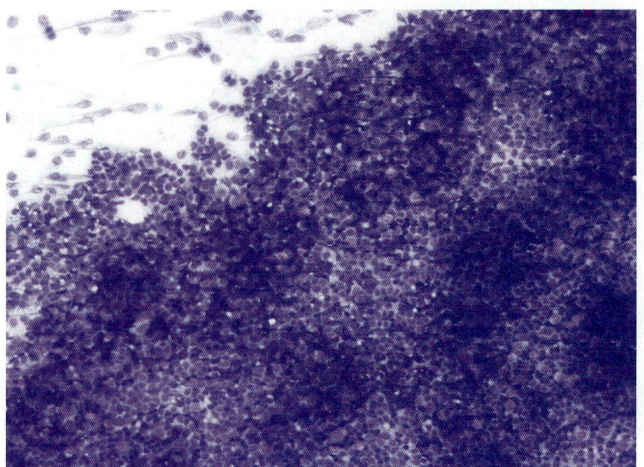

Figure 1.77 — Parotid Gland, Extranodal Marginal Zone Lymphoma of Mucosa-Associated Lymphoid Tissue (MALT Lymphoma). A markedly cellular aspirate is shown here consisting of a monotonous population of small- to intermediate-sized lymphocytes. On-site evaluation of this material should prompt collection of additional material for immunophenotyping (flow cytometry) studies. (Diff Quik stain, medium power)

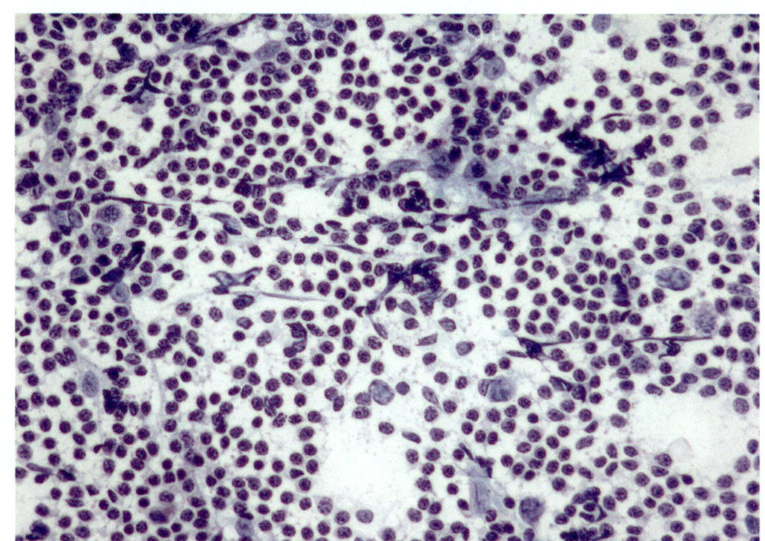

Figure 1.78 — Parotid Gland, Extranodal Marginal Zone Lymphoma of Mucosa-Associated Lymphoid Tissue (MALT Lymphoma). A population of monotonous-appearing lymphocytes is present. The malignant lymphocytes show scant cytoplasm, round to slightly irregular nuclear contours, and dispersed chromatin and rare small nucleoli. Scattered larger cells consistent with immunoblasts are seen. (Papanicolaou stain, high power)

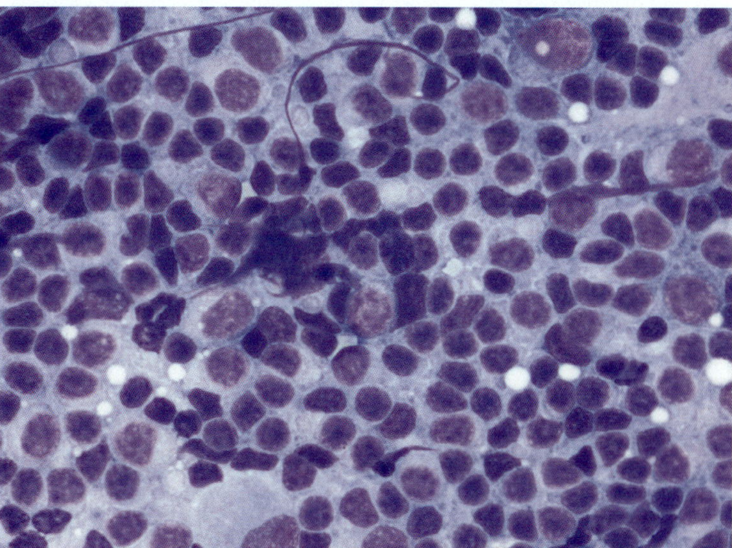

Figure 1.79 — Parotid Gland, Extranodal Marginal Zone Lymphoma of Mucosa-Associated Lymphoid Tissue (MALT Lymphoma). Malignant lymphocytes with round to slightly irregular nuclear contours are seen at high power. MALT lymphomas are distinguished from other lymphomas, particularly follicular and mantle cell lymphomas, by their immunophenotype. MALT lymphomas are positive for CD20 and bcl2, and negative for CD5, CD10, CD23, bcl6, and cyclin D1. (Diff Quik stain, high power)

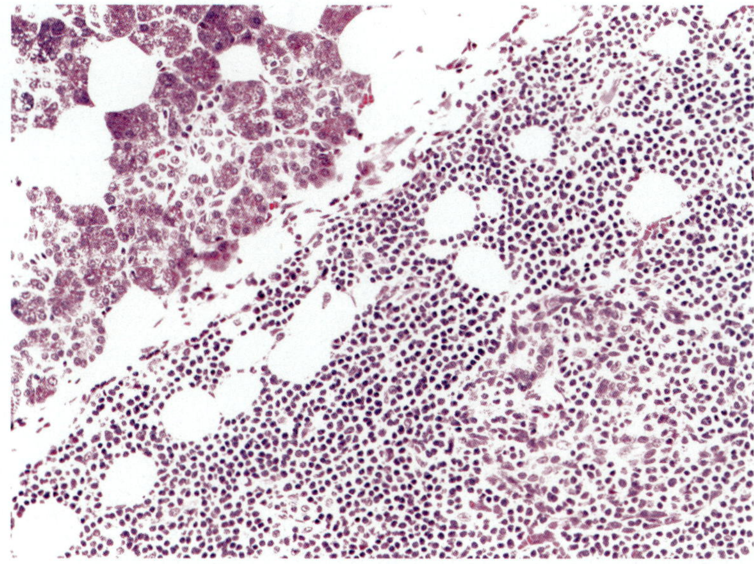

Figure 1.80 — Parotid Gland, Extranodal Marginal Zone Lymphoma of Mucosa-Associated Lymphoid Tissue (MALT Lymphoma) (Histology). The normal parotid gland tissue is replaced by a mononuclear infiltrate of neoplastic lymphocytes surrounding nests of epithelial cells and infiltrating in fat. This characteristic infiltration and destruction of epithelial structures by neoplastic lymphoid cells is a key histological finding. Immunostains may be useful if flow cytometry is not performed or is unsuccessful. The neoplastic lymphocytes cells of marginal zone lymphoma are positive for bcl2 and lack expression of CD5, CD10, CD23, and cyclin D1. (Hematoxylin and eosin stain, medium power)

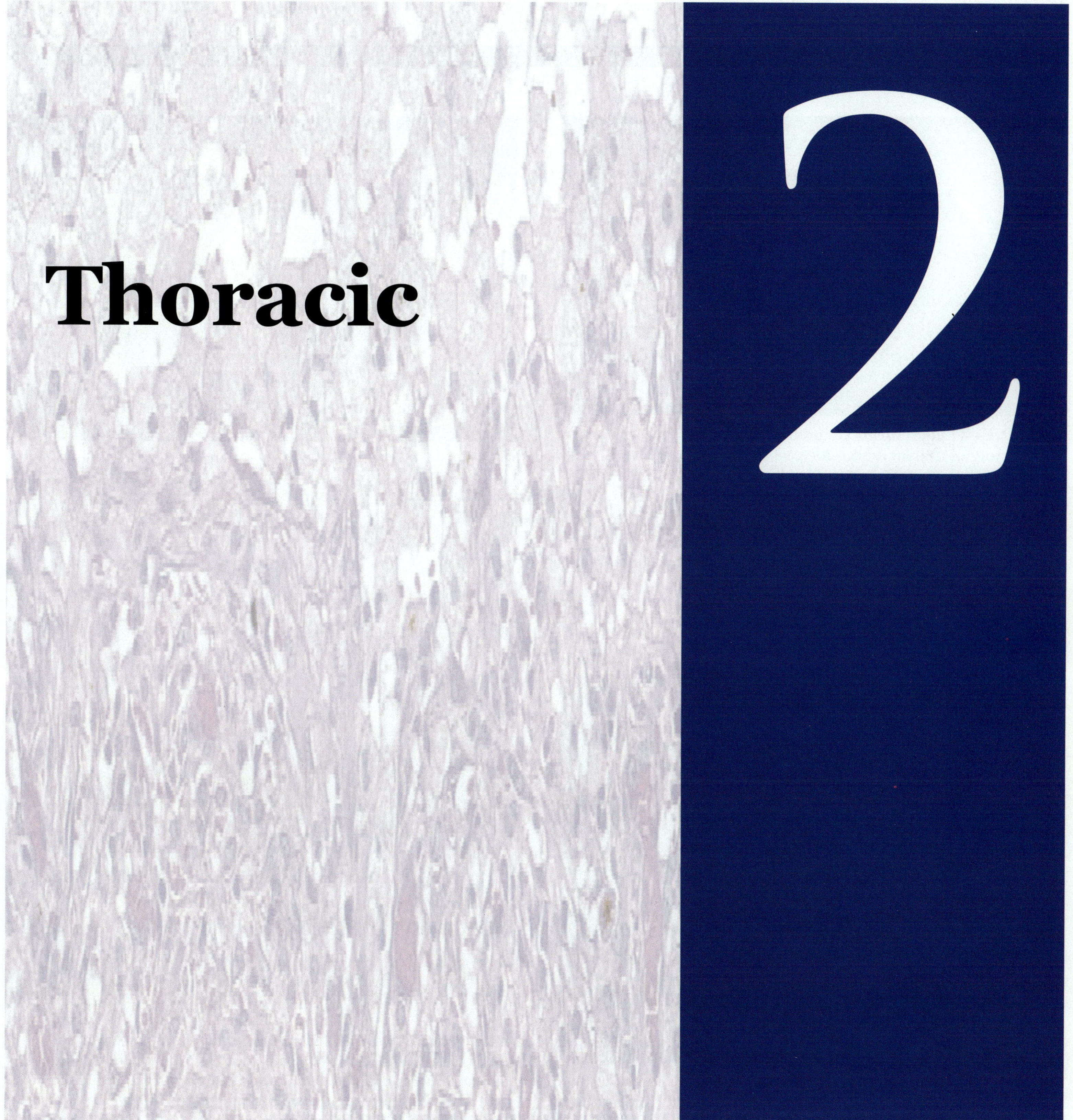

2 Thoracic

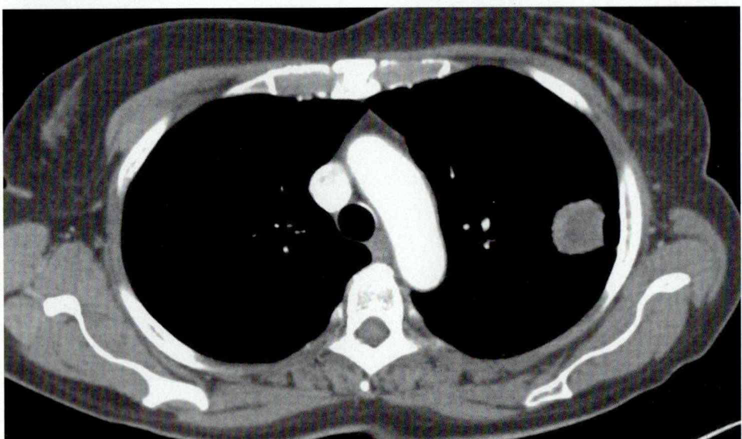

Figure 2.1 — Lung, Adenocarcinoma. This 77-year-old woman had a history of ovarian cancer 20 years ago. Axial contrast-enhanced CT image of the chest in soft tissue windows shows a 2.5-cm spiculated left upper lobe nodule.

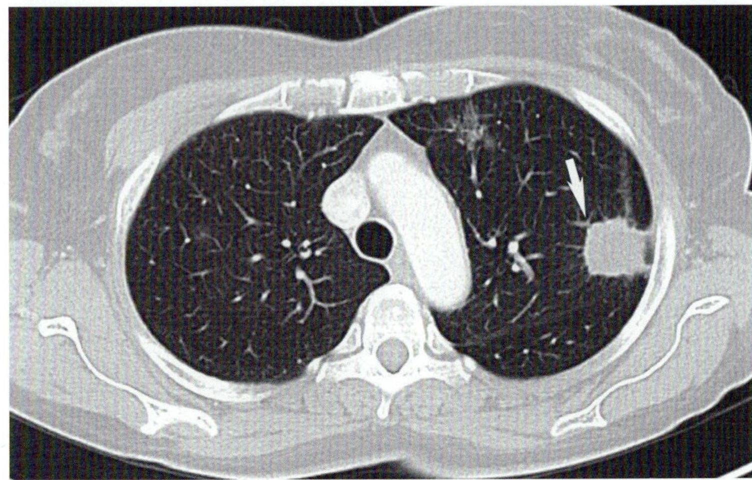

Figure 2.2 — Lung, Adenocarcinoma. Spiculated left upper lobe nodule is well depicted on lung windows. Its size and irregular, spiculated margins (arrow) are suggestive of malignancy.

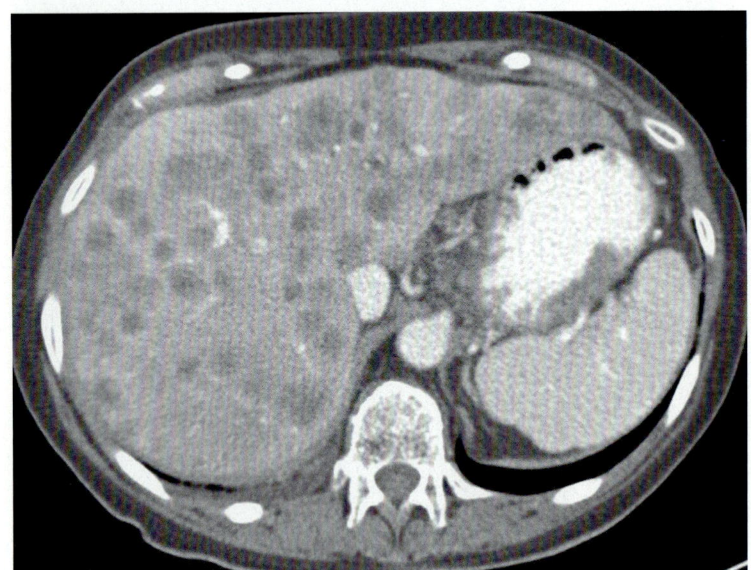

Figure 2.3 — Lung, Adenocarcinoma (Metastatic to the Liver). Multiple hypodense lesions, compatible with metastatic disease, are also present in the liver of the same patient.

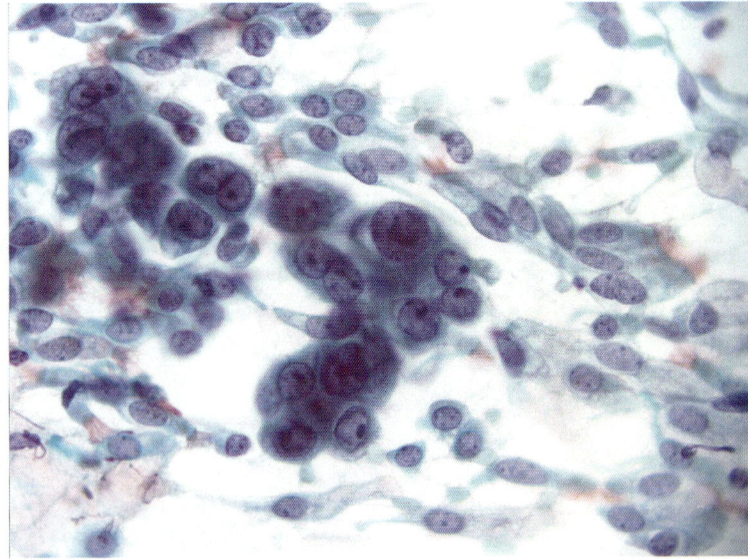

Figure 2.4 — Lung, Adenocarcinoma. A loosely cohesive group of malignant cells showing a glandular architecture is seen in the center of the field. The nuclei are enlarged and hyperchromatic with prominent nucleoli. Numerous benign ciliated bronchial epithelial cells are present surrounding the tumor cells. (Papanicolaou stain, high power)

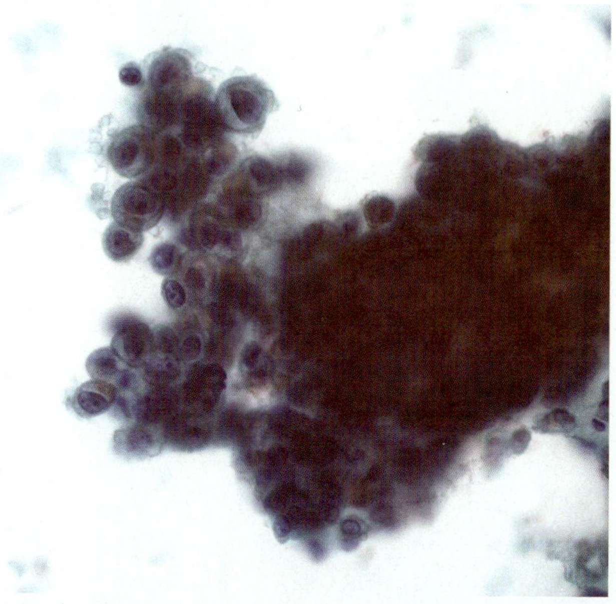

Figure 2.5 — Lung, Adenocarcinoma. A fragment of tumor cells is present showing high N/C ratios, nuclear hyperchromasia, and the presence of cytoplasmic mucin. A mucin stain can be performed on direct smears to confirm that a non-small cell carcinoma is an adenocarcinoma. (Papanicolaou stain, high power)

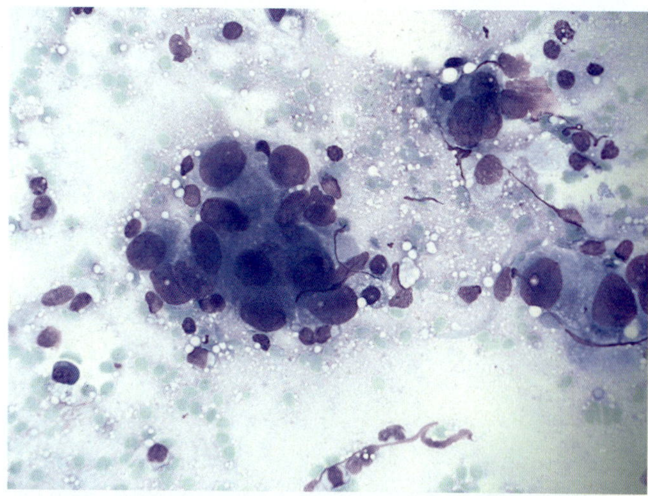

Figure 2.6 — Lung, Adenocarcinoma. A fragment of malignant epithelium is shown with the tumor cells forming small glandular structures. The nuclei are markedly enlarged when compared to scattered background lymphocytes, and have variably prominent nucleoli. (Diff Quik stain, high power)

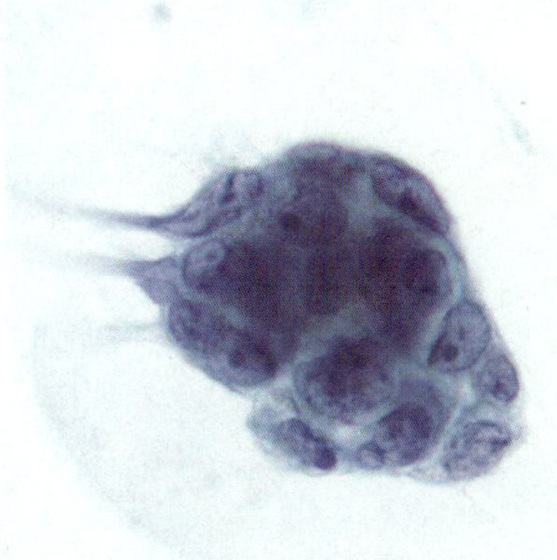

Figure 2.7 — Lung, Adenocarcinoma. This tumor fragment shows enlarged nuclei with very irregular nuclear contours, coarse chromatin, and prominent nucleoli. It is of particular importance in practice to obtain material for cell block preparation when pulmonary adenocarcinoma is considered, as molecular studies for EGFR, KRAS, and EML4/ALK are routinely used to triage patients for chemotherapeutics. (Papanicolaou stain, high power)

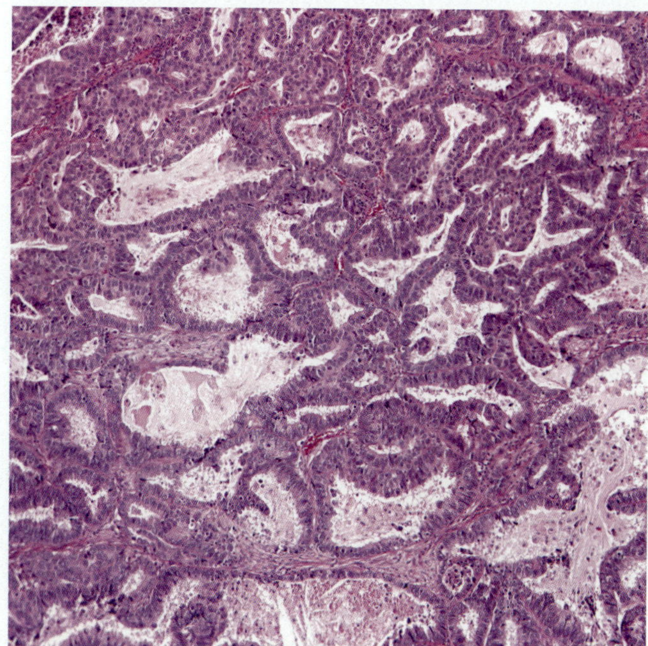

Figure 2.8 — Lung, Adenocarcinoma (Histology). Moderately differentiated adenocarcinoma of the lung with abundant, back-to-back neoplastic glandular structures and luminal mucin. (Hematoxylin and eosin stain, low power)

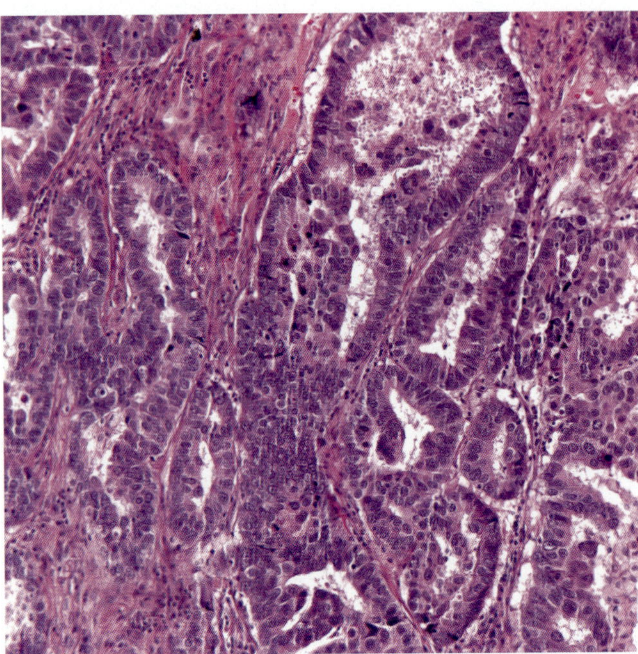

Figure 2.9 — Lung, Adenocarcinoma (Histology). Moderately differentiated adenocarcinoma of the lung. Neoplastic glands are made up of cells with a basophilic cytoplasm and a central nucleus with a prominent nucleolus. The neoplastic cells were CK7 and TTF-1 positive. (Hematoxylin and eosin stain, medium power)

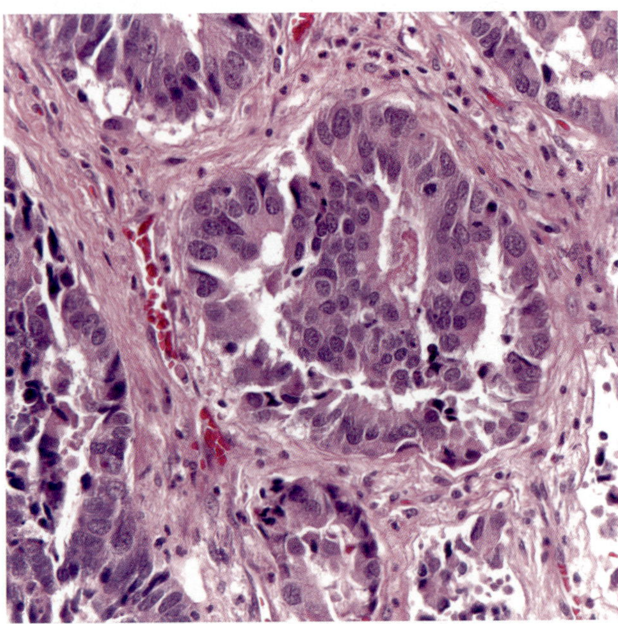

Figure 2.10 — Lung, Adenocarcinoma (Histology). The neoplastic cells have dense cytoplasm and mildly pleomorphic nuclei with irregular contours, coarse chromatin, and prominent nucleoli. There is brisk mitotic activity. (Hematoxylin and eosin stain, high power)

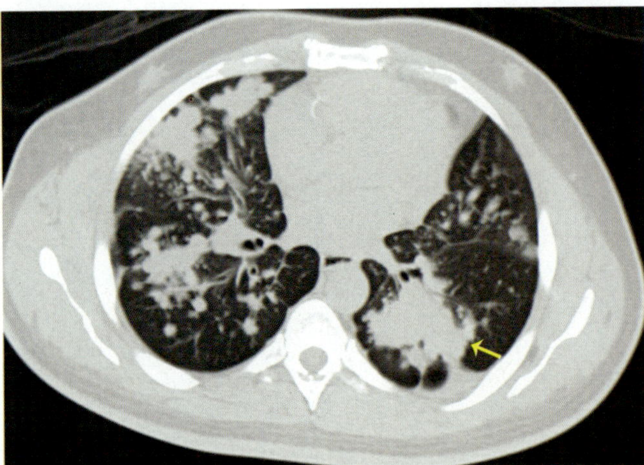

Figure 2.11 — Lung, Adenocarcinoma with Bronchioloalveolar Features. Axial CT of the chest in lung windows shows multiple bilateral pulmonary nodules and masses randomly distributed in the lungs. The appearance mimics metastatic disease. The largest mass in the left lower lobe (arrow) was targeted for biopsy.

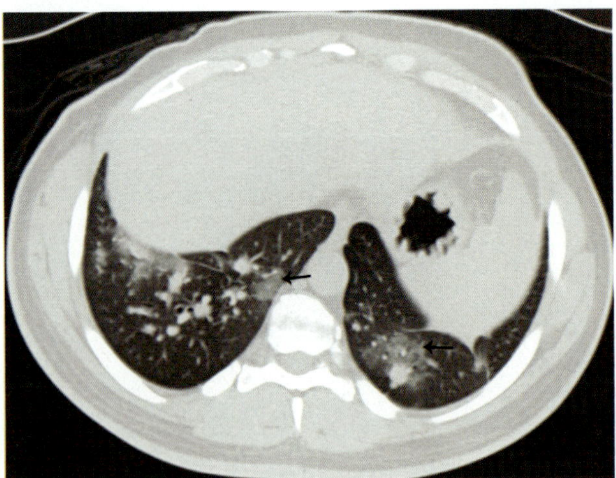

Figure 2.12 — Lung, Adenocarcinoma with Bronchioloalveolar Features. More inferiorly in the chest, large areas of peripheral ground-glass opacity (arrows) are associated with several of the masses. Bronchioloalveolar carcinoma (BAC) usually appears as ground glass opacity on CT. The development of soft tissue density solid component with a ground-glass nodule is concerning for the development of invasive adenocarcinoma.

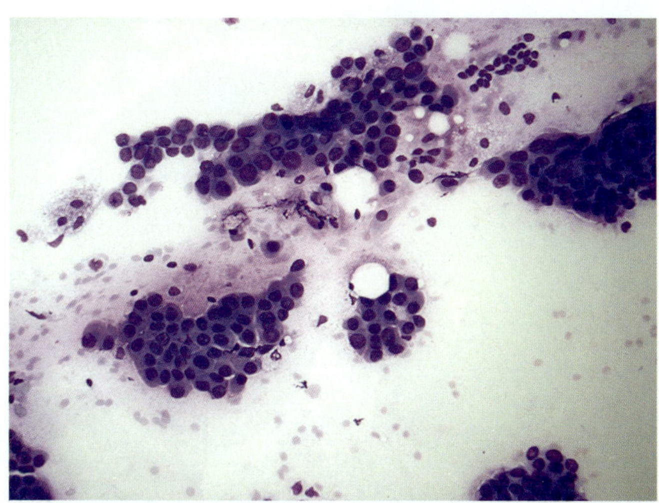

Figure 2.13 — Lung, Adenocarcinoma with Bronchioloalveolar Features. Non-mucinous BAC, also termed adenocarcinoma *in situ*, is a subtype of pulmonary adenocarcinoma which shows distinct cytologic characteristics. Definitive diagnosis of BAC, though, requires the exclusion of an invasive component and therefore can only be made on tissue excision. Flat sheets of tumor cells with mild to moderate nuclear enlargement and disorganization suggest BAC. (Diff Quik stain, medium power)

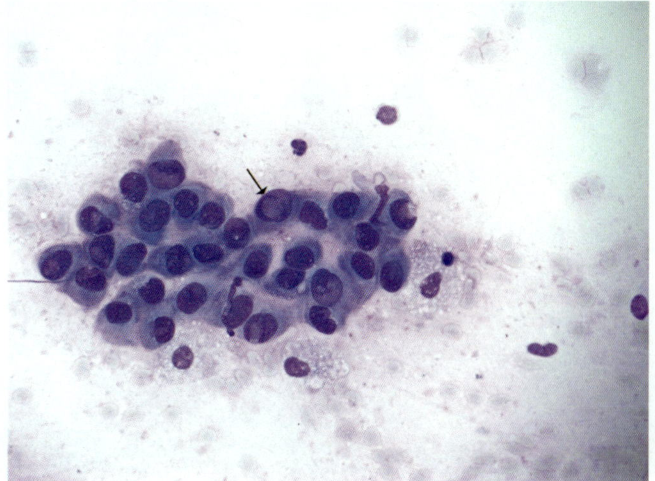

Figure 2.14 — Lung, Adenocarcinoma with Bronchioloalveolar Features. BAC shares many features with papillary thyroid carcinoma, including intranuclear pseudoinclusions, pale chromatin, and a flat sheet arrangement of tumor cells. A sheet of tumor cells is present demonstrating nuclear enlargement, nuclear border irregularities, and an intranuclear inclusion (arrow). (Diff Quik stain, high power)

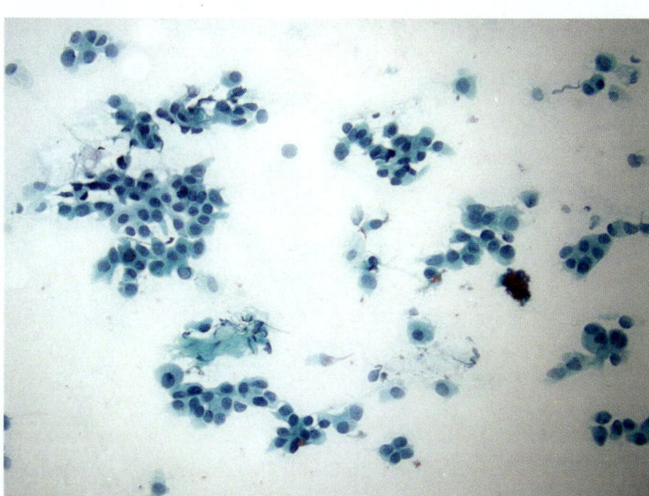

Figure 2.15 — Lung, Adenocarcinoma with Bronchioloalveolar Features. A cellular aspirate is shown with numerous fragments of neoplastic cells and scattered single cells. The neoplastic cells show moderate anisonucleosis, slightly increased nuclear-to-cytoplasmic ratios, and slightly pale chromatin, all features of BAC. (Papanicolaou stain, medium power)

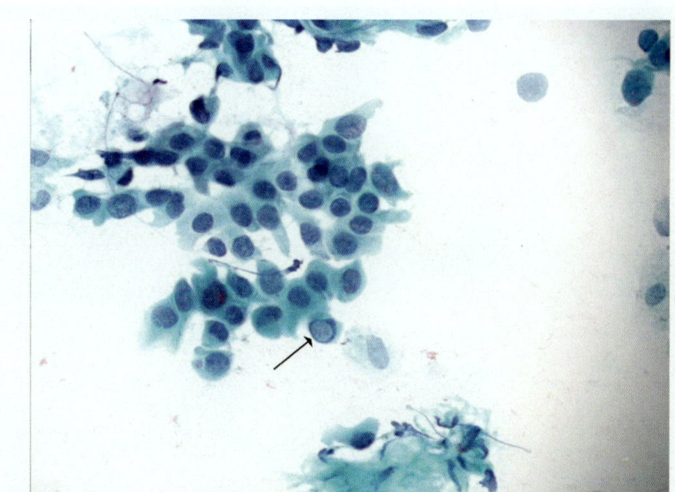

Figure 2.16 — Lung, Adenocarcinoma with Broncioloalveolar Features. A flat sheet of tumor cells with nuclear enlargement, pale chromatin, and an intranuclear inclusion (arrow) is shown. Because BACs typically have a diffuse radiographic appearance, the differential diagnosis is often an infectious or reactive nonneoplastic process. Presence of intranuclear inclusions would exclude a mesothelial process which is often in the differential diagnosis of a peripheral lung lesion. (Papanicolaou stain, high power)

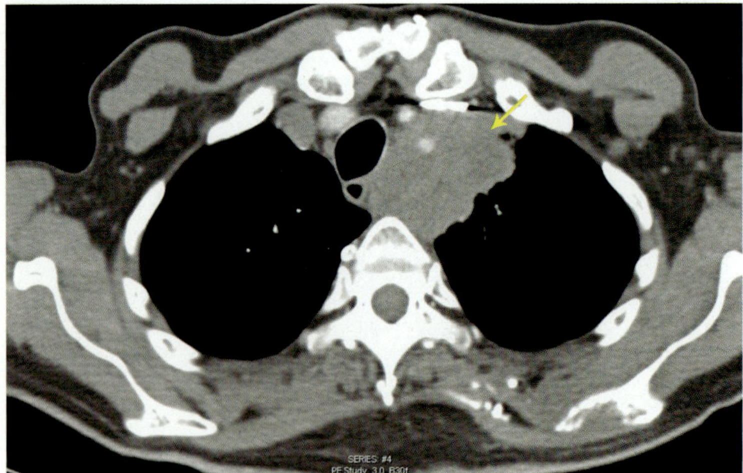

Figure 2.17 — Lung, Squamous Cell Carcinoma. A 73-year-old man presented to the ED with left shoulder pain and dyspnea. Axial contrast-enhanced CT image shows a soft tissue mass in the medial left upper chest encasing the origin of the great vessels (arrow).

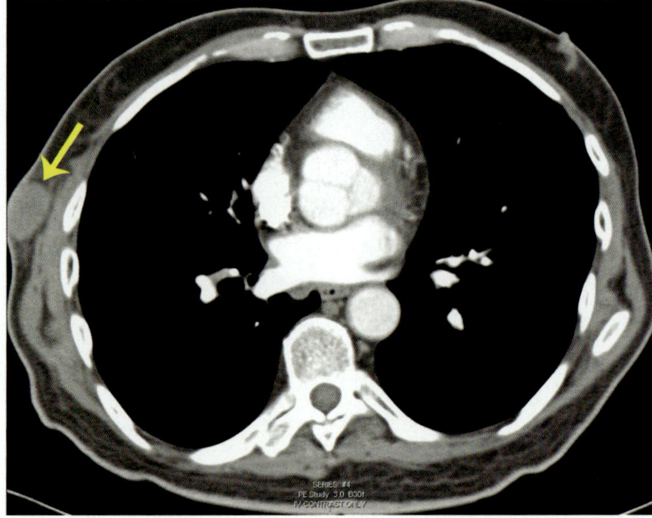

Figure 2.18 — Lung, Squamous Cell Carcinoma. Axial contrast-enhanced CT image at the level of the mid chest in the same patient shows a subcutaneous mass in the right chest wall (arrow). Squamous cell carcinomas of the lung most often arise centrally and are seen more often in male smokers.

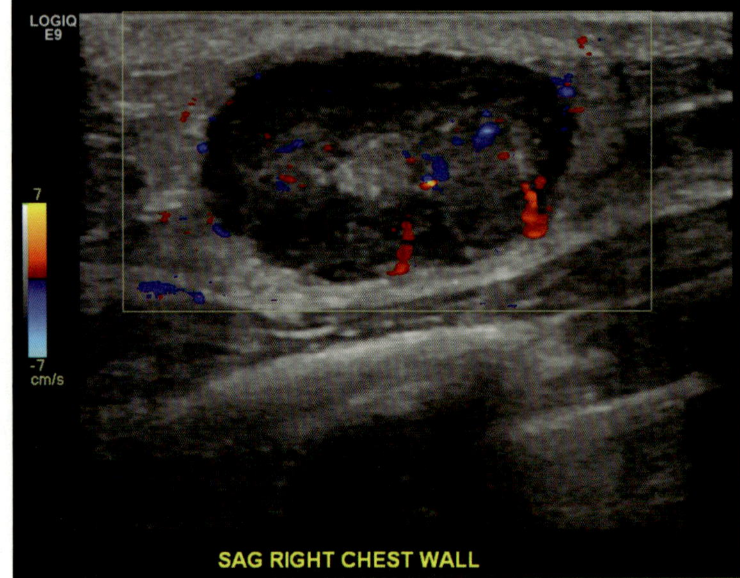

Figure 2.19 — Lung, Squamous Cell Carcinoma. Sonographic image confirms the presence of a hypoechoic chest wall mass with internal vascularity which was targeted for biopsy. The nodule was found to represent metastatic squamous cell carcinoma from lung primary.

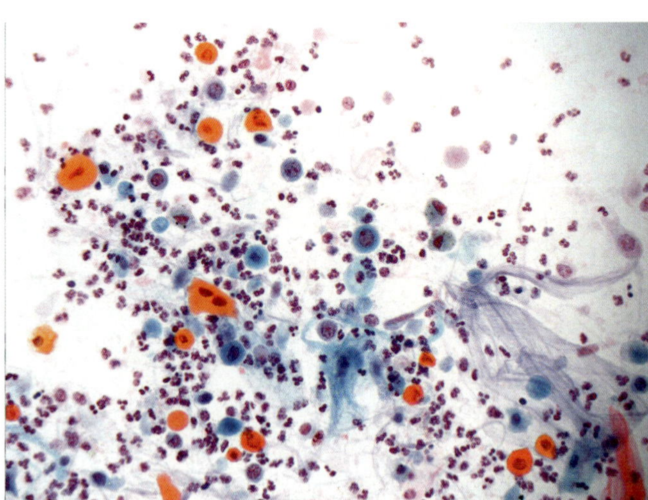

Figure 2.20 — Lung, Squamous Cell Carcinoma. Numerous single malignant squamous cells are present. The cytoplasm ranges from deep blue to bright orange (keratinized cells). The nuclear-to-cytoplasmic ratio is increased in the tumor cells and nuclei appear hyperchromatic and coarse. Numerous neutrophils, indicative of necrosis, are scattered in the background, a characteristic finding of squamous cell carcinoma. (Papanicolaou stain, medium power)

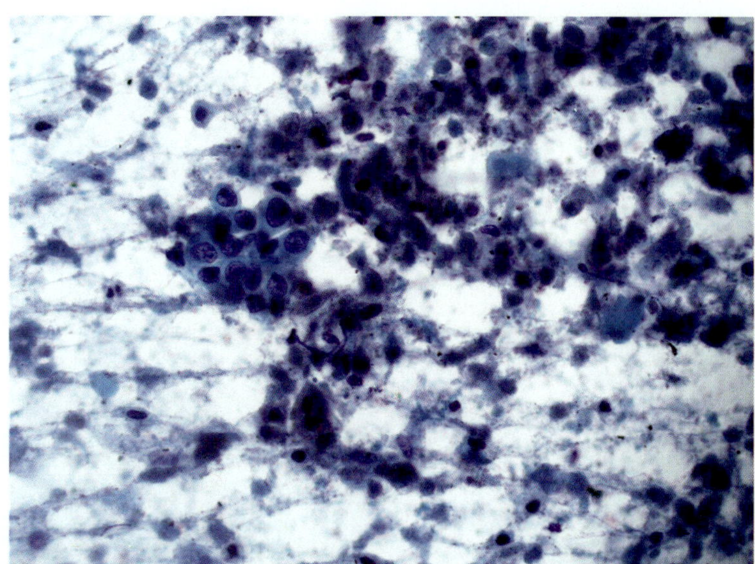

Figure 2.21 — Lung, Squamous Cell Carcinoma. A single fragment of malignant squamous cells (non-keratinized) is present in a background of extensive necrotic debris. The tumor cells show dense, opaque blue cytoplasm with hyperchromatic, irregularly shaped nuclei. Necrotic smears must be carefully examined for tumor cells, as they can be sparse. (Papanicolaou stain, medium power)

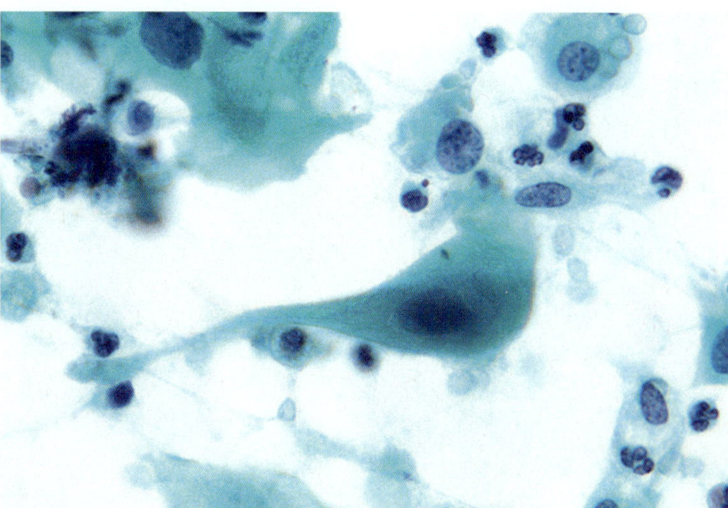

Figure 2.22 — Lung, Squamous Cell Carcinoma. A single malignant squamous cell is present in the center of the field showing dense cytoplasm and a "tadpole" shape that is characteristic of squamous cell carcinoma. Neutrophils are present in the background. (Papanicolaou stain, high power)

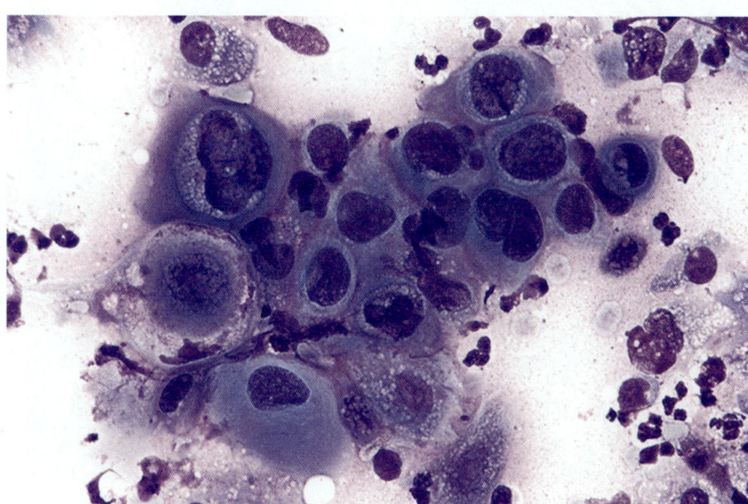

Figure 2.23 — Lung, Squamous Cell Carcinoma. On Diff Quik stain, squamous cells appear a distinct "robin's egg" blue color. The cytoplasm is dense and the malignant cells have distinct cell borders. Occasionally, intercellular bridges can be seen connecting adjacent squamous cells (not shown). (Diff Quik stain, high power)

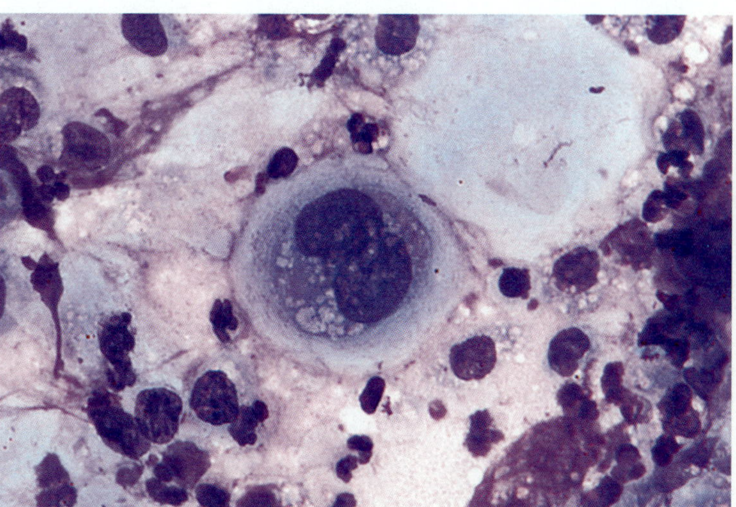

Figure 2.24 — Lung, Squamous Cell Carcinoma. Squamous cell carcinoma is most often centrally located and diagnostic material may be obtained by FNA, sputum collection, bronchial brushing, washing, or lavage. A malignant squamous cell is shown with pale blue cytoplasm and an enlarged, bilobed nucleus. (Diff Quik stain, high power)

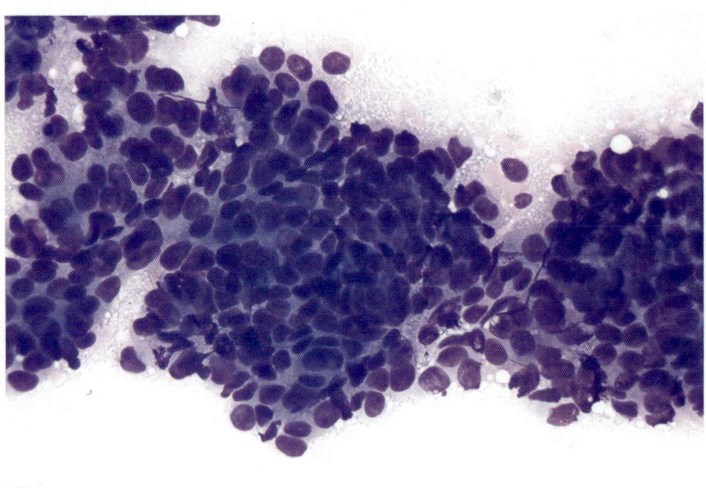

Figure 2.25 — Lung, Squamous Cell Carcinoma. Poorly-differentiated squamous cell carcinoma (basaloid-type) may resemble high-grade large cell neuroendocrine carcinoma (as seen here). Immunostaining with p63, TTF-1, and neuroendocrine markers may help differentiate the two as the management approaches are quite different for these two tumor types. (Diff Quik stain, medium power)

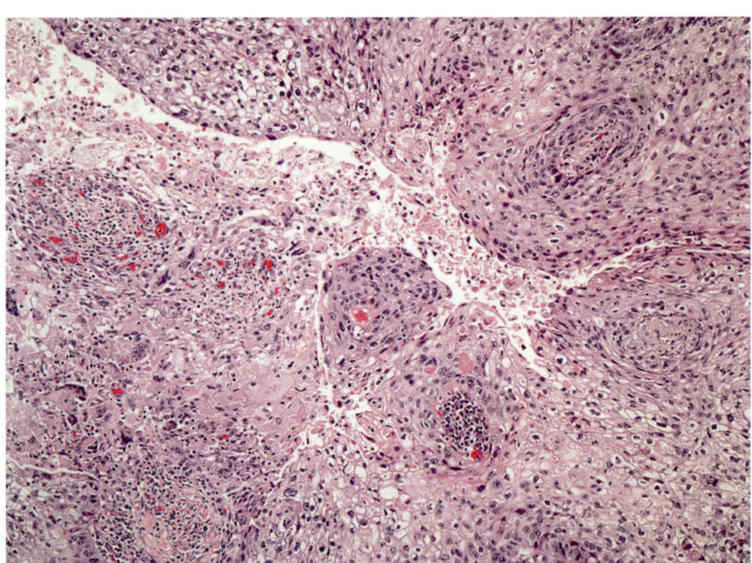

Figure 2.26 — Lung, Squamous Cell Carcinoma (Histology). Sheets of neoplastic cells show dense, eosinophilic, and glassy cytoplasm and distinct cell borders and pleomorphic nuclei. Granular debris consistent with necrosis is present in the center of the field. (Hematoxylin and eosin stain, medium power)

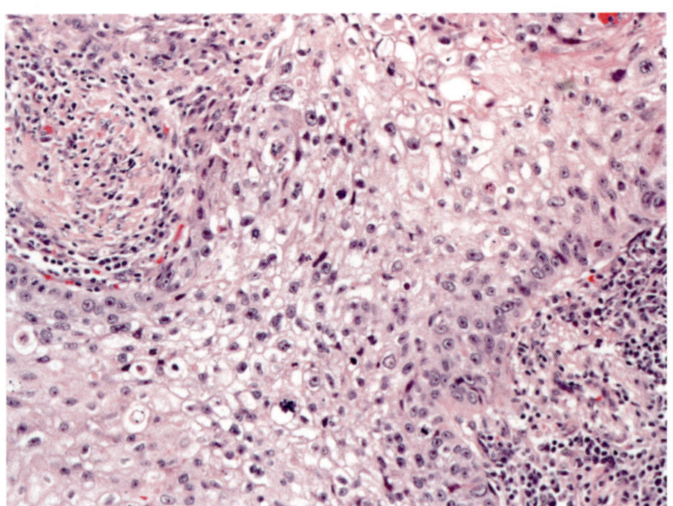

Figure 2.27 — Lung, Squamous Cell Carcinoma (Histology). The neoplastic cells have distinct cytoplasmic borders. The nuclei are pleomorphic and have variably sized nucleoli. There are numerous mitoses and apoptotic bodies. (Hematoxylin and eosin stain, high power)

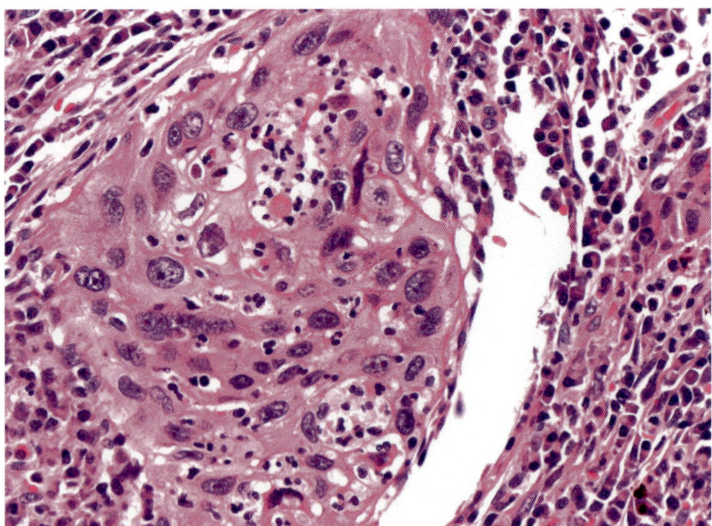

Figure 2.28 — Lung, Squamous Cell Carcinoma (Histology). Moderately to poorly differentiated squamous cell carcinoma. The neoplastic cells are polygonal, pink, and have distinct cell borders. The cytoplasm is dense and eosinophilic reflecting keratinization of the tumor cells. Bizarrely shaped nuclei are abundant. (Hematoxylin and eosin stain, high power)

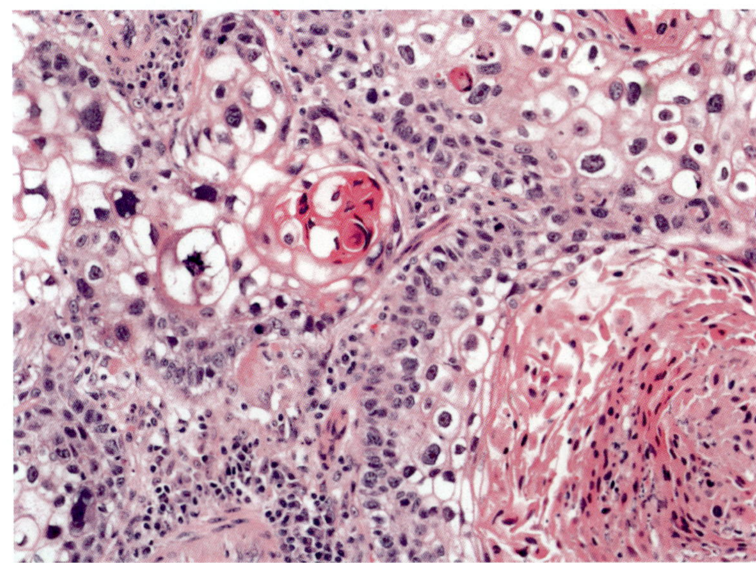

Figure 2.29 — Lung, Squamous Cell Carcinoma (Histology). Poorly differentiated squamous cell carcinoma showing distinct cell borders, dense cytoplasm, and hyperchromatic nuclei with occasional prominent nucleoli. Focal keratinization is still evident. (Hematoxylin and eosin stain, high power)

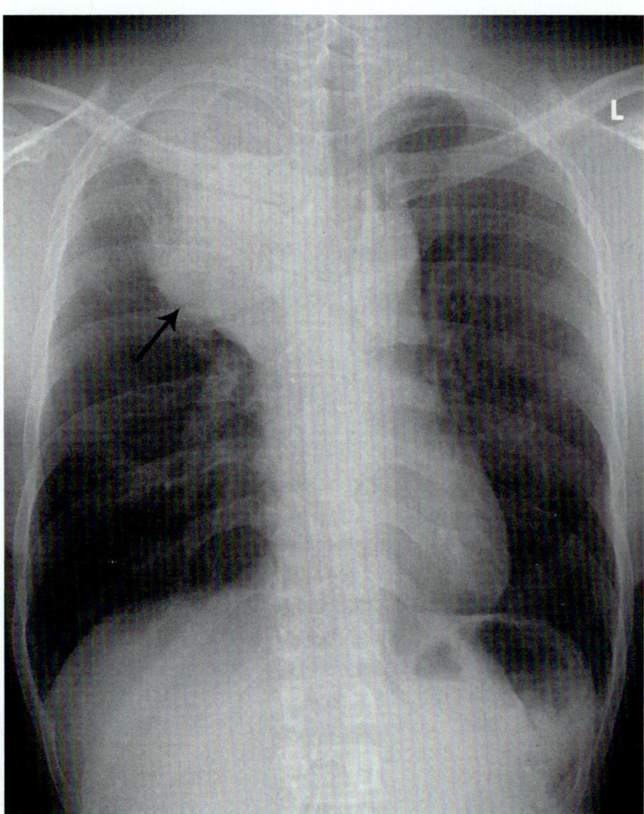

Figure 2.30 — Lung, Small Cell Carcinoma. X-ray of the chest shows a large mass in the medial right upper lobe (arrow). Small cell carcinoma is a very aggressive tumor and often presents with mediastinal lymph node involvement.

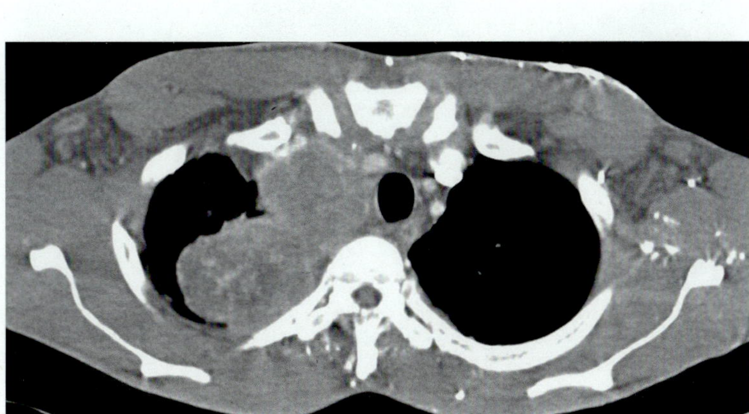

Figure 2.31 — Lung, Small Cell Carcinoma. Axial contrast-enhanced CT confirms a large heterogeneous mass in the mediastinum in the right paratracheal region. Small cell carcinoma is seen almost exclusively in smokers, and most often in men.

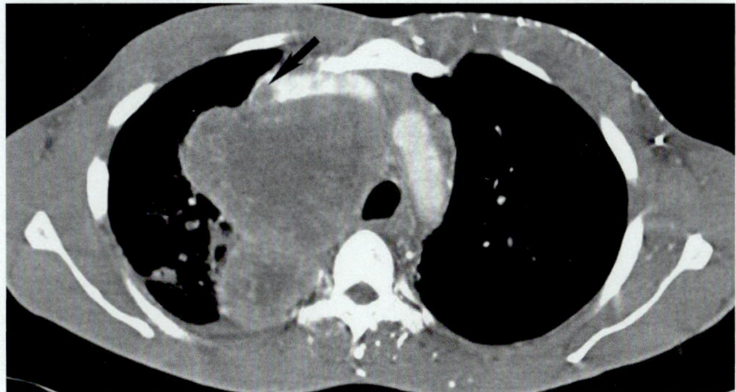

Figure 2.32 — Lung, Small Cell Carcinoma. Axial contrast-enhanced CT slightly more inferiorly shows further extension of the heterogeneous, necrotic mass. Note the mass is invading the left innominate vein (arrow).

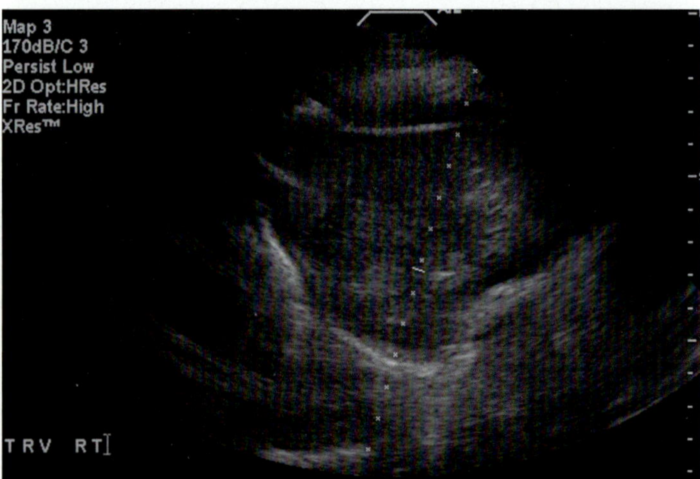

Figure 2.33 — Lung, Small Cell Carcinoma. Sonographic image obtained during ultrasound-guided biopsy shows the large right-sided mass. Small cell carcinoma is typically treated with chemotherapy and radiation rather than surgery and the prognosis is very poor.

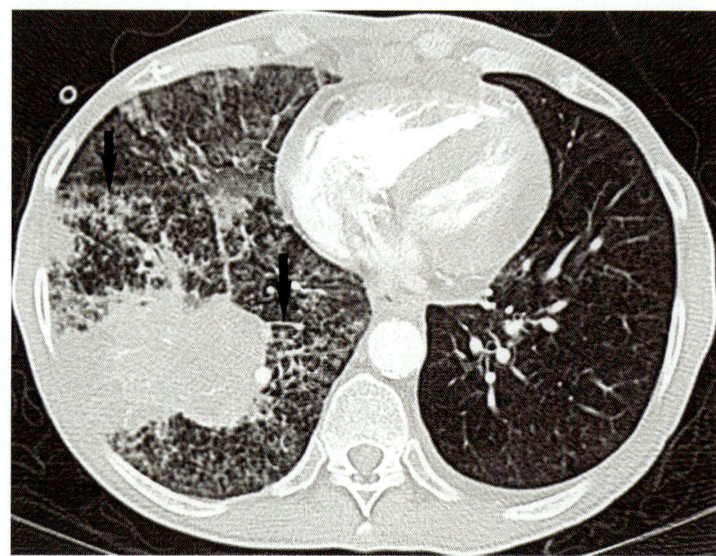

Figure 2.34 — Lung, Small Cell Carcinoma. Axial CT of the chest in lung windows demonstrates a large mass in the right lower lobe. There is also extensive adjacent interstitial thickening (arrows) which represents lymphangitic spread of cancer.

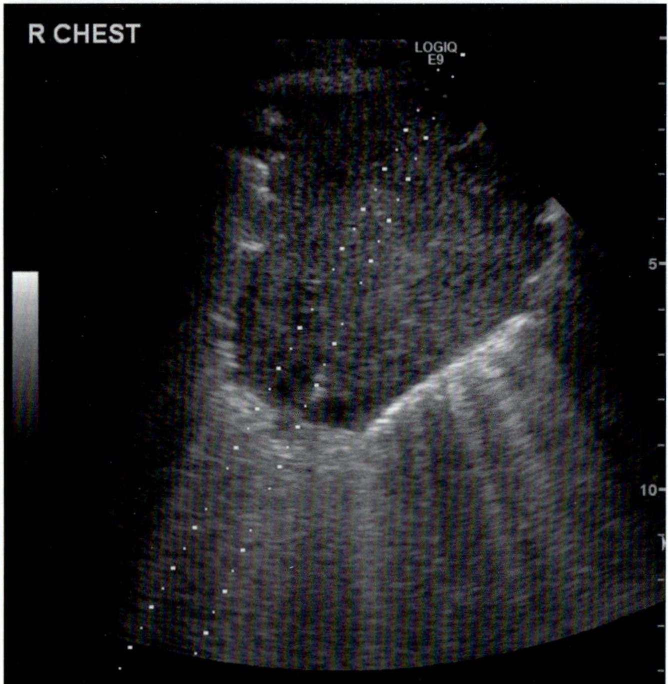

Figure 2.35 — Lung, Small Cell Carcinoma. Sonographic image obtained during the ultrasound-guided biopsy shows the large right lower lobe mass found to represent a small cell carcinoma.

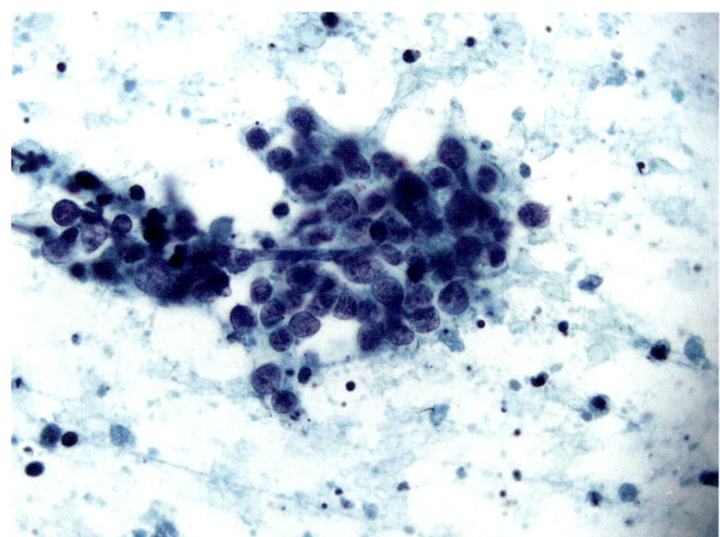

Figure 2.36 — Lung, Small Cell Carcinoma. This fragment of malignant cells shows enlarged nuclei with very scant cytoplasm. Chromatin is finely granular and nucleoli are inconspicuous or absent, characteristic of cells of neuroendocrine origin. Numerous apoptotic bodies are seen within the fragment and in the background. (Papanicolaou stain, high power)

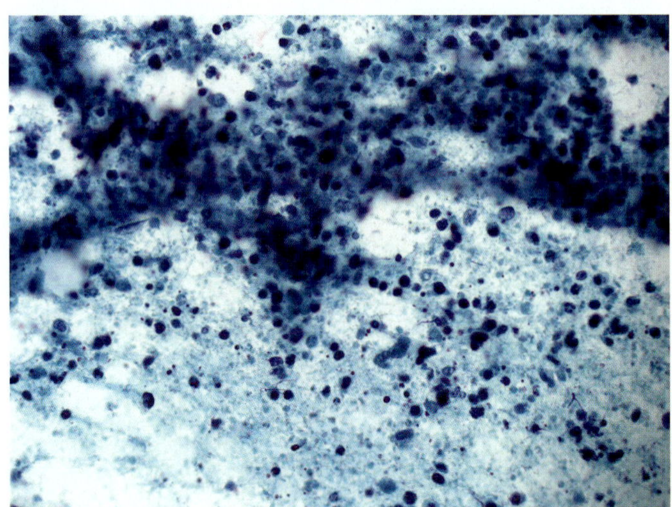

Figure 2.37 — Lung, Small Cell Carcinoma. A background of extensive necrosis, including cellular debris and numerous apoptotic bodies reflects the high cell turnover in small cell carcinoma. Viable tumor cells may be sparse. The presence of neoplastic neuroendocrine type cells without mitotic figures, apoptotic bodies, or necrosis should prompt consideration of another diagnosis, such as carcinoid tumor. (Papanicolaou stain, medium power)

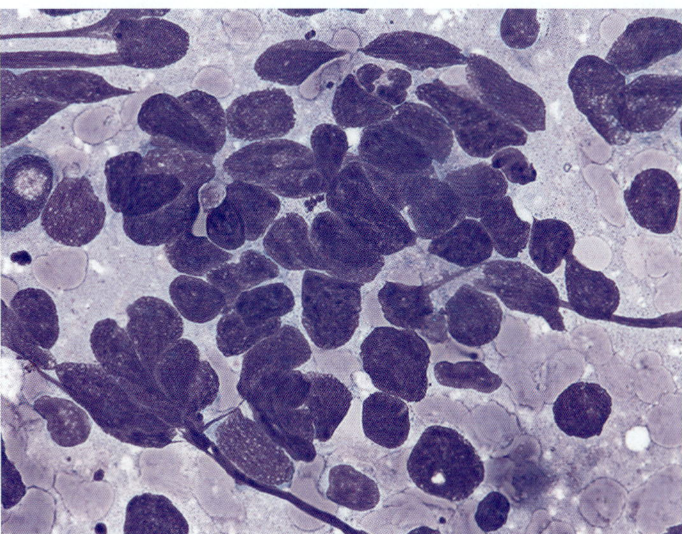

Figure 2.38 — Lung, Small Cell Carcinoma. Tumor cells show nuclear molding or deformation of nuclei due to compression by adjacent nuclei. Occasional nuclear streaks, termed crush artifact, are seen here and are indicative of the fragility of the tumor cells. Vague rosette formations are also evident. (Diff Quik stain, high power)

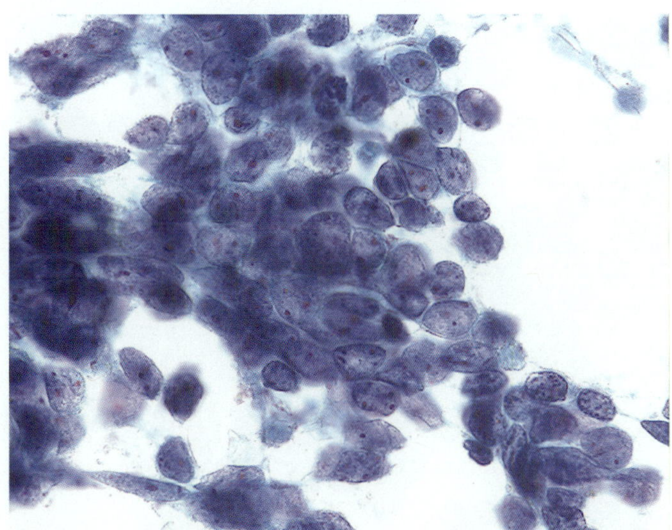

Figure 2.39 — Lung, Small Cell Carcinoma. Tumor cells in small cell carcinoma may be present in sheets, fragments, or dispersed singly. Even when present in a sheet, the cells show loose cohesion. Finely granular chromatin is evident in these tumor cells, which also demonstrate single or multiple small nucleoli. (Papanicolaou stain, high power)

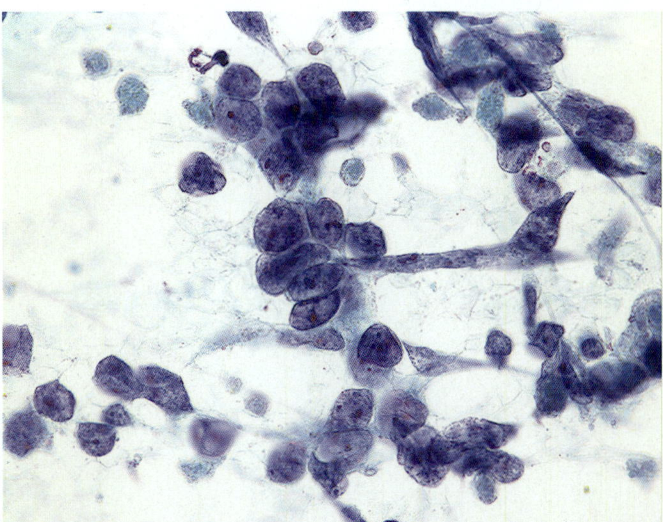

Figure 2.40 — Lung, Small Cell Carcinoma. Nuclear molding is evident in the tumor cells in the center of the field. Cytoplasm is scant to absent. The pathologic differential diagnosis for small cell carcinoma often includes a high-grade lymphoma or poorly differentiated non-small cell carcinoma. (Papanicolaou stain, high power)

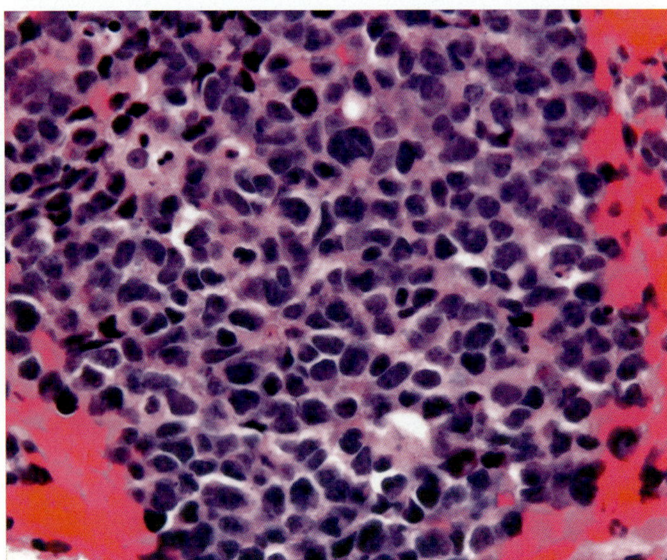

Figure 2.41 — Lung, Small Cell Carcinoma (Histology). A sheet of tumor cells shows small- to medium-sized angulated nuclei with finely granular chromatin and inconspicuous nuclei. Mitotic figures and apoptotic bodes are readily identified. (Hematoxylin and eosin stain, high power)

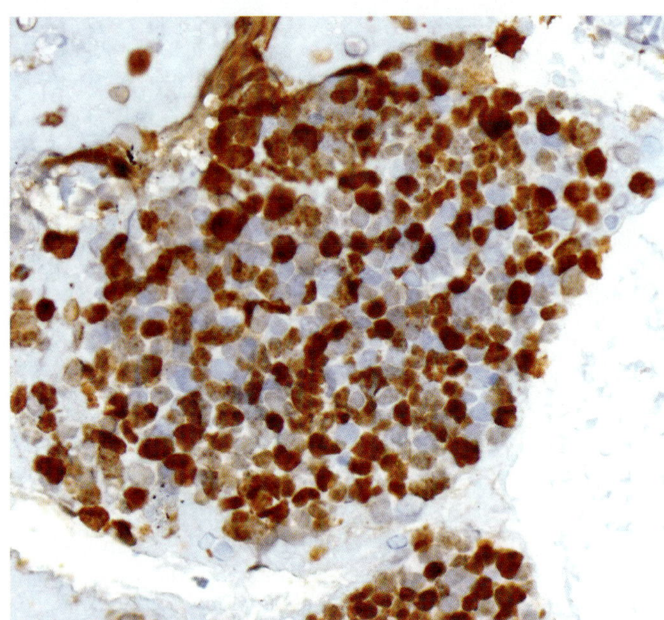

Figure 2.42 — Lung, Small Cell Carcinoma (Histology). A Ki-67 (Mib-1) immunostain highlights most of the tumor nuclei. This reflects the very high proliferative rate of the tumor. (Ki-67 immunostain, high power)

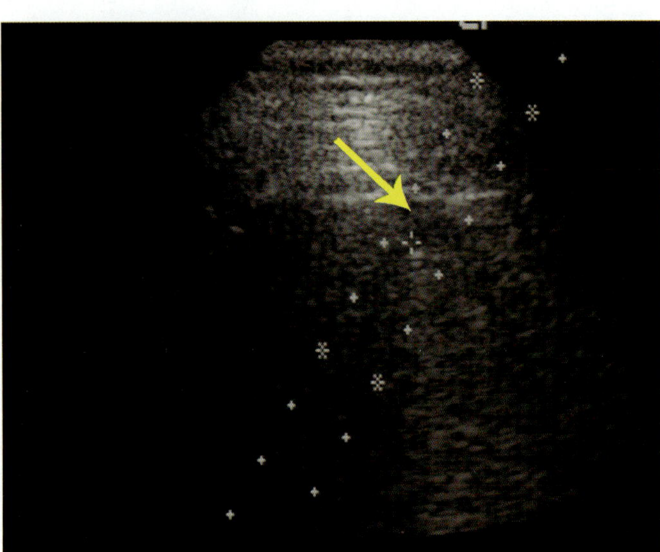

Figure 2.43 — Lung, Pulmonary Hamartoma. Sonographic image demonstrates a subtle 1.0-cm mass in the left lower lobe abutting the pleura (arrow). The appearance is nonspecific, though pulmonary hamartomas are typically solitary and subpleural.

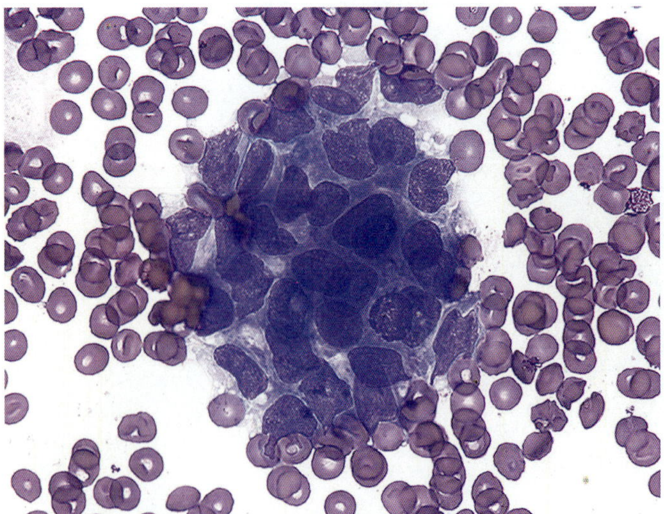

Figure 2.44 — Lung, Pulmonary Hamartoma. A fragment of epithelial cells is present showing slightly increased nuclear-to-cytoplasmic ratio. These cells raised concern for a metastasis in this patient with a history of mammary carcinoma and in the absence of other cellular components of hamartoma. (Diff Quik stain, high power)

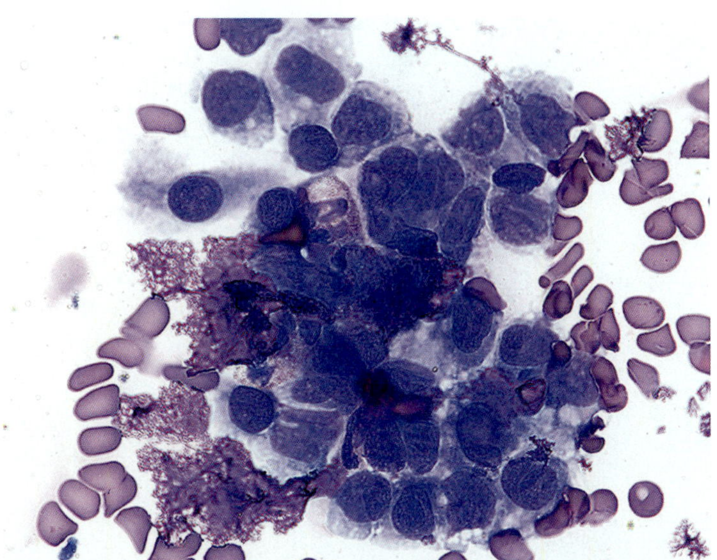

Figure 2.45 — Lung, Pulmonary Hamartoma. Epithelial cells with slightly increased nuclear-to-cytoplasmic ratio and mildly irregular nuclear contours are pictured. These cells represent reactive bronchial epithelial cells that are a part of this rare benign tumor. (Diff Quik stain, high power)

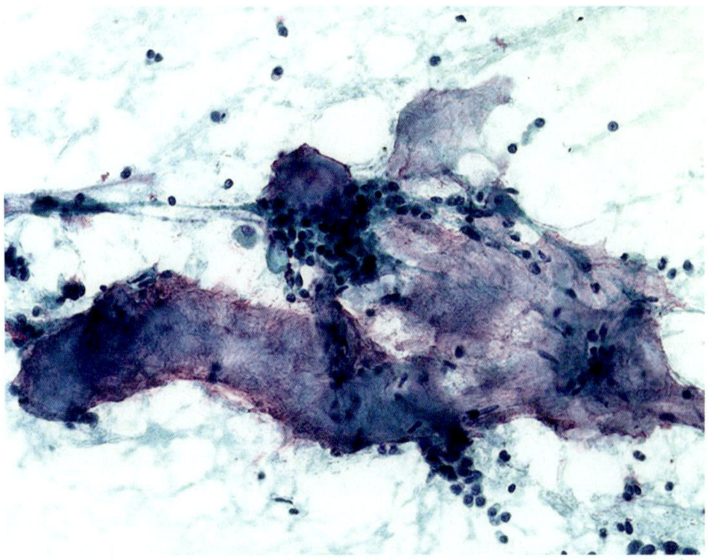

Figure 2.46 — Lung, Pulmonary Hamartoma. A polymorphous admixture of epithelium with abundant chondroid matrix may be seen in aspirates of pulmonary hamartoma (seen here). Alternatively, aspirates may be sparsely cellular, depending on the area of the tumor sampled. (Papanicolaou stain, low power)

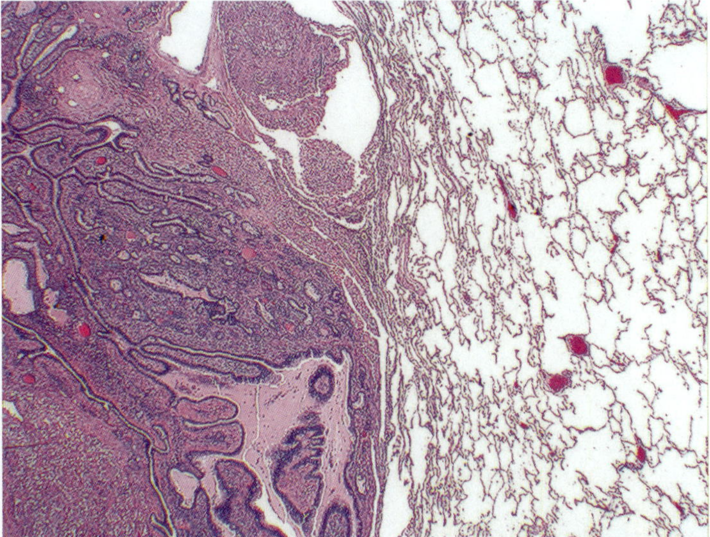

Figure 2.47 — Lung, Pulmonary Hamartoma (Histology). A well-circumscribed mass is seen in the left of the field adjacent to benign pulmonary parenchyma at the right of the field. Islands of disorganized respiratory epithelium are admixed with mesenchymal elements and fibrous tissue. (Hematoxylin and eosin stain, medium power)

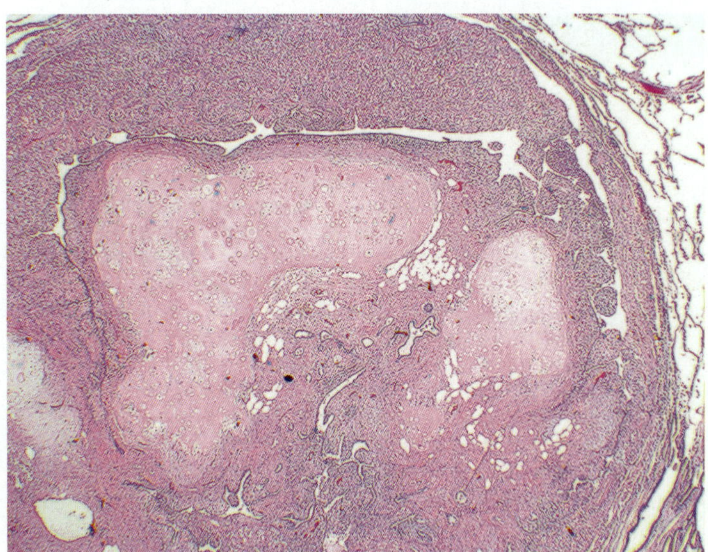

Figure 2.48 — Lung, Pulmonary Hamartoma (Histology). Benign-appearing chondroid material is surrounded by bronchial epithelium and fibrous tissue. These lesions may calcify or ossify and thus may yield only scant diagnostic material on FNA. (Hematoxylin and eosin stain, medium power)

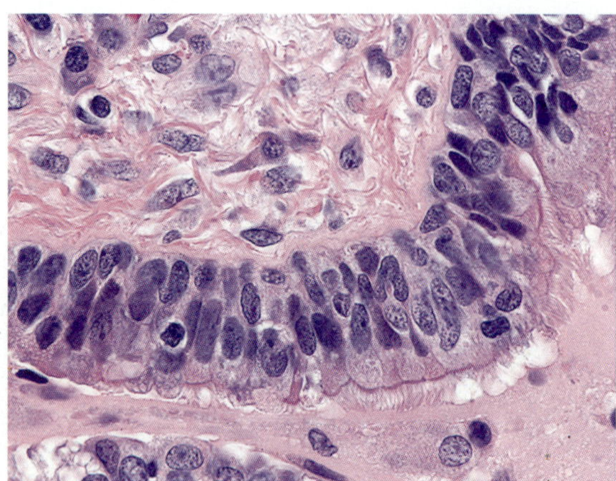

Figure 2.49 — Lung, Pulmonary Hamartoma (Histology). Bronchial epithelial cells comprising one component of the pulmonary hamartoma. Terminal bars and cilia are evident. The nuclei are slightly enlarged, hyperchromatic, and show moderate architectural disorganization. (Hematoxylin and eosin stain, high power)

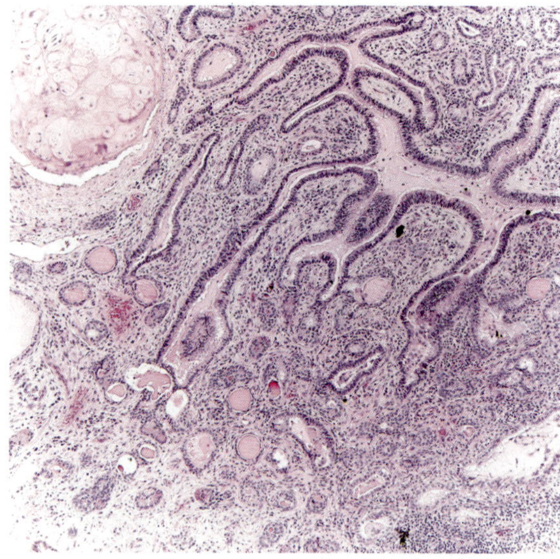

Figure 2.50 — Lung, Pulmonary Hamartoma (Histology). Hamartomas are rare lesions that occur more commonly in adult males. The lesion shows both mesenchymal and epithelial differentiation. The lesion is composed of mature bronchial epitheliumas well as cartilage, mature fat, and spindle cells without any cytological atypia. (Hematoxylin and eosin stain, medium power)

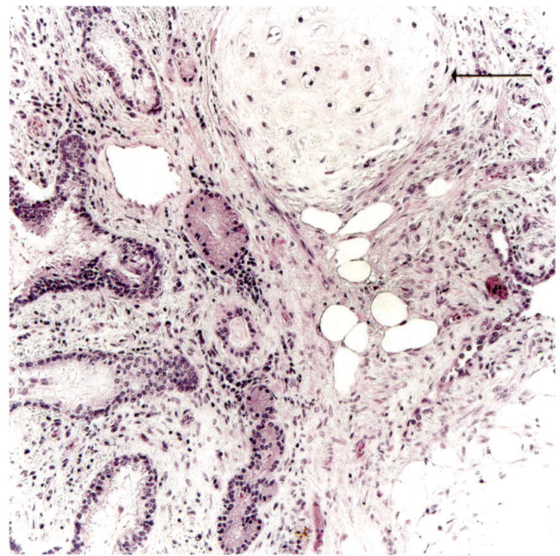

Figure 2.51 — Lung, Pulmonary Hamartoma (Histology). The lesion demonstrates benign respiratory epithelium admixed with benign appearing spindle cells in a myxoid background. Note the presence of benign cartilage (arrow). Small epithelial tubules are present at the periphery of the lesion admixed with chronic inflammation. There is no cytological atypia or any other features worrisome for malignancy. (Hematoxylin and eosin stain, high power)

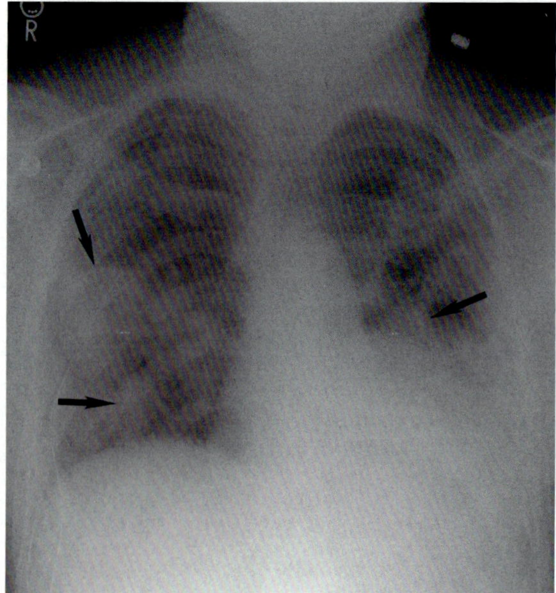

Figure 2.52 — Lung, Squamous Papillomatosis. This 27-year-old male complained of chronic shortness of breath. X-ray of the chest shows multiple bilateral lung masses, several of which are cavitary (arrows).

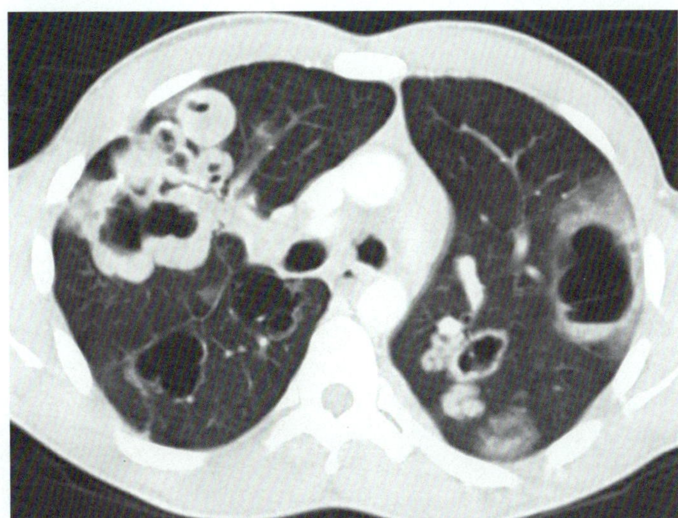

Figure 2.53 — Lung, Squamous Papillomatosis. Axial CT image of the chest in lung windows shows multiple thick-walled cavitary lesions in the lungs bilaterally. Papillomatosis results from infection of the upper respiratory tract by the human papillomavirus and can spread to the trachea and lung parenchyma. Parenchymal nodules are usually cavitary.

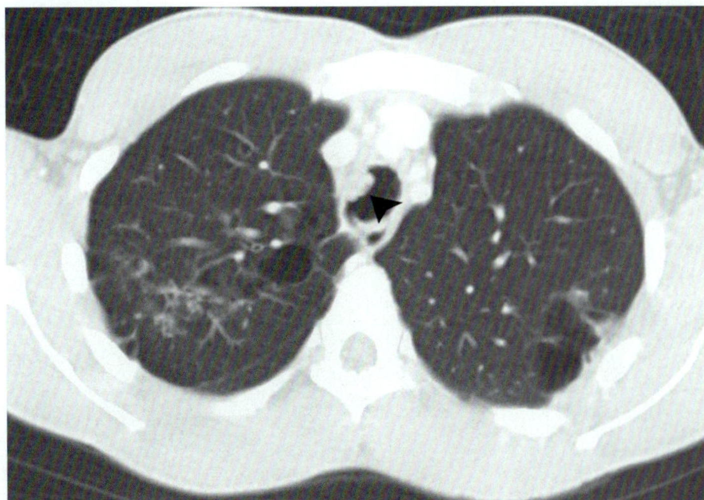

Figure 2.54 — Lung, Squamous Papillomatosis. There are also small masses in the trachea (arrowhead). Patients with squamous papillomatosis often have multiple lesions in the trachea and bronchi.

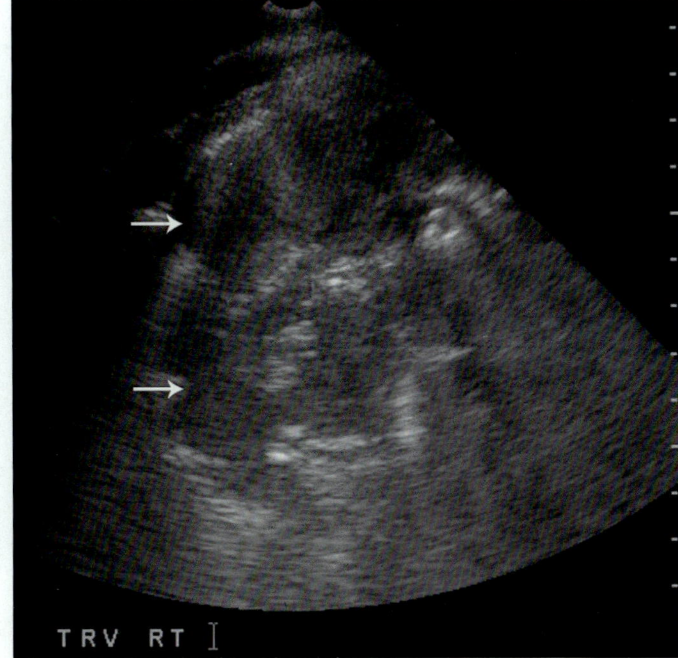

Figure 2.55 — Lung, Squamous Papillomatosis. Sonographic image confirms echogenic masses in the right chest (arrows).

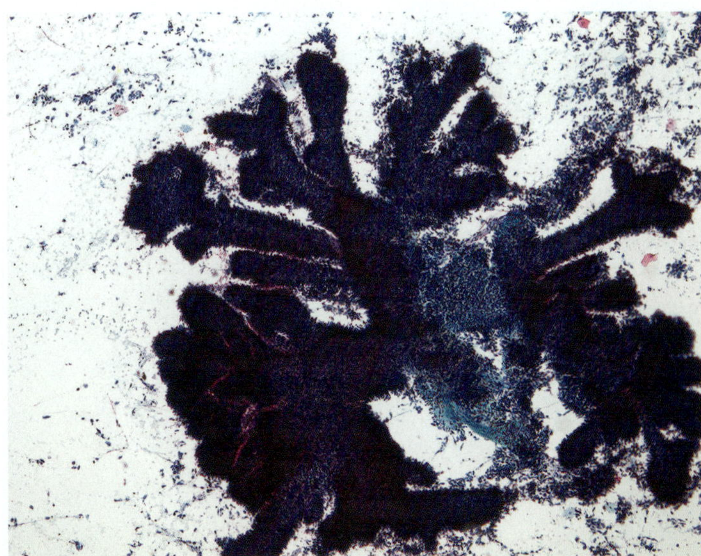

Figure 2.56 — Lung, Squamous Papillomatosis. Pulmonary papillomas most commonly occur in large bronchi. They are often associated with laryngeal (as in this patient) or tracheal lesions, and are related to low-risk types of human papillomavirus (HPV). At low power, the papillary architecture of this lesion is readily apparent with variably shaped papillae radiating out from a central fibrovascular core. (Papanicolaou stain, low power)

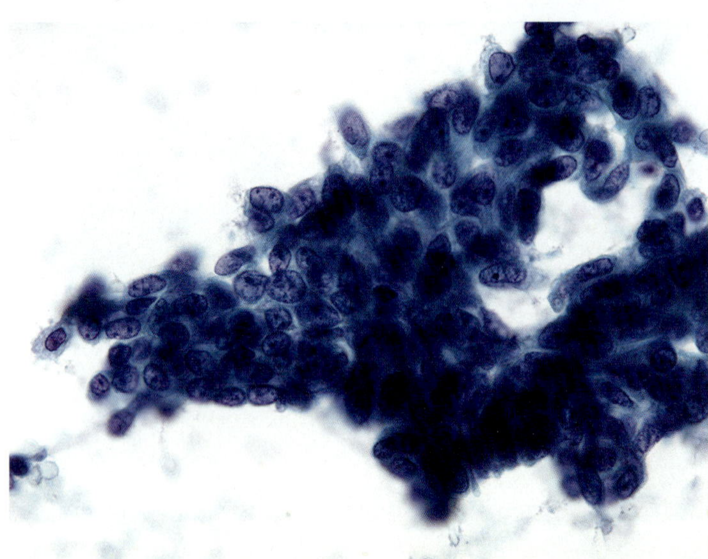

Figure 2.57 — Lung, Squamous Papillomatosis. This cellular fragment shows cytologic atypia with nuclear overlap and mild anisonucleosis. Dysplasia and squamous cell carcinoma may rarely develop in a squamous papilloma. (Papanicolaou stain, high power)

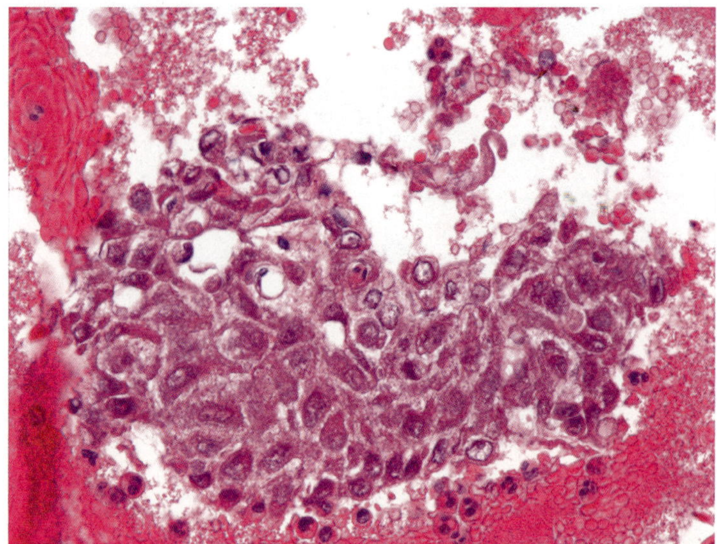

Figure 2.58 — Lung, Squamous Papillomatosis (Cell Block). This cell block preparation shows atypical squamous cells with well-defined cell borders and focally increased nuclear-to-cytoplasmic ratio, raising concern for dysplasia. HPV *in situ* hybridization may be used to confirm that the lesion is related to HPV infection. (Hematoxylin and eosin stain, high power)

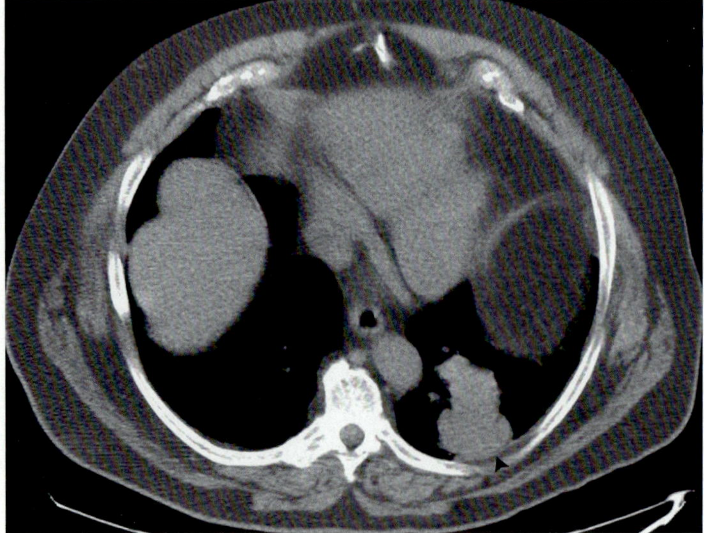

Figure 2.59 — Lung, Metastatic Papillary Thyroid Carcinoma. This 71-year-old man with a distant history of a total thyroidectomy and radioiodine ablation presented with elevated thyroglobulin. Axial unenhanced CT of the chest shows a large left lower lobe mass (arrowhead). Although the appearance is nonspecific, a primary lung neoplasm is in the differential.

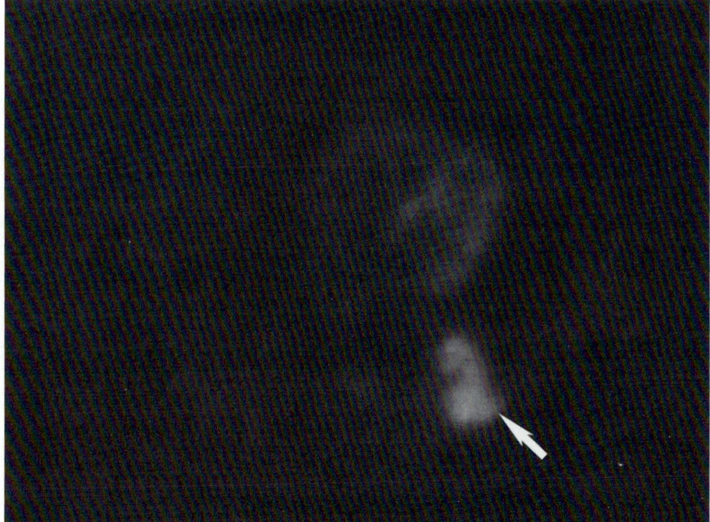

Figure 2.60 — Lung, Metastatic Papillary Thyroid Carcinoma. PET scan shows the left lower lobe mass is FDG-avid (arrow). This finding was concerning given the patient's history of papillary thyroid carcinoma, although typically metastases are multiple rather than solitary.

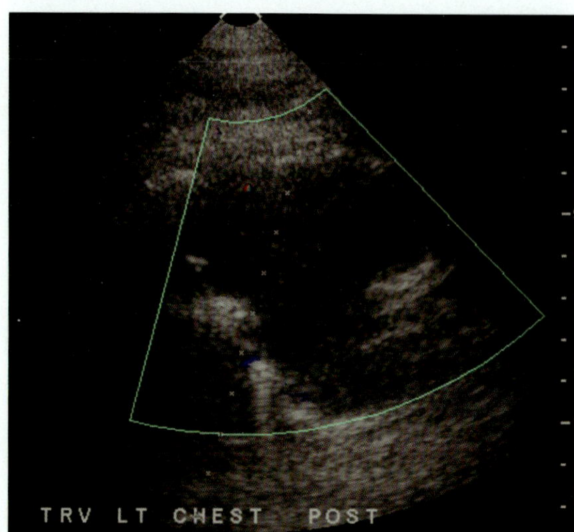

Figure 2.61 — Lung, Metastatic Papillary Thyroid Carcinoma. Sonographic image confirms the presence of a hypoechoic left chest mass. The lung is a common site for metastatic lesions and metastases are more commonly multiple, round, located in the periphery, and of varying size. Virtually any type of tumor can metastasize to the lung.

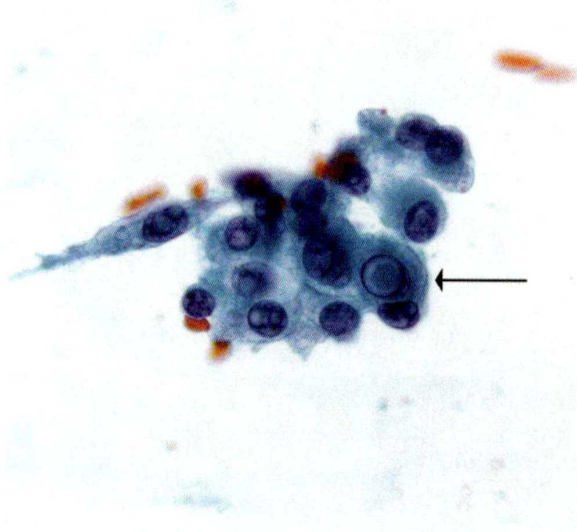

Figure 2.62 — Lung, Metastatic Papillary Thyroid Carcinoma. Among carcinomas that metastasize to the lung, the most common primary sites include colon, breast, pancreas, and stomach. In this case, scant tumor material was present on the aspirate smears. This fragment of tumor cells shows anisonucleosis with clear pale chromatin and a large intranuclear inclusion (arrow). (Papanicolaou stain, high power)

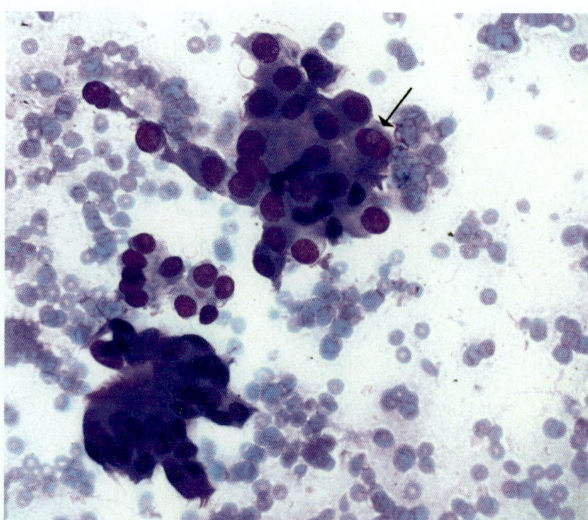

Figure 2.63 — Lung, Metastatic Papillary Thyroid Carcinoma. The neoplastic cells show oval-shaped nuclei and a single intranuclear inclusion (arrow). Papillary thyroid carcinoma shares many morphologic features with bronchioloalveolar carcinoma of the lung, so the radiographic and clinical impression is important in distinguishing the two. A group of benign, ciliated bronchial epithelial cells is present in the bottom left portion of the field. (Diff Quik stain, high power)

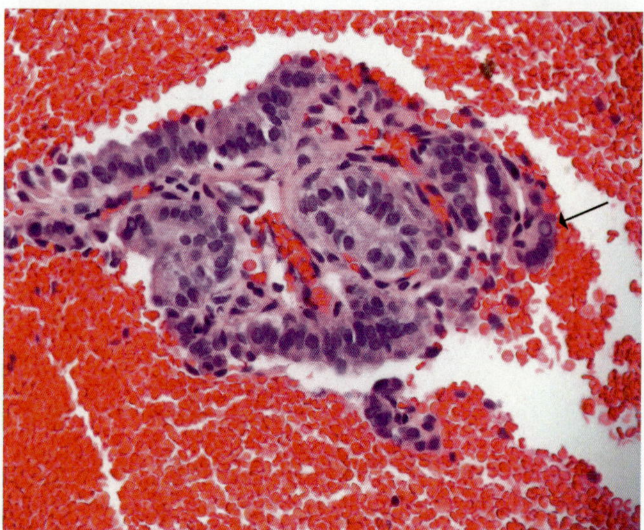

Figure 2.64 — Lung, Metastatic Papillary Thyroid Carcinoma (Cell Block). Material was available in the cell block for confirmatory immunostains. Tumor cells show focal intranuclear inclusions (arrow). Although a TTF-1 was positive, this does not distinguish primary lung tumors from metastatic thyroid carcinoma. (Hematoxylin and eosin stain, high power)

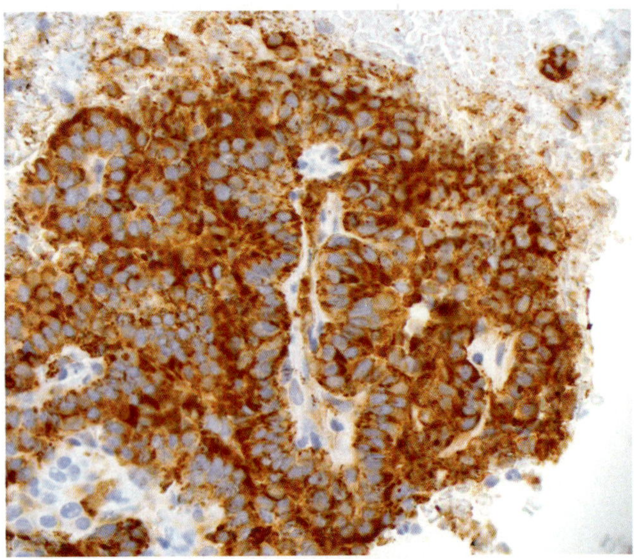

Figure 2.65 — Lung, Metastatic Papillary Thyroid Carcinoma (Cell Block). A thyroglobulin stain is strongly positive in the tumor cells. PAX-8 was also performed and was positive, consistent with a thyroid primary. (Thyroglobulin immunostain, high power)

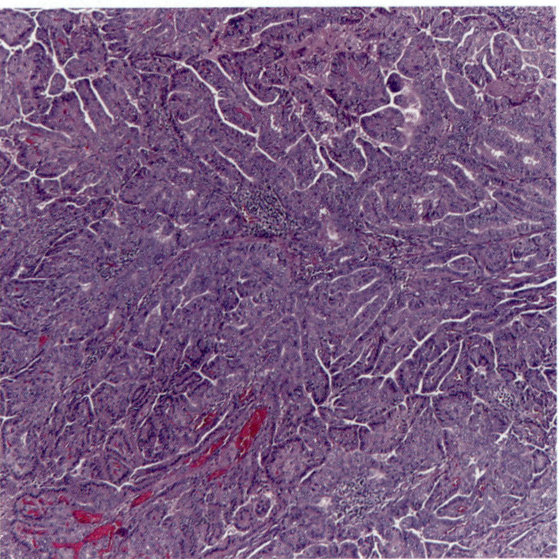

Figure 2.66 — Lung, Metastatic Papillary Thyroid Carcinoma (Histology). Metastatic papillary thyroid carcinoma involving the lung shows characteristic complex papillae and elongated follicles. At low power, a primary adenocarcinoma of the lung is considered in the differential. (Hematoxylin and eosin stain, low power)

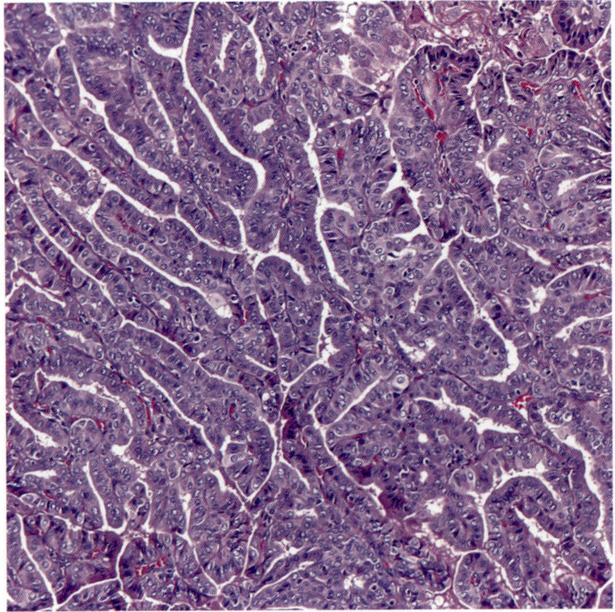

Figure 2.67 — Lung, Metastatic Papillary Thyroid Carcinoma (Histology). The combination of architectural and cytological features is characteristic of metastatic papillary thyroid carcinoma. The nuclei are overlapping and demonstrate pale, "open" chromatin. (Hematoxylin and eosin stain, medium power)

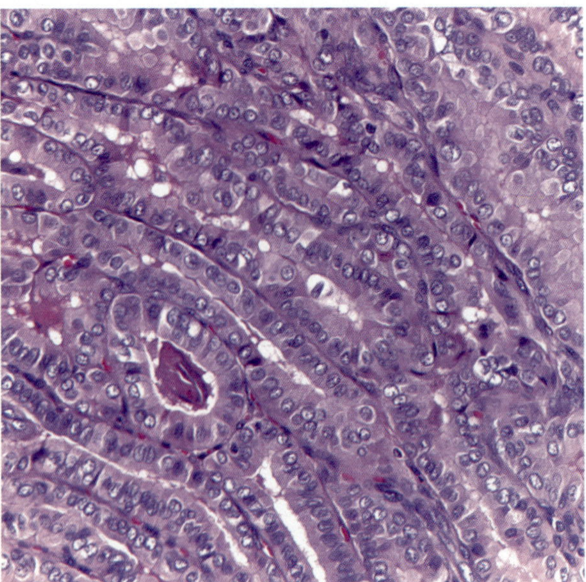

Figure 2.68 — Lung, Metastatic Papillary Thyroid Carcinoma (Histology). The tumor has a distinct papillary. The nuclei are enlarged, overlapping, and crowded. Optically clear nuclei with a ground-glass appearance are noted and nuclear grooves are numerous. (Hematoxylin and eosin stain, high power)

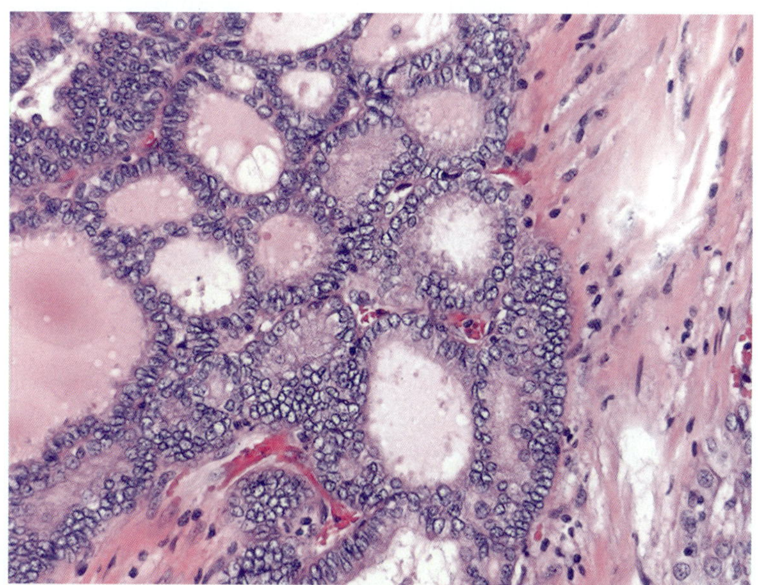

Figure 2.69 — Lung, Metastatic Papillary Thyroid Carcinoma (Histology). Although the neoplasm in this case forms a follicular architecture, the nuclear features are classic for papillary thyroid carcinoma. (Hematoxylin and eosin stain, high power)

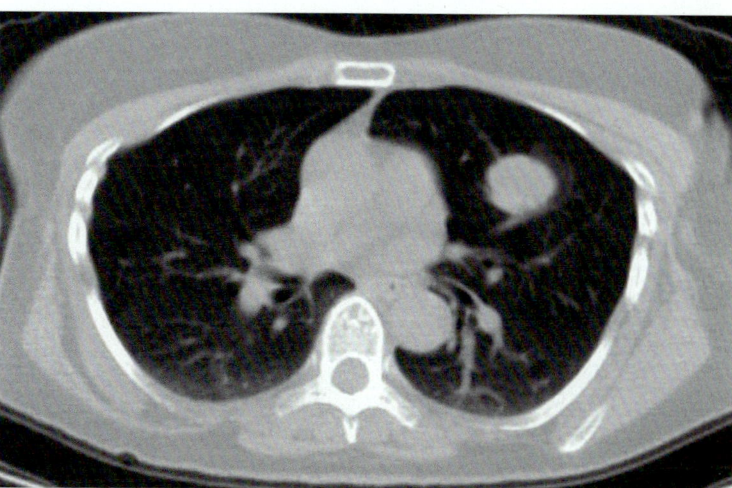

Figure 2.70 — Lung, Metastatic Melanoma. This 64-year-old woman had a history of melanoma excised from her back 2 years prior, and a history of multiple basal cell carcinomas and a cutaneous squamous cell carcinoma. Axial CT image in lung windows show a left upper lobe pulmonary nodule.

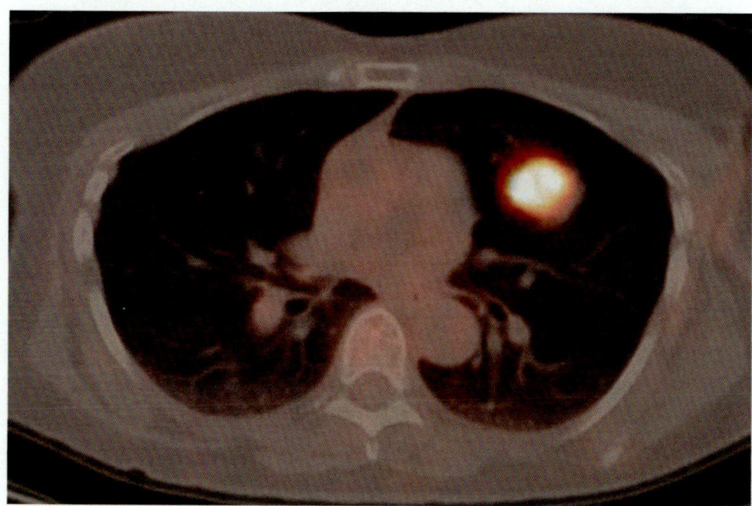

Figure 2.71 — Lung, Metastatic Melanoma. Fused PET/CT scan shows the nodule is FDG-avid. The patient has a history of melanoma and the mass was found to be metastatic melanoma. Included in the differential is a primary lung cancer.

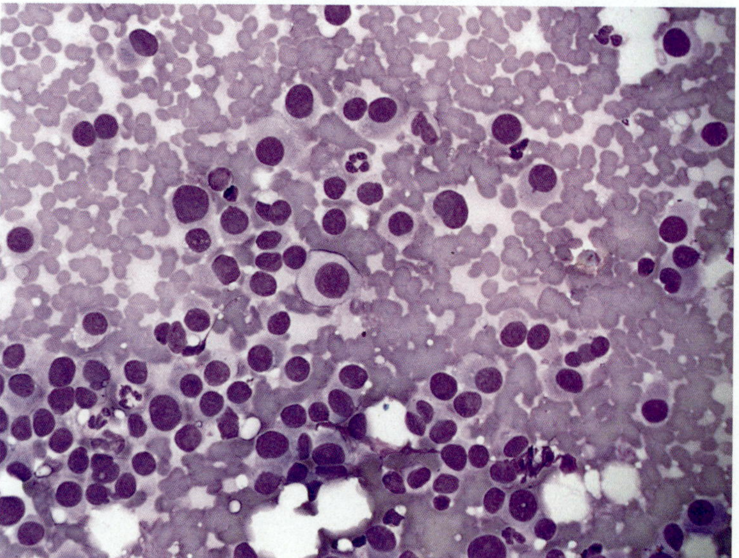

Figure 2.72 — Lung, Metastatic Melanoma. A population of singly dispersed neoplastic cells is shown. The tumor cells are fairly monotonous with round to oval nuclei and a moderate amount of cytoplasm. Occasional larger cells are seen and some cells show an eccentric nucleus (plasmacytoid appearance) often encountered in malignant melanoma. (Diff Quik stain, high power)

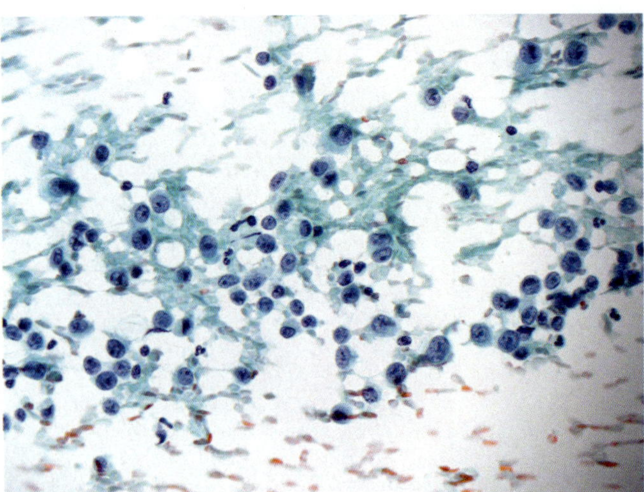

Figure 2.73 — Lung, Metastatic Melanoma. Malignant melanoma can look like many other neoplasms, including carcinoma and lymphoma, hence its moniker "the great imitator." Tumor cells may form sheets and fragments, or may be dispersed, as seen in this image. The nuclei are round to oval with occasional prominent nucleoli. (Papanicolaou stain, medium power)

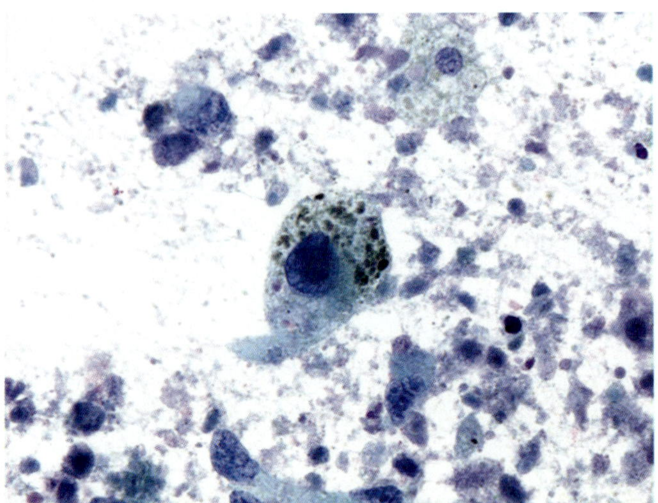

Figure 2.74 — Lung, Metastatic Melanoma. Malignant melanomas frequently metastasize to the lung. The presence of melanin pigment in the cytoplasm as seen here is practically diagnostic, but is often not present. Melanin pigment needs to be differentiated from the more common anthracosis and hemosiderosis. (Papanicolaou stain, high power)

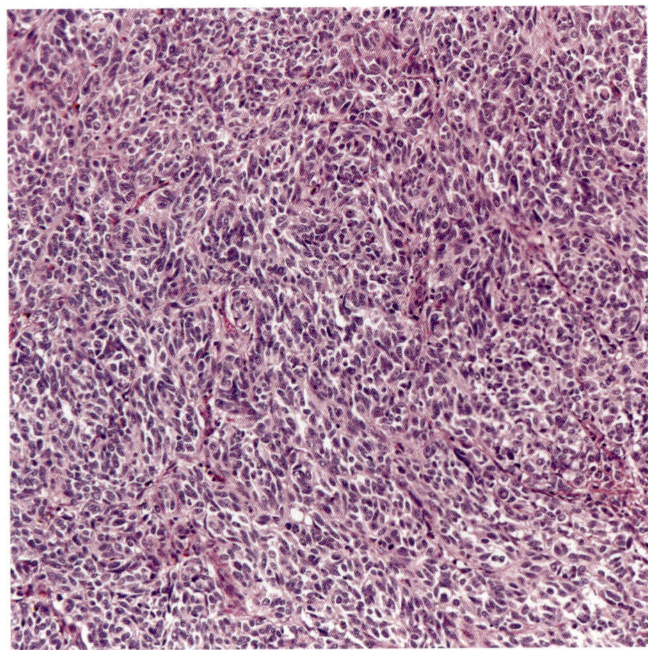

Figure 2.75 — Lung, Metastatic Melanoma (Histology). The patient has a prior posterior neck melanoma. The neoplasm consists of nests of large, spindle-shaped cells with large nuclei with prominent nucleoli. (Hematoxylin and eosin stain, low power)

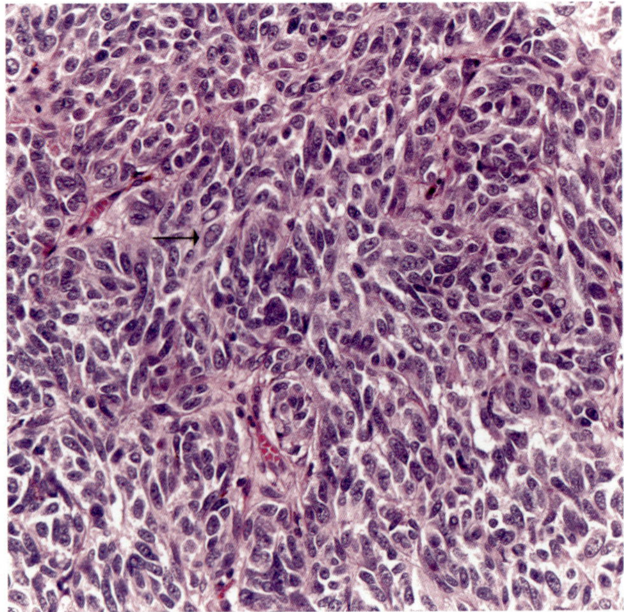

Figure 2.76 — Lung, Metastatic Melanoma (Histology). The neoplastic cells have pink cytoplasm with oval to round nuclei and prominent nucleoli. Distinct pseudoinclusions (arrow) can be seen in some of the nuclei. (Hematoxylin and eosin stain, medium power)

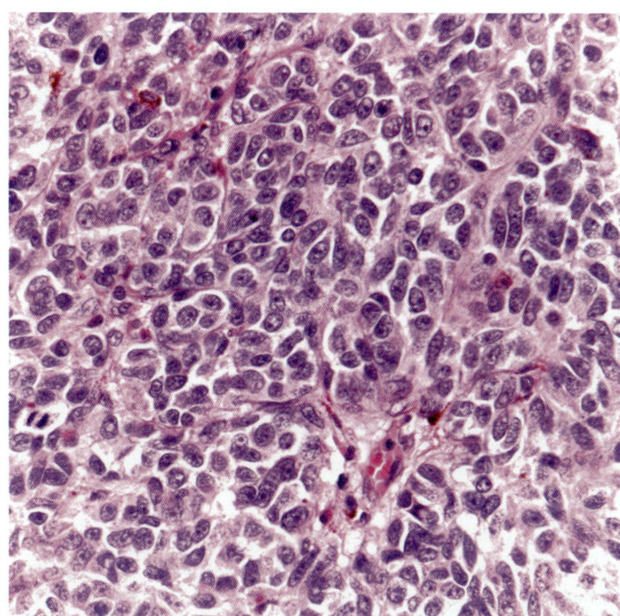

Figure 2.77 — Lung, Metastatic Melanoma (Histology). The neoplastic nuclei have oval- to spindle-shaped nuclei and are arranged in nests. Note some focal deposits of brown pigment, characteristic of melanoma. (Hematoxylin and eosin stain, high power)

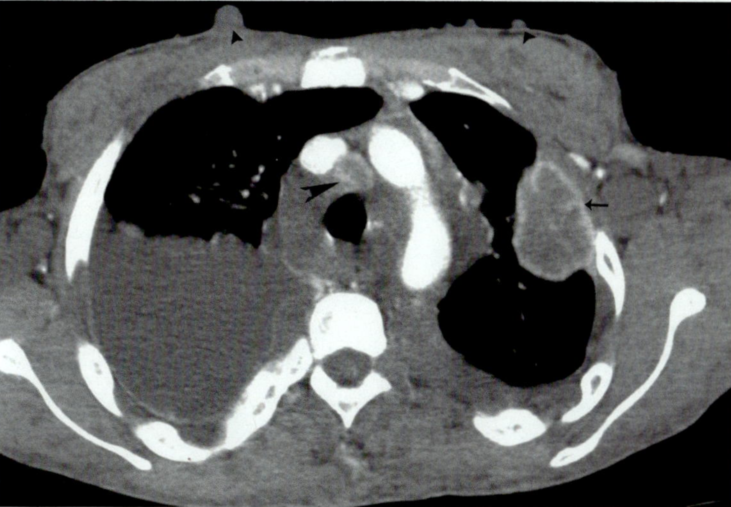

Figure 2.78 — Lung, Metastatic Malignant Peripheral Nerve Sheath Tumor. This 32-year-old man had neurofibromatosis type 1 and a history of malignant peripheral nerve sheath tumor of the left leg. Axial contrast-enhanced CT shows an enhancing pleural-based mass in the left upper lobe (arrow) and a right pleural effusion. Enhancing mediastinal adenopathy (arrowhead) and multiple subcutaneous neurofibromas (arrowheads) are also present.

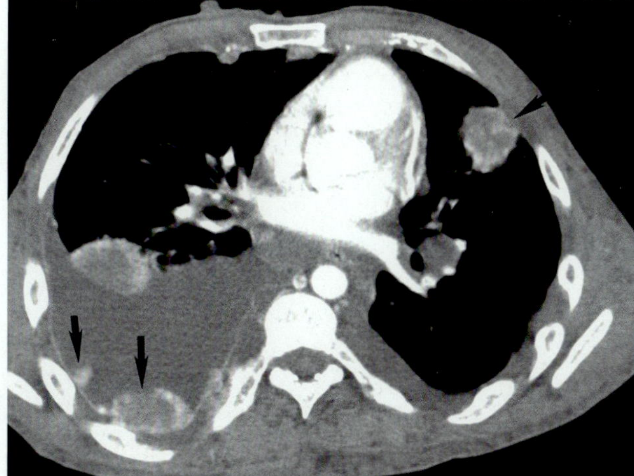

Figure 2.79 — Lung, Metastatic Malignant Peripheral Nerve Sheath Tumor. Axial contrast-enhanced CT slightly more inferiorly shows enhancing masses, mostly pleural based (arrows), in the lungs bilaterally. There is an associated moderate right and small left pleural effusion. These enhancing masses were found to represent metastatic malignant peripheral nerve sheath tumor.

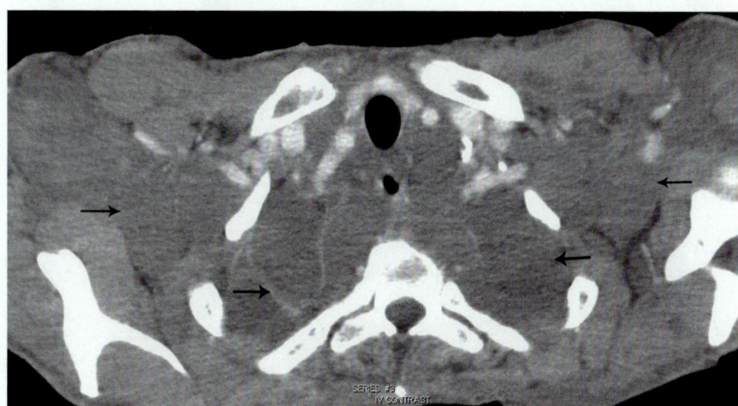

Figure 2.80 — Lung, Metastatic Malignant Peripheral Nerve Sheath Tumor. Axial contrast-enhanced CT image of the upper chest shows extensive low-density masses in the lung apices and axillary regions bilaterally compatible with neurofibromas (arrows).

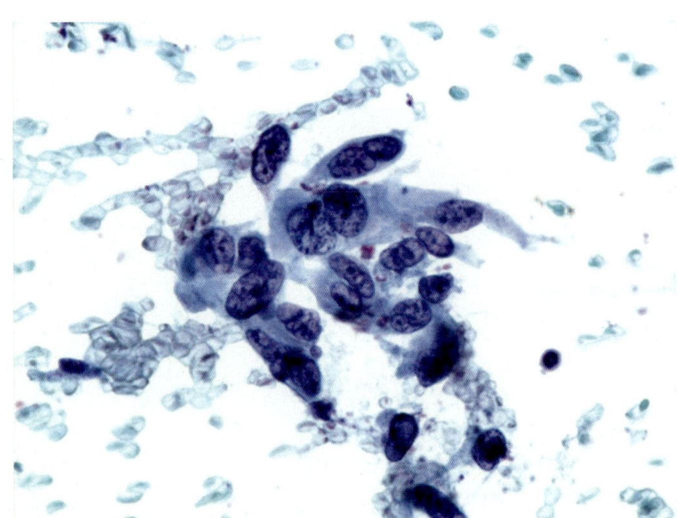

Figure 2.81 — Lung, Metastatic Malignant Peripheral Nerve Sheath Tumor. Due to their hematogenous dissemination, lung is a common site for metastases from sarcomas. The malignant cells shown here show oval- to spindle-shaped nuclei with a moderate amount of cytoplasm. The nuclei are hyperchromatic with irregular nuclear contours and occasional nucleoli. (Papanicolaou stain, high power)

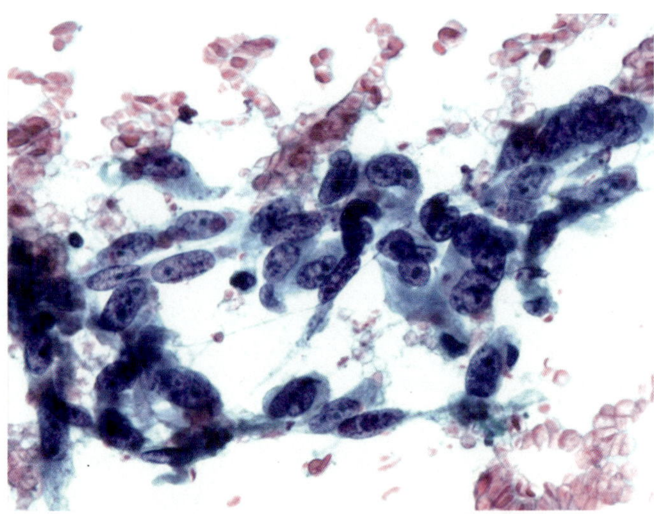

Figure 2.82 — Lung, Metastatic Malignant Peripheral Nerve Sheath Tumor. Malignant spindle cells are shown in a loosely cohesive fragment. The nuclei show tapered ends, characteristic of neural origin. Chromatin is unevenly dispersed and nucleoli are variably present. (Papanicolaou stain, high power)

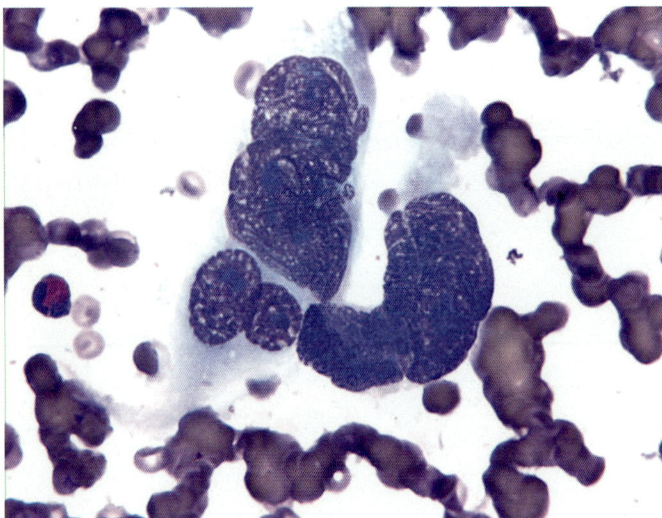

Figure 2.83 — Lung, Metastatic Malignant Peripheral Nerve Sheath Tumor. These few malignant cells are markedly enlarged when compared to the background red blood cells and a single inflammatory cell. The nuclei show bizarre shapes and prominent nucleoli. (Diff Quik stain, high power)

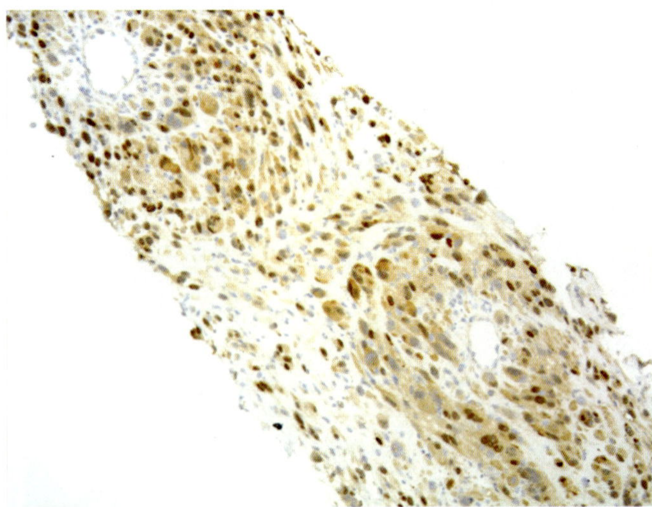

Figure 2.84 — Lung, Metastatic Malignant Peripheral Nerve Sheath Tumor (Core Biopsy). A core biopsy of the lesion shows densely packed malignant spindle cells with bizarre nuclear shapes. An immunostain for S-100 protein is positive (nuclear stain), consistent with the patient's known history of malignant peripheral nerve sheath tumor. It should be noted that S-100 is characteristically focal and can be negative in these tumors. (S-100 protein immunostain, medium power)

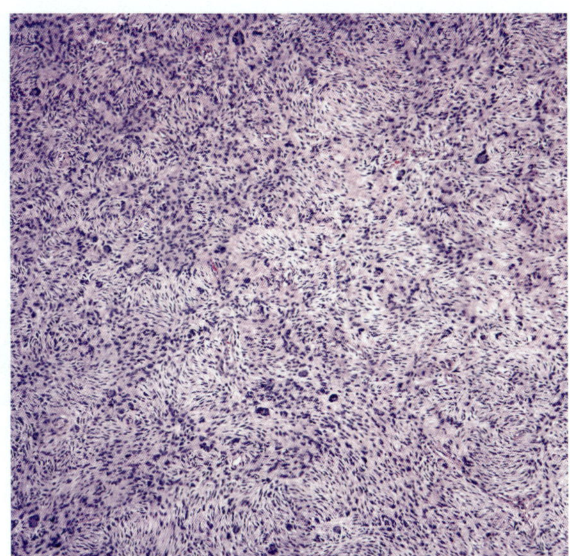

Figure 2.85 — Lung, Metastatic Malignant Peripheral Nerve Sheath Tumor (Histology). This cellular neoplasm shows a prominent spindle cell component with numerous bizarre, multinucleated cells. There are numerous mitoses. (Hematoxylin and eosin stain, low power)

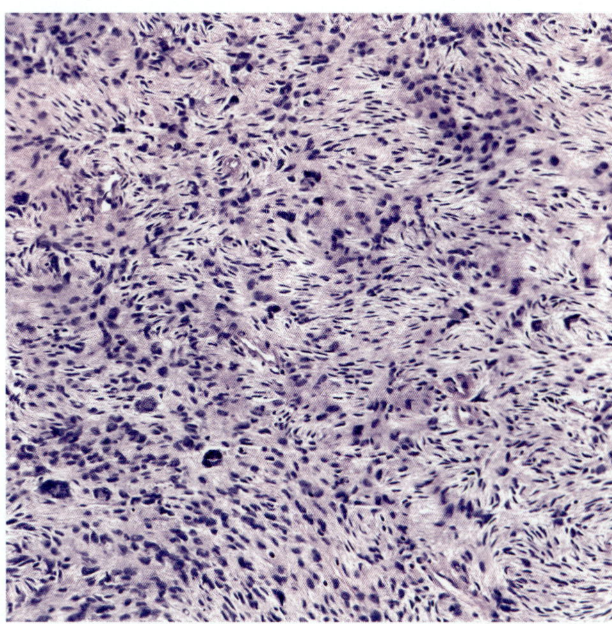

Figure 2.86 — Lung, Metastatic Malignant Peripheral Nerve Sheath Tumor (Histology). A spindle cell neoplasm with high cellularity, pleomorphism, and a high mitotic rate is shown. Note the presence of numerous multinucleated giant cells. (Hematoxylin and eosin stain, medium power)

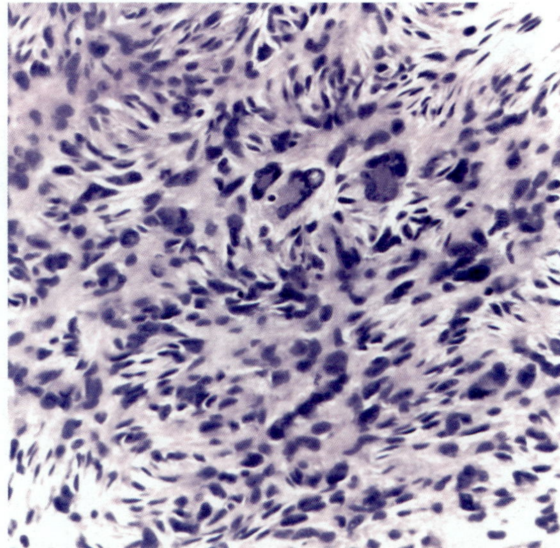

Figure 2.87 — Lung, Metastatic Malignant Peripheral Nerve Sheath Tumor (Histology). Spindle cells are admixed with plump bizarre tumor cells showing multinucleation. Neoplastic cells show nuclear positivity with S-100 protein. The diagnosis can be firmly established if the tumor occurs in a patient with NF-1. (Hematoxylin and eosin stain, high power)

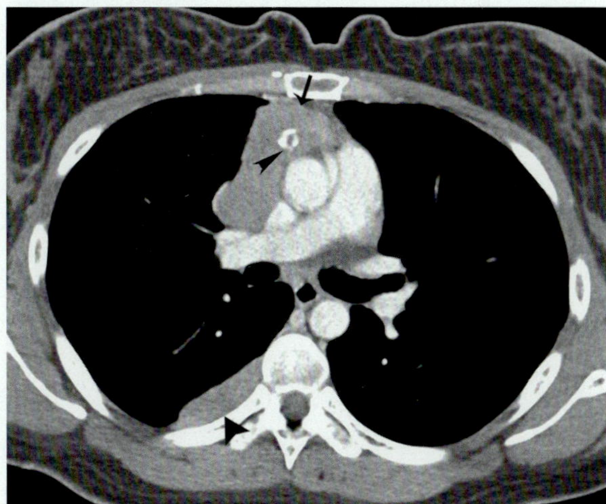

Figure 2.88 — Mediastinum, Thymoma. Axial contrast-enhanced CT shows a lobulated, homogenous anterior mediastinal mass (arrow) containing a small coarse calcification (arrowhead). This mass was resected and found to be a thymoma. A pleural-based mass is also present in the right posterior lung from a drop metastasis (arrowhead).

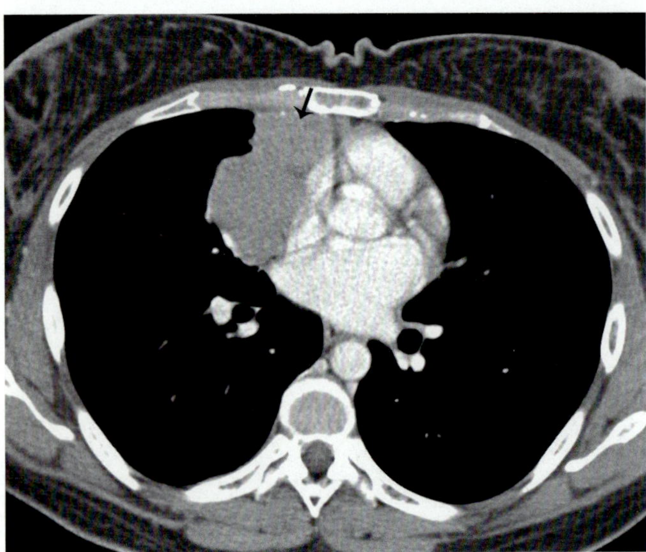

Figure 2.89 — Mediastinum, Thymoma. Axial CT slightly more inferiorly at the level of the heart shows the soft tissue mass in the anterior mediastinum (arrow) and further extent of thymoma. Most thymomas are found in the anterior mediastinum.

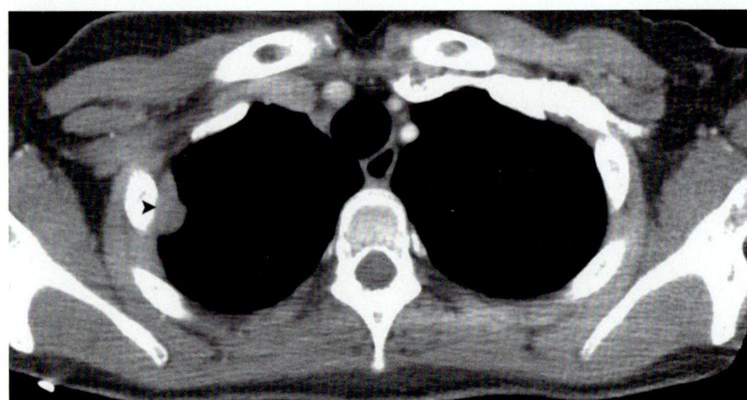

Figure 2.90 — Mediastinum, Thymoma. Several years later, the patient developed a new pleural-based mass, representing a metastatic pleural lesion, in the right upper lobe (arrowhead).

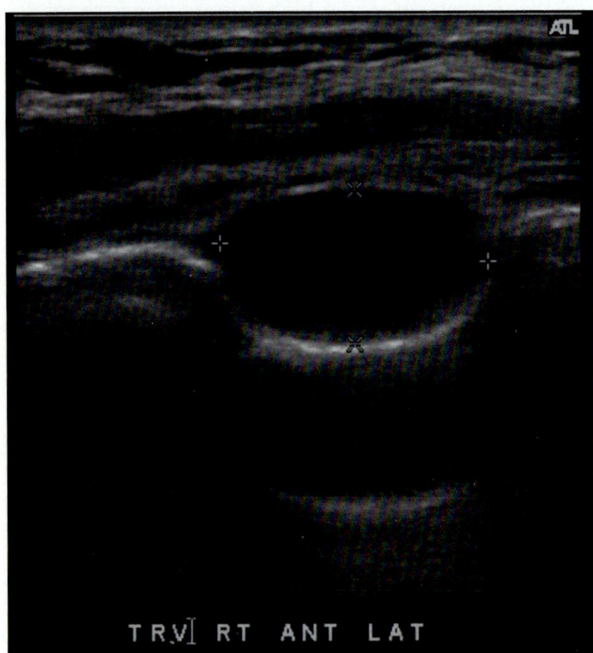

Figure 2.91 — Mediastinum, Thymoma. Sonography during ultrasound-guided biopsy shows a hypoechoic, pleural-based mass compatible with recurrent thymoma. Thymomas frequently metastasize to the pleura.

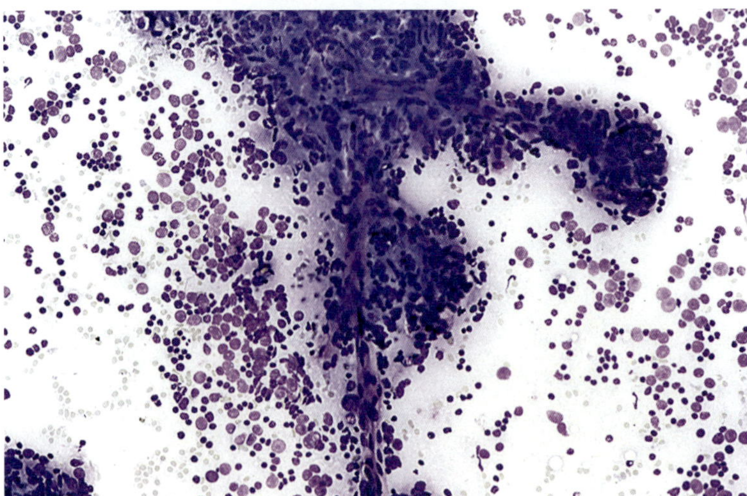

Figure 2.92 — Mediastinum, Thymoma. Thymomas typically consist of two cell populations, lymphocytes and epithelial cells. Scattered small lymphocytes are seen here dispersed singly in the background. The fragment in the center of the field shows spindle-shaped epithelial cells with small- to intermediate-sized nuclei with small blood vessels traversing the fragment. (Diff Quik stain, medium power)

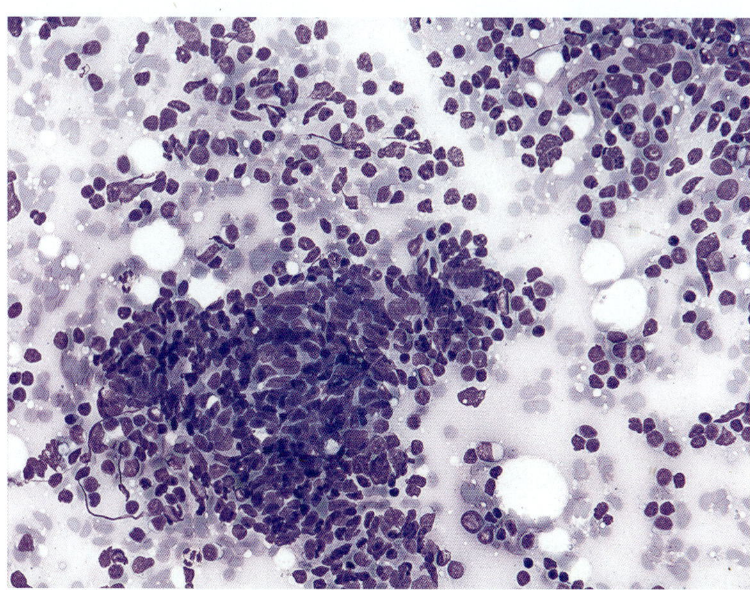

Figure 2.93 — Mediastinum, Thymoma. Although overall an uncommon tumor, thymoma is the most common primary tumor of the anterior mediastinum. A group of neoplastic epithelial cells is admixed with scattered small lymphocytes in the background. (Diff Quik stain, medium power)

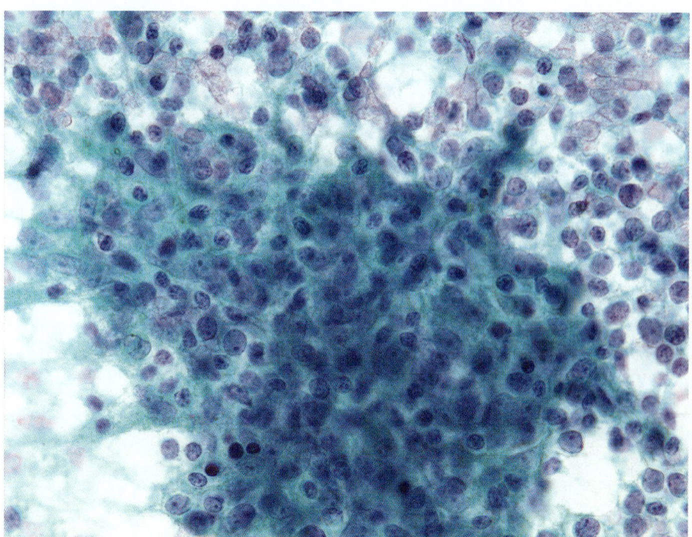

Figure 2.94 — Mediastinum, Thymoma. This fragment shows epithelial cells admixed with small lymphocytes. The epithelial cells have a moderate amount of cytoplasm, ill-defined cell borders, and pale chromatin with small- to moderate-sized nucleoli. (Papanicolaou stain, high power)

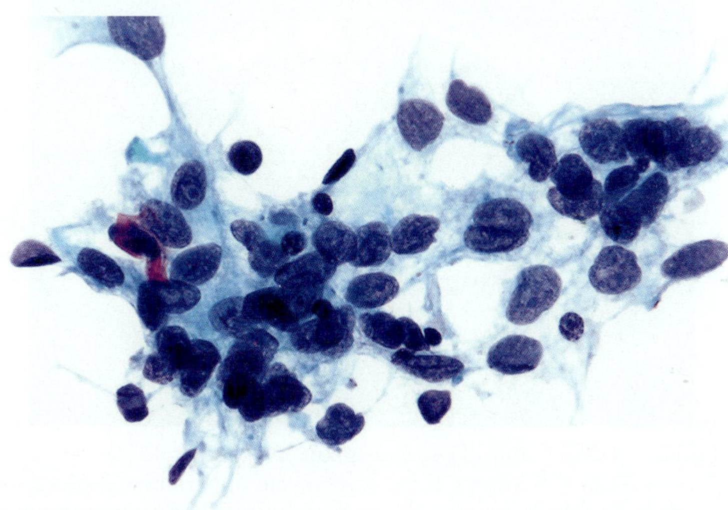

Figure 2.95 — Mediastinum, Thymoma. The epithelial cells shown here have a moderate amount of cytoplasm and oval-shaped nuclei with occasional nucleoli. Thymic carcinomas show marked nuclear atypia, mitotic figures, and necrosis. They most often show squamous cell differentiation. (Papanicolaou stain, high power)

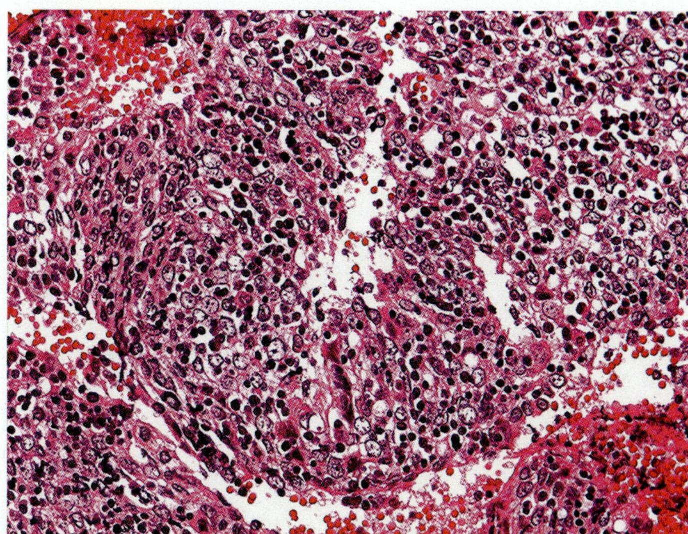

Figure 2.96 — Mediastinum, Thymoma. This cell block preparation shows the two populations of cells characteristic of thymoma. Epithelial cells show round to oval nuclei with pale chromatin and moderate amounts of cytoplasm with ill-defined cell borders. Lymphocytes with small, dark round nuclei and scant cytoplasm are admixed. (Hematoxylin and eosin stain, medium power)

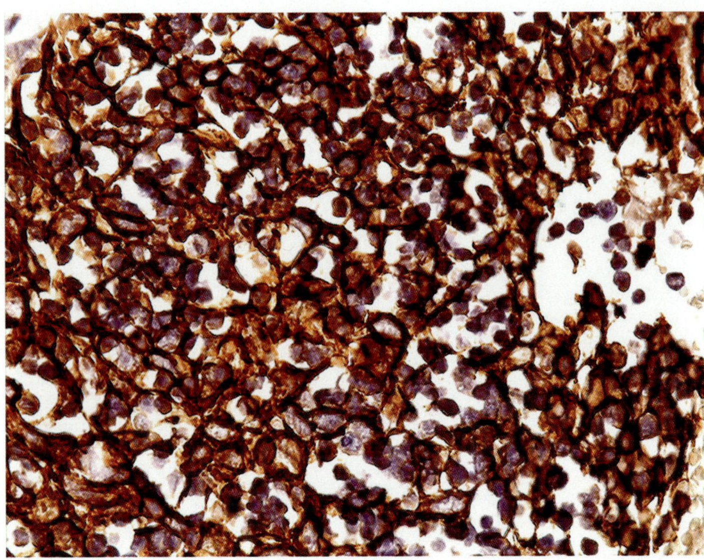

Figure 2.97 — Mediastinum, Thymoma. A cytokeratin immunostain performed on the cell block highlights the epithelial nature of the majority of the cells in this thymoma. Few small lymphocytes present at 3 o'clock are negative for keratin. (Cytokeratin AE1/3 immunostain, high power)

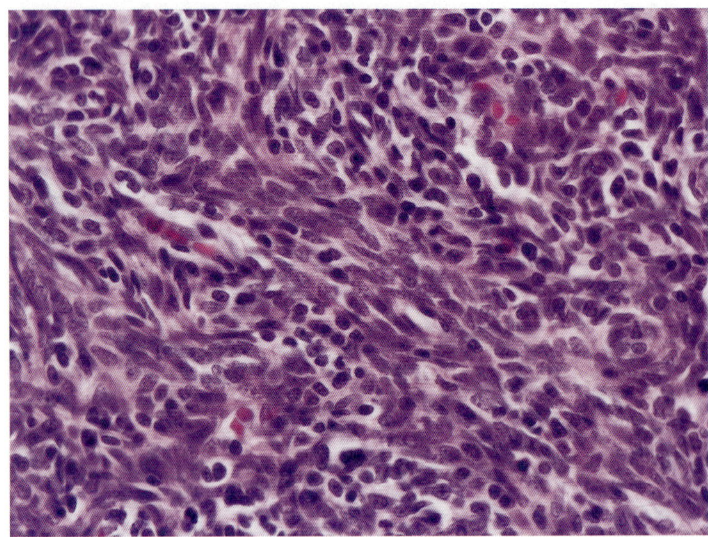

Figure 2.99 — Mediastinum, Thymoma (Histology). The epithelial component is predominant here with spindle to oval-shaped nuclei. Scattered lymphocytes are present, which are T-lymphocytes of thymic origin. (Hematoxylin and eosin stain, high power)

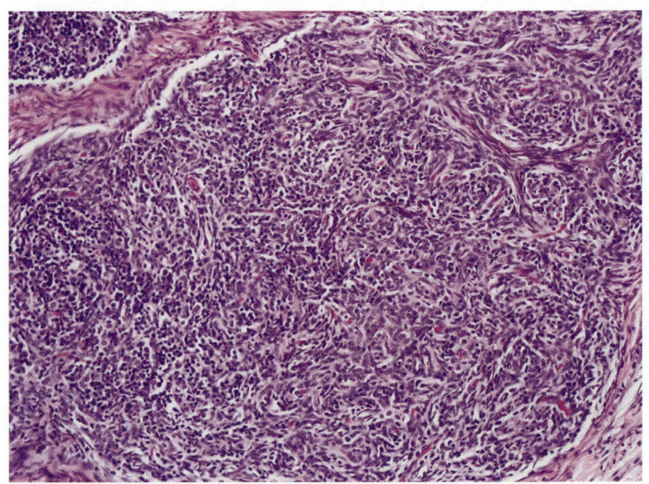

Figure 2.98 — Mediastinum, Thymoma (Histology). Cytologically bland spindle to epithelioid cells are admixed with small lymphocytes. This tumor was classified as a type AB thymoma, showing variable areas of epithelial and lymphocyte-dense tumor. (Hematoxylin and eosin stain, medium power)

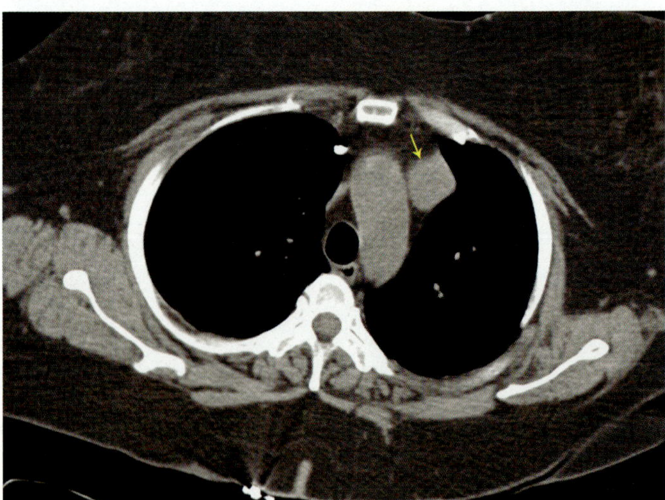

Figure 2.100 — Lung, Post-transplant Lymphoproliferative Disease. Axial CT images at the level of the upper chest shows a well-defined soft tissue mass in the anterior mediastinum anterior to the aortic arch (arrow). This is a 50-year-old woman status post-bilateral lung transplants 8 years prior for pulmonary hypertension with increasing fatigue, dyspnea, and night sweats. Post-transplant lymphoproliferative disease in the chest occurs most commonly with lung transplant patients. Biopsy is often necessary to confirm the diagnosis.

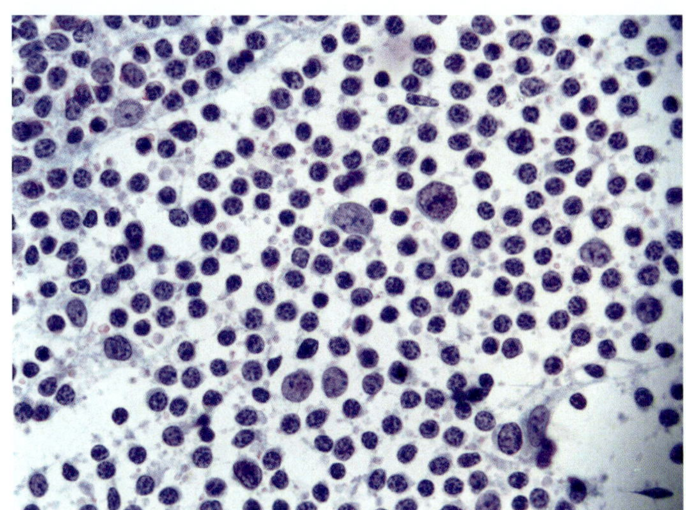

Figure 2.101 — Lung, Post-transplant Lymphoproliferative Disease. This patient underwent a lung transplant several years prior to this biopsy. The aspirate smear shows a predominant population of small lymphocytes with occasional larger cells consistent with immunoblasts. (Papanicolaou stain, high power)

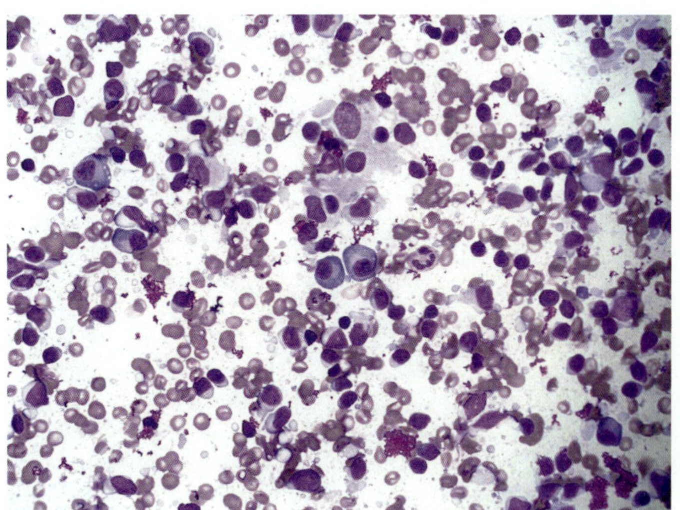

Figure 2.102 — Lung, Post-transplant Lymphoproliferative Disease. A range of small- and intermediate-sized lymphocytes are present. Several plasma cells are shown, including two in the center of the field. Plasma cells are recognized by their deep blue cytoplasm, eccentrically placed nuclei, and perinuclear clearing of the cytoplasm (hof). (Diff Quik stain, medium power)

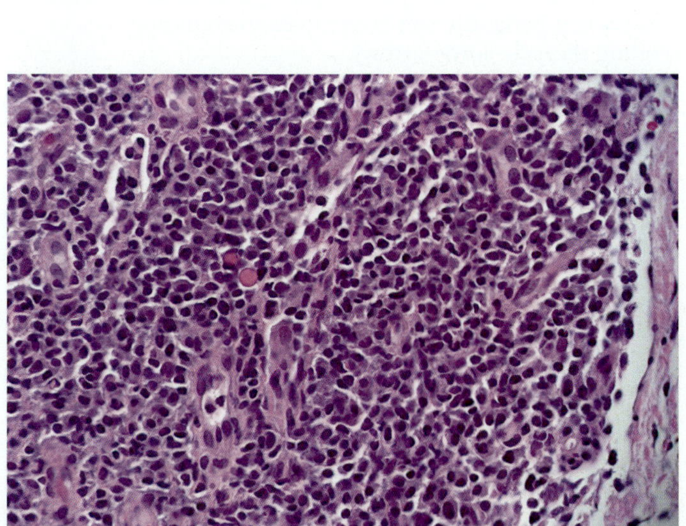

Figure 2.103 — Lung, Post-transplant Lymphoproliferative Disease (Core Biopsy). The core biopsy sample showed a polymorphous population of small lymphocytes, immunoblasts, and plasma cells. Flow cytometry performed on this sample was limited by small sample, but showed a population of B-cells with an increased ratio of kappa to lambda light chains, suggestive of a clonal process. (Hematoxylin and eosin stain, high power)

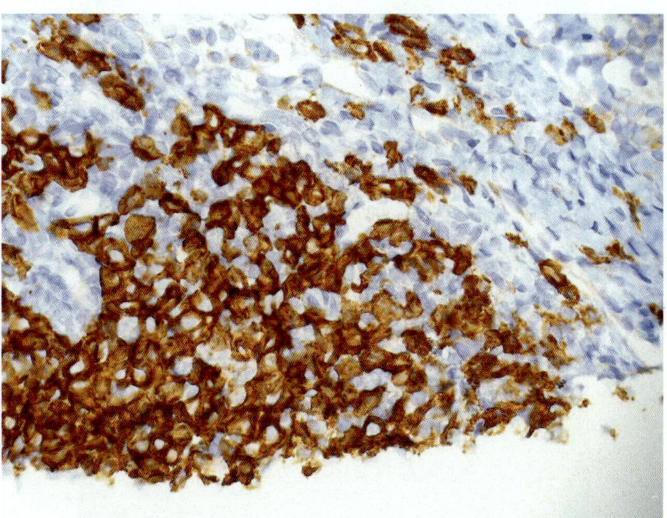

Figure 2.104 — Lung, Post-transplant Lymphoproliferative Disease (Core Biopsy). An immunostain for CD138, a marker of plasma cells, is positive in many of the cells. Immunostains for kappa and lambda light chain confirmed the clonality of the lesion, as virtually all of the plasma cells marked for kappa light chain (not shown). (CD138immunostain, high power)

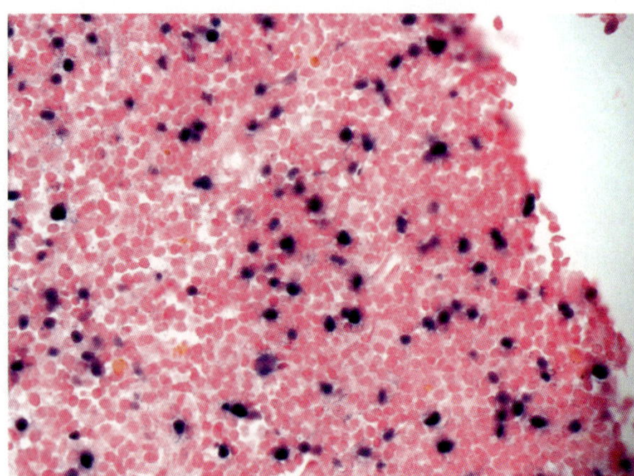

Figure 2.105 — Lung, Post-transplant Lymphoproliferative Disease (Core Biopsy). Post-transplant lymphoproliferative disease is due to the immunosuppression associated with organ or bone marrow transplantation. Most cases are related to Epstein–Barr virus (EBV) infection. In this case, an *in situ* hybridization studies for EBV is positive, with the clonal hematopoietic cells showing dark blue nuclei. (EBV *in situ* hybridization, high power)

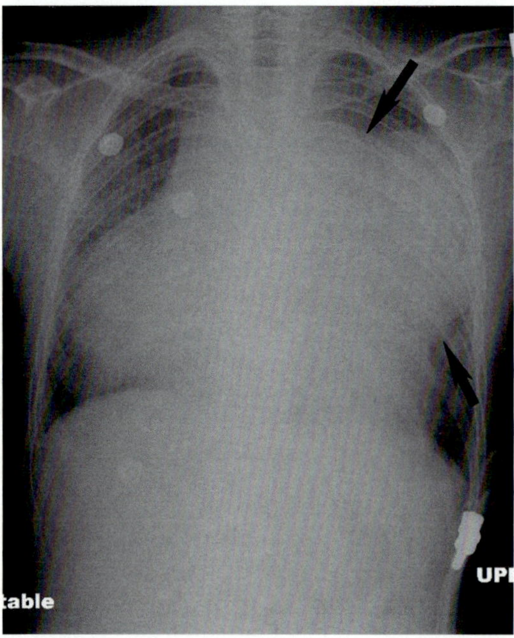

Figure 2.107 — Mediastinum, Diffuse Large B-Cell Lymphoma. This 11-year-old girl presented with a 2-week history of progressive cough and dyspnea. AP view of the chest demonstrates a large mediastinal mass (arrows).

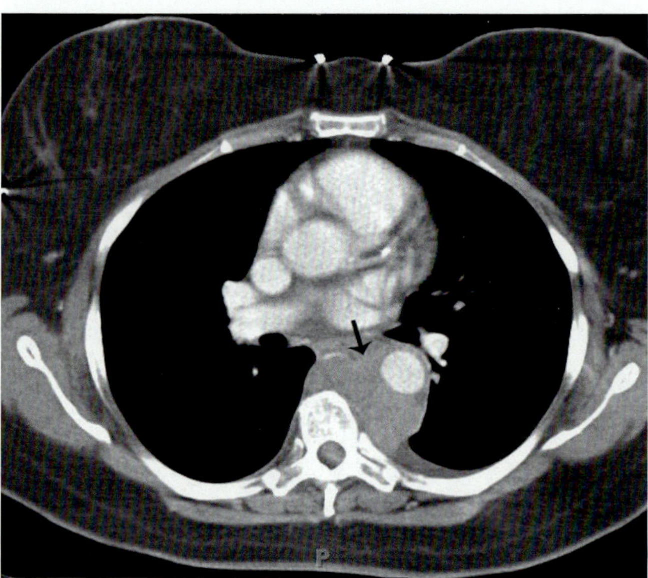

Figure 2.106 — Mediastinum, Diffuse Large B-Cell Lymphoma. This 57-year-old woman had a history of lymphoma treated with bone marrow transplant. Her last CT 1 month ago was normal, but now she complains of chest pain. Axial contrast-enhanced CT demonstrates a periaortic soft tissue mass surrounding the descending thoracic aorta (arrow).

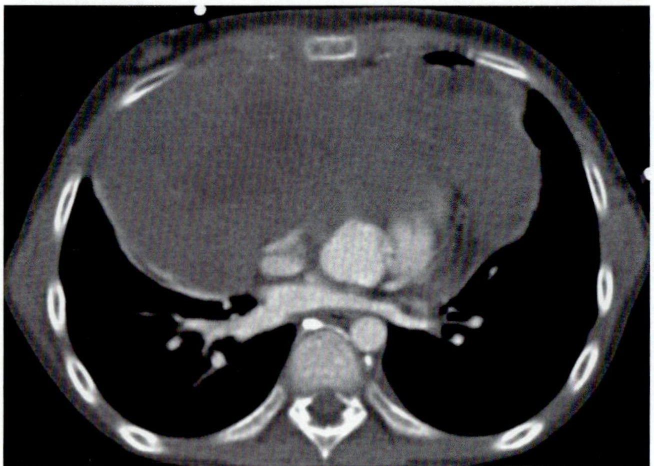

Figure 2.108 — Mediastinum, Diffuse Large B-Cell Lymphoma. Axial CT image confirms a large mass in the anterior mediastinum with mass effect, displacing the aorta and pulmonary arteries posteriorly. Diffuse large B-cell lymphoma is the second most common malignancy of the mediastinum, after Hodgkin lymphoma.

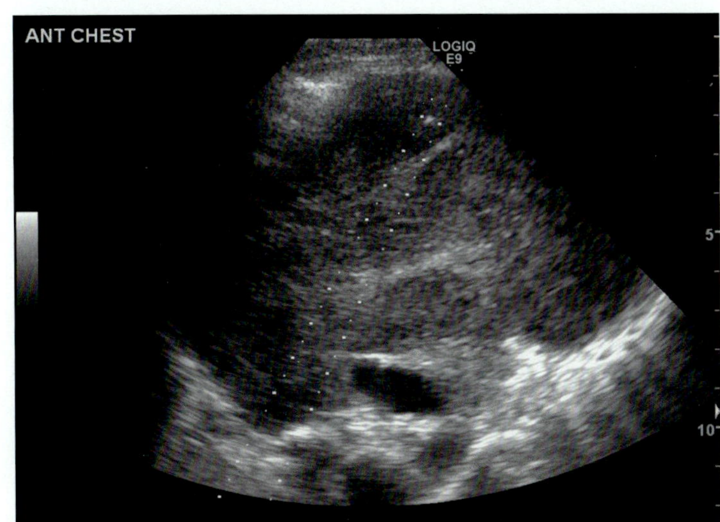

Figure 2.109 — Mediastinum, Diffuse Large B-Cell Lymphoma. Sonographic image obtained during ultrasound-guided biopsy shows the large heterogeneous mass in the anterior chest. The anterior mediastinum is the second most common site of non-Hodgkin lymphoma following the abdomen.

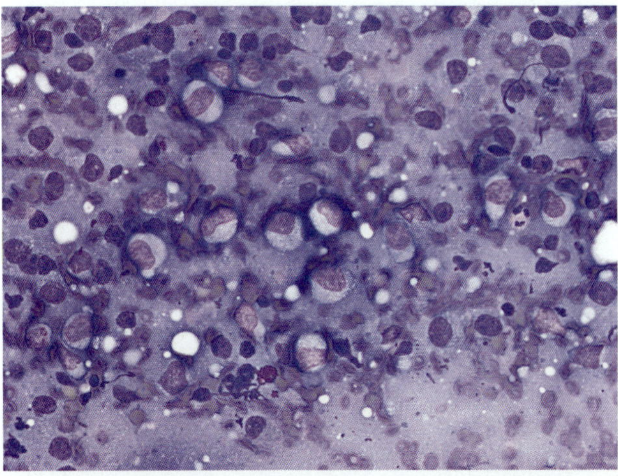

Figure 2.110 — Mediastinum, Diffuse Large B-Cell Lymphoma. Scattered, large, atypical lymphoid cells are present showing irregular nuclear contours and a small to moderate amount of basophilic cytoplasm. Nucleoli are present in most of the neoplastic cells. Aspirates may be sparsely cellular due to stromal sclerosis. (Diff Quik stain, medium power)

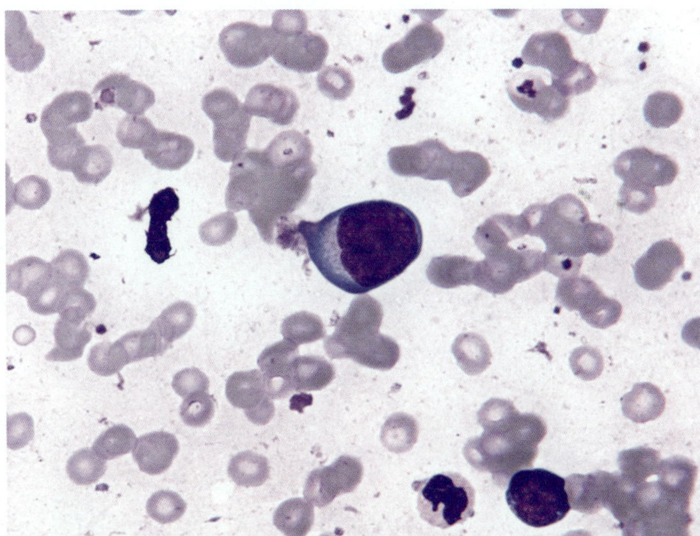

Figure 2.111 — Mediastinum, Diffuse Large B-Cell Lymphoma. Two malignant single cells with high nuclear to cytoplasmic ratio and scant basophilic cytoplasm are shown. The differential diagnosis includes Hodgkin lymphoma, anaplastic large cell lymphoma, and germ cell tumors. Tissue studies confirmed a large B-cell lymphoma. (Diff Quik stain, high power)

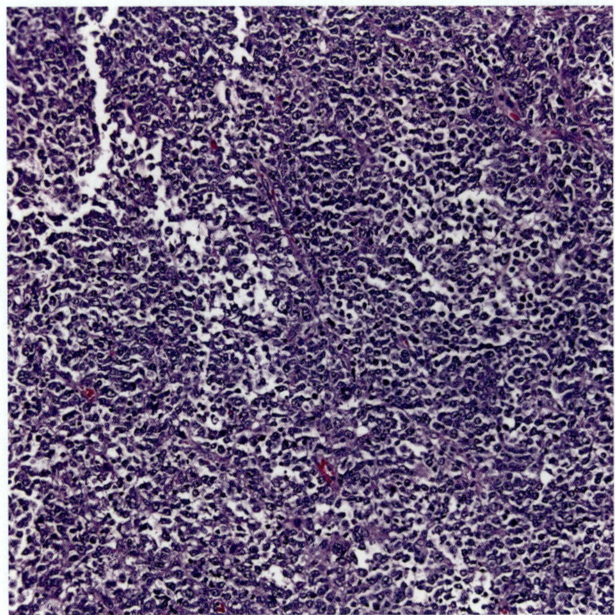

Figure 2.112 — Mediastinum, Diffuse Large B-Cell Lymphoma (Histology). This lymphocytic population is forming sheets with no normal lymph node architecture apparent. The lymphocytes are large and have indistinct cellular borders. (Hematoxylin and eosin stain, low power)

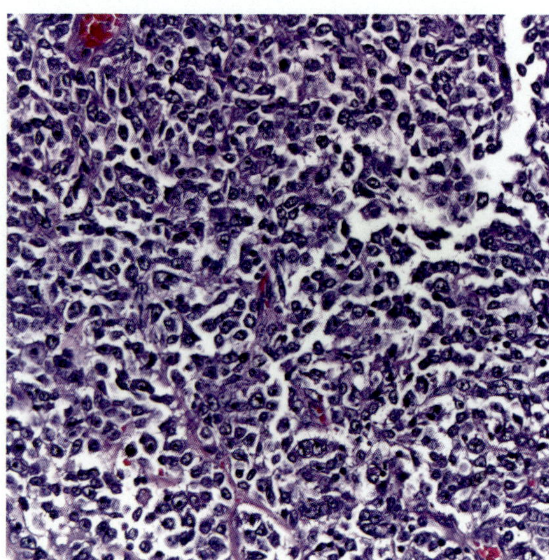

Figure 2.113 — Mediastinum, Diffuse Large B-Cell Lymphoma (Histology). A monotonous population of atypical large lymphocytes is shown. The nuclei are round to oval, but may have irregular nuclear contours and variably prominent nucleoli. Apoptosis is often abundant. (Hematoxylin and eosin stain, medium power)

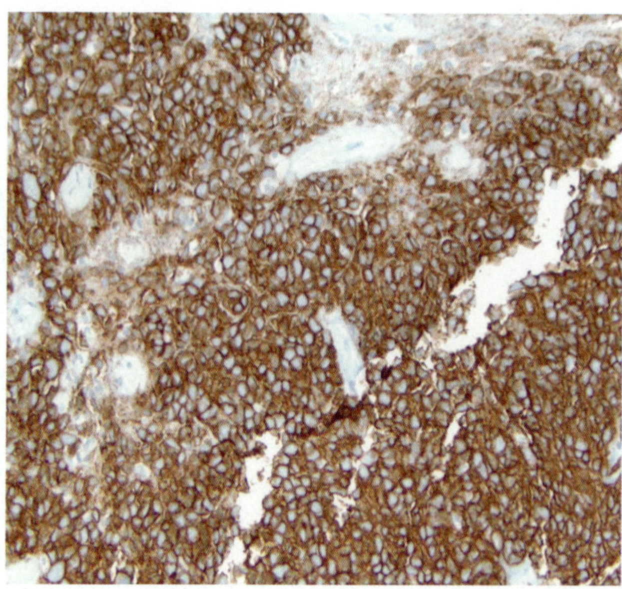

Figure 2.114 — Mediastinum, Diffuse Large B-Cell Lymphoma (Histology). The neoplastic cells are positive for CD20, consistent with a B-cell neoplasm. A Ki-67 immunostain may be performed to illustrate the proliferative rate for the tumor. (CD20 immunostain, medium power)

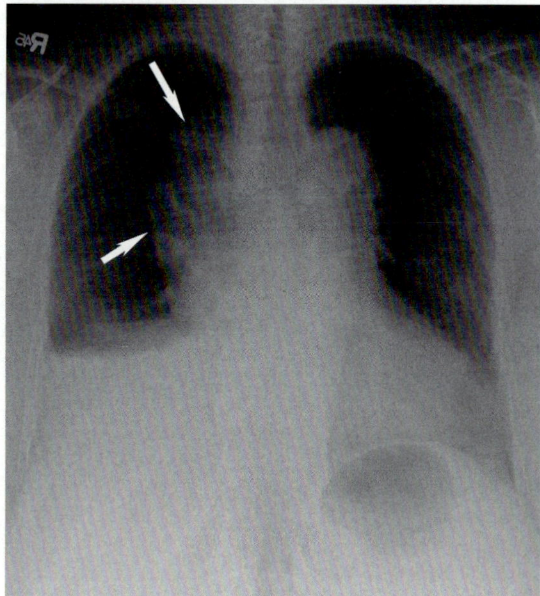

Figure 2.115 — Anterior Mediastinum, Hodgkin Lymphoma. This 55-year-old woman had a history of chronic sinusitis and presented with hoarseness. PA x-ray of the chest shows a lobulated mediastinal mass (arrows). A right pleural effusion is also present.

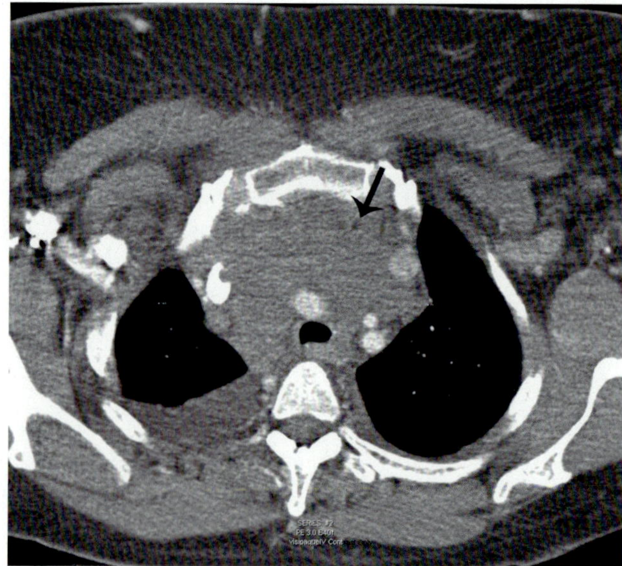

Figure 2.116 — Anterior Mediastinum, Hodgkin Lymphoma. Axial contrast-enhanced CT image shows a large anterior mediastinal mass representing coalescent lymph nodes encasing the great vessels (arrow).

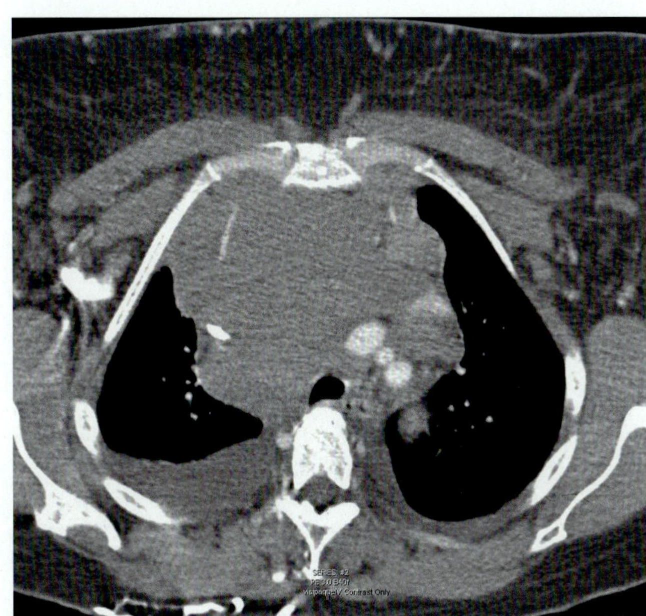

Figure 2.117 — Anterior Mediastinum, Hodgkin Lymphoma. The mass extends further inferiorly in the anterior mediastinum encasing the great vessels. Hodgkin lymphoma is the most common malignant mediastinal tumor and is seen more often in young women.

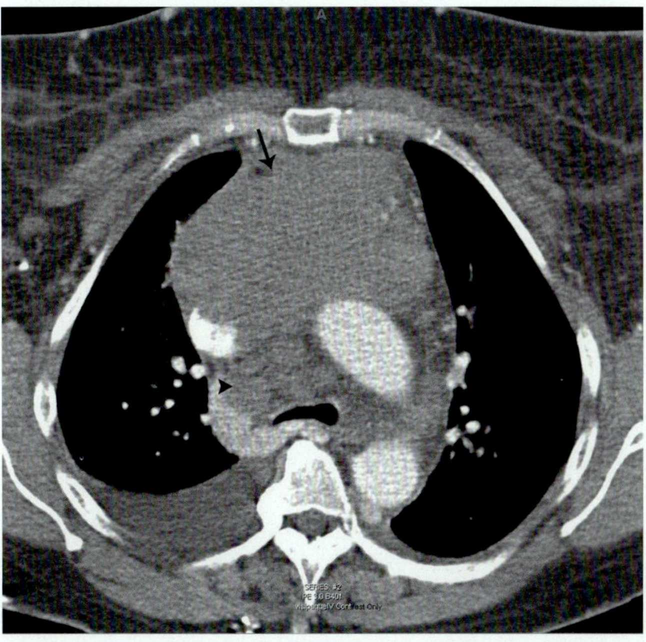

Figure 2.118 — Anterior Mediastinum, Hodgkin Lymphoma. Anterior mediastinal mass (arrow) extends to the level of the aortic arch. There is also precarinal adenopathy (arrowhead). Patients often present with fever, weight loss, and night sweats.

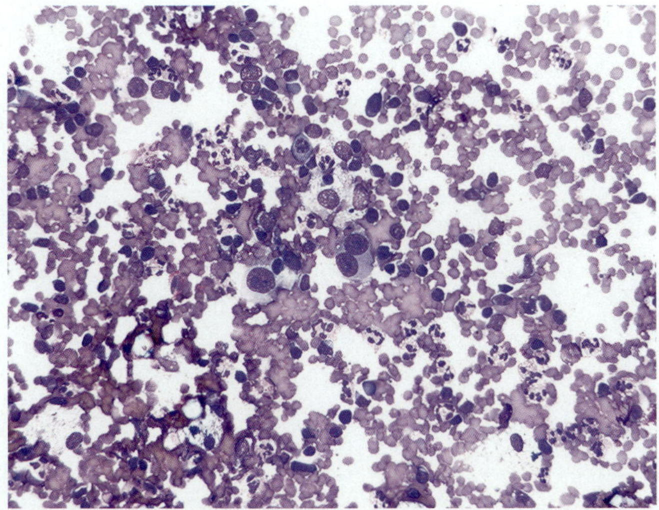

Figure 2.119 — Anterior Mediastinum, Hodgkin Lymphoma. Two large, atypical cells, one binucleated, are present in a background of mixed inflammation. The inflammatory infiltrate includes neutrophils, eosinophils, small lymphocytes, and plasma cells. Aspirates of Hodgkin lymphoma may be sparsely cellular due to fibrotic stroma. (Diff Quik stain, medium power)

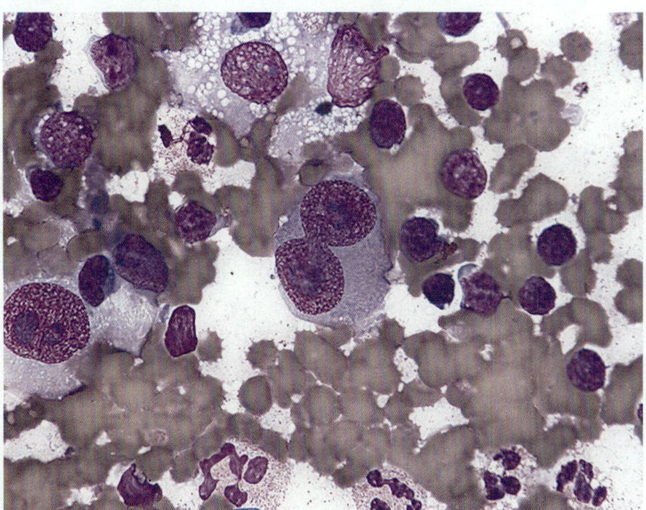

Figure 2.120 — Anterior Mediastinum, Hodgkin Lymphoma. A large cell with a bilobed nucleus, consistent with a classical Reed–Sternberg cell, is present in the center of the field. There are prominent nucleoli and a moderate amount of cytoplasm. (Diff Quik stain, high power)

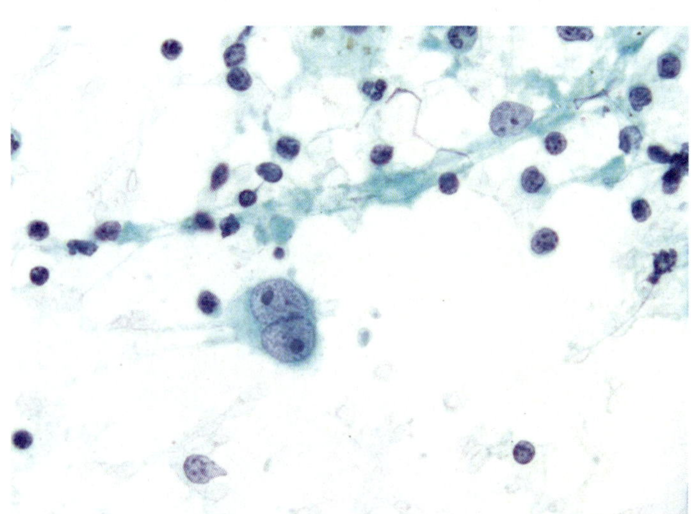

Figure 2.121 — Anterior Mediastinum, Hodgkin Lymphoma. A Reed–Sternberg cell is present in a background of predominantly small lymphocytes. Reed–Sternberg type cells may be seen in other hematopoietic neoplasms (e.g., chronic lymphocytic leukemia) and nonneoplastic conditions (e.g., infectious mononucleosis), so care must be taken in confirming the diagnosis of Hodgkin lymphoma. (Papanicolaou stain, high power)

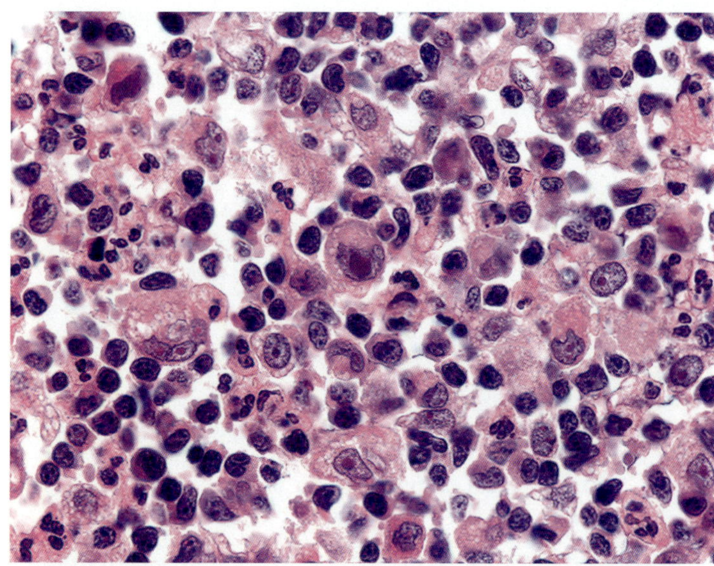

Figure 2.122 — Anterior Mediastinum, Hodgkin Lymphoma (Cell Block). Several Reed–Sternberg cells are present in this field, some mononuclear and others binucleated. All show prominent nucleoli which appear bright red or magenta on routine hematoxylin and eosin staining. (Hematoxylin and eosin stain, high power)

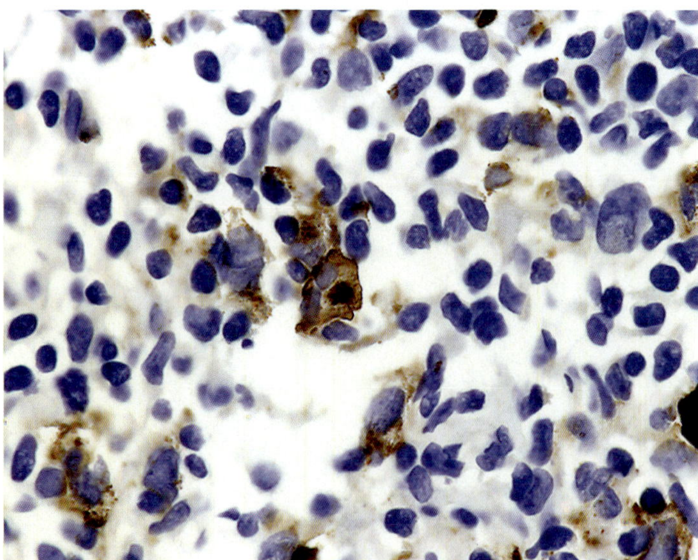

Figure 2.123 — Anterior Mediastinum, Hodgkin Lymphoma (Cell Block). CD30 immunostaining shows a characteristic perinuclear dot-like positivity. Reed–Sternberg cells are typically positive for CD30 and CD15 but negative for CD45. (CD30 stain, high power)

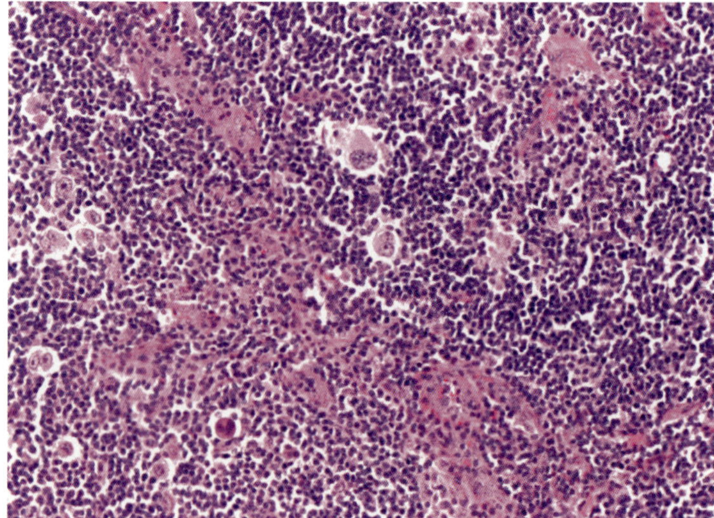

Figure 2.124 — Anterior Mediastinum, Hodgkin Lymphoma. Diffuse infiltrate of mixed inflammatory cells with the prominent presence of scattered large cells with binucleation characteristic of Reed–Sternberg cells. The large atypical cells in this case stained for CD30 and CD15. (Hematoxylin and eosin stain, medium power)

Abdomen

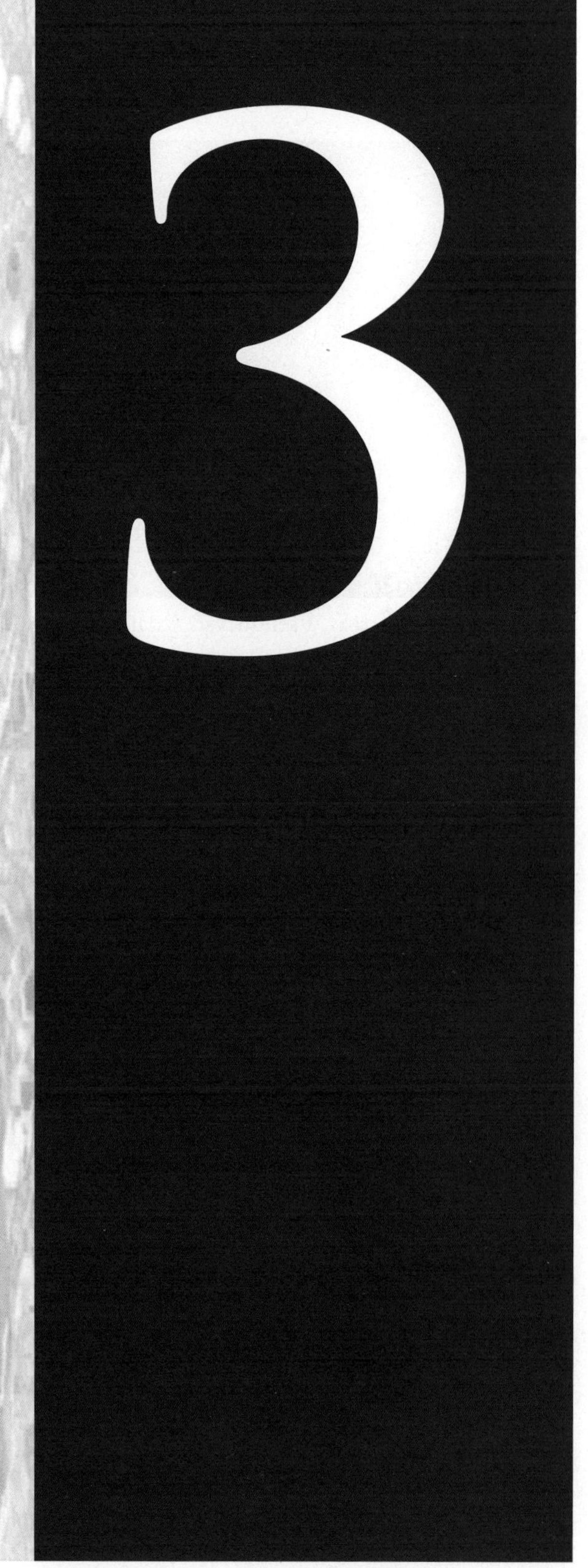

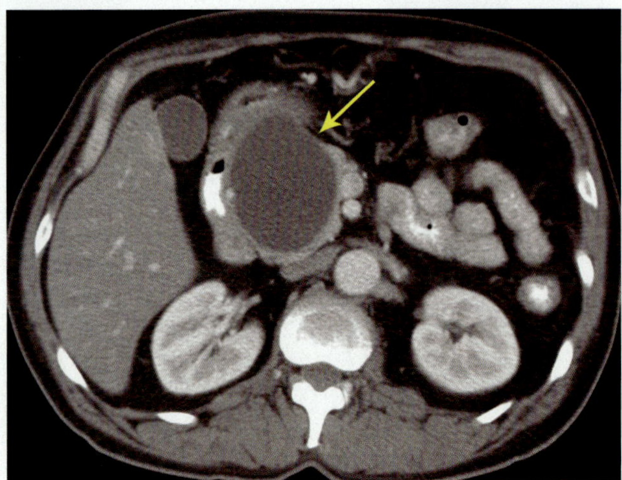

Figure 3.1 — Pancreas, Pseudocyst. Axial contrast-enhanced CT of the upper abdomen demonstrates a smoothly marginated, well-defined cystic lesion in the region of the pancreatic head (arrow). Pseudocysts are one of the complications of acute or chronic pancreatitis. Mural nodularity or an enhancing component, which can be indicative of malignancy, was not seen in this lesion. A pseudocyst was favored and this lesion markedly decreased in size on follow-up imaging (not shown).

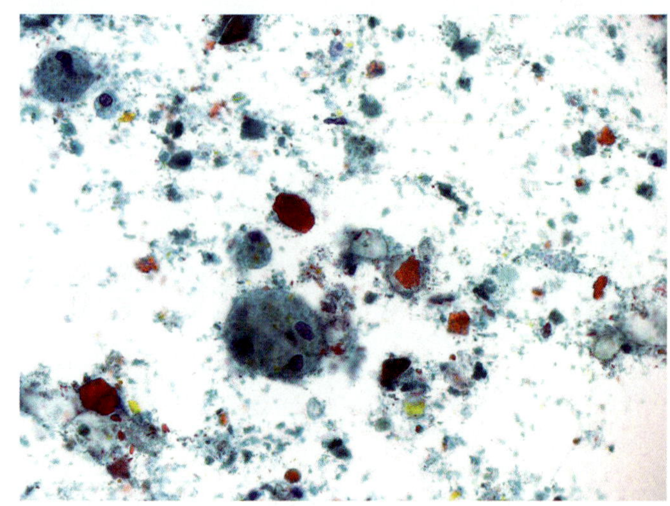

Figure 3.2 — Pancreas, Pseudocyst. Pseudocysts often arise in a setting of chronic pancreatitis, as in this patient. The aspirate smear consists of numerous macrophages, few inflammatory cells, and proteinaceous debris, including bile pigment. A pseudocyst does not have an epithelial lining. (Papanicolaou stain, medium power)

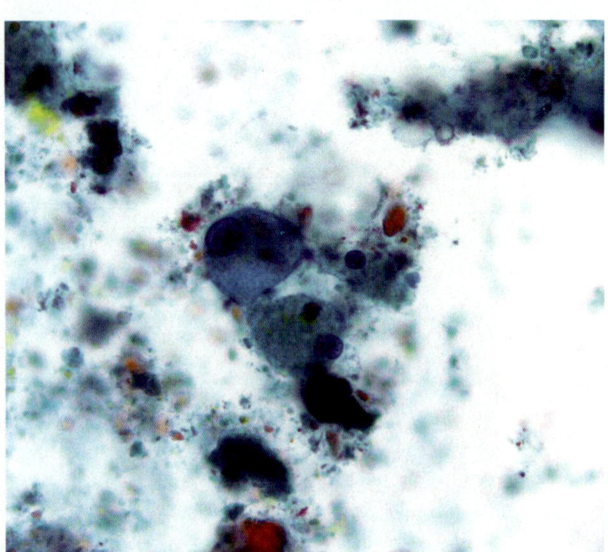

Figure 3.3 — Pancreas, Pseudocyst. Two macrophages are shown in the center of the field with cytoplasm packed with debris. A portion of the FNA sample may be sent for chemical analysis, which typically shows a high amylase and low CEA in a pseudocyst. (Papanicolaou stain, high power)

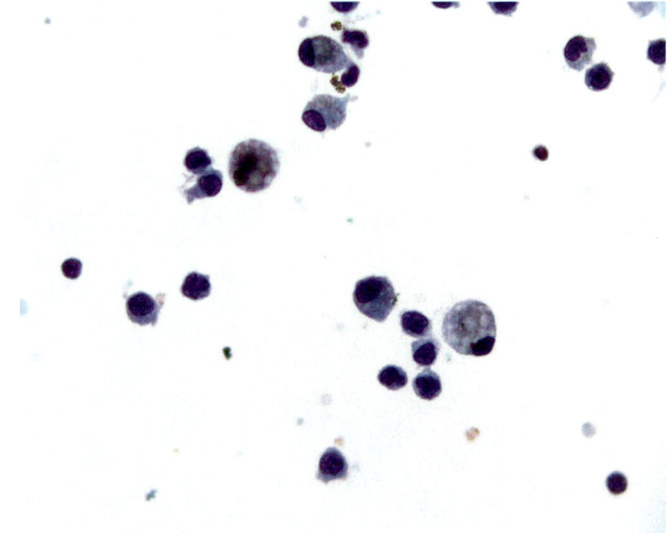

Figure 3.4 — Pancreas, Pseudocyst. A few macrophages are admixed with small lymphocytes from this cystic lesion. A liquid-based preparation, as seen here, removes some of the obscuring debris from the background. (Papanicolaou stain, high power)

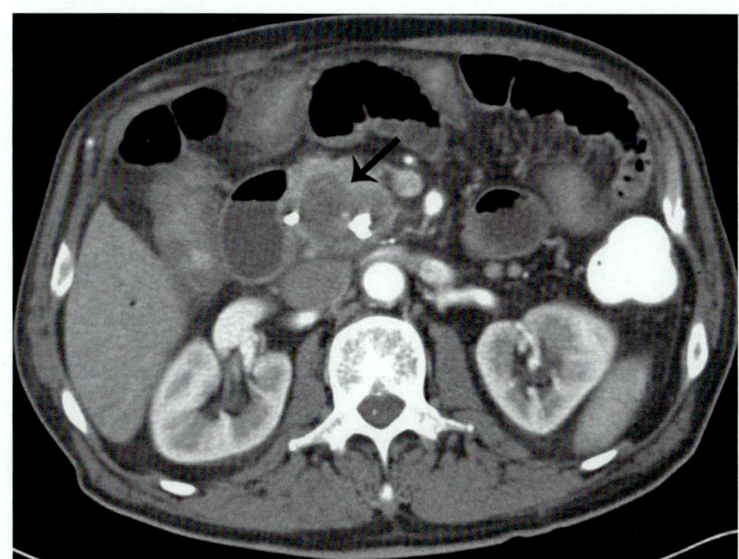

Figure 3.5 — Pancreas, Adenocarcinoma. This patient was an 80-year-old man who presented with obstructive jaundice, a common presenting complaint for pancreatic adenocarcinoma. Axial contrast-enhanced CT in the arterial phase shows an irregular hypoechoic mass in the pancreatic head and uncinate process (arrow).

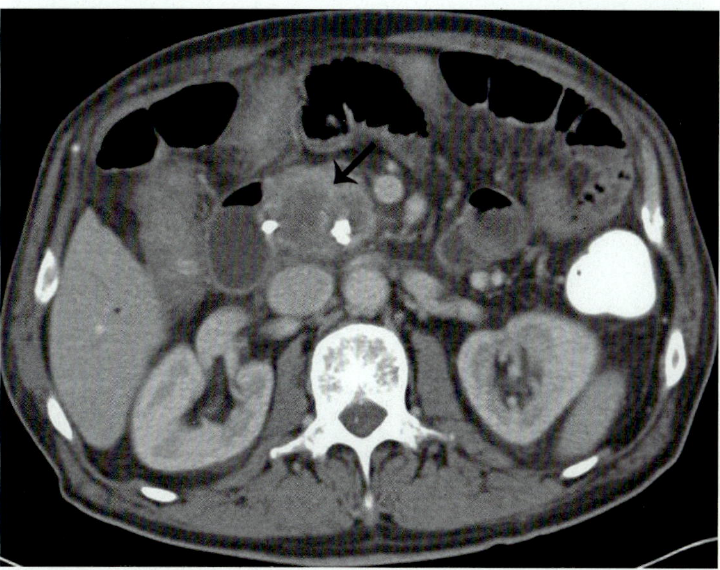

Figure 3.6 — Pancreas, Adenocarcinoma. Axial contrast-enhanced CT in the venous phase confirms the hypoechoic mass in the pancreatic head and uncinate process (arrow).

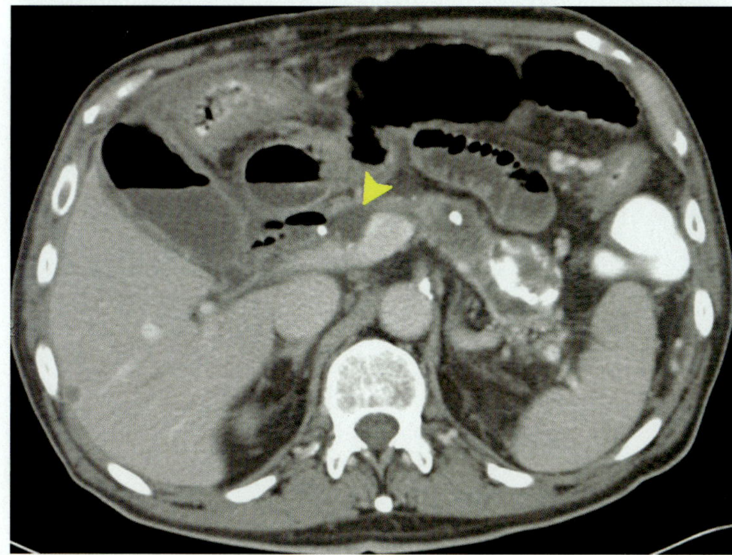

Figure 3.7 — Pancreas, Adenocarcinoma. There is resultant pancreatic ductal dilatation (arrowhead). Pancreatic adenocarcinoma is typically irregular and hypovascular, as in this case. Desmoplastic reaction is common, resulting in pancreatic ductal dilation.

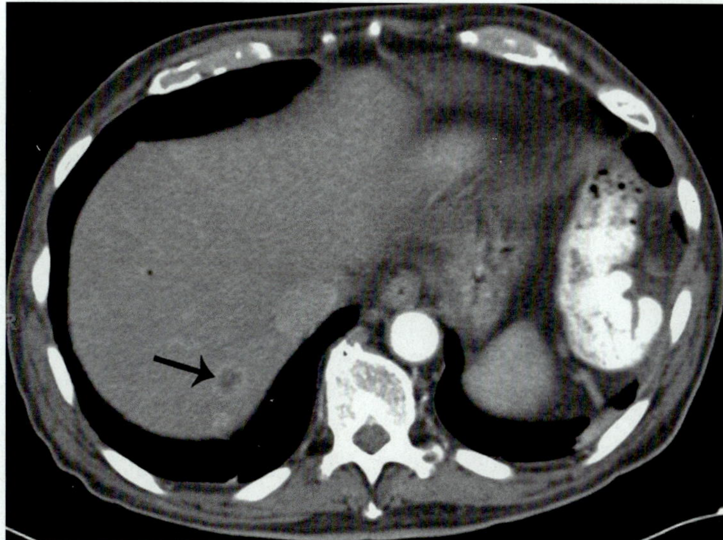

Figure 3.8 — Pancreas, Adenocarcinoma. Axial contrast-enhanced CT in the venous phase shows a small hypodense liver lesion with peripheral enhancement that is suspicious for metastatic disease (arrow). Pancreatic adenocarcinomas are considered unresectable when liver metastases or significant vascular invasion (i.e., celiac axis, superior mesenteric artery, portal or superior mesenteric vein), or carcinomatosis are present.

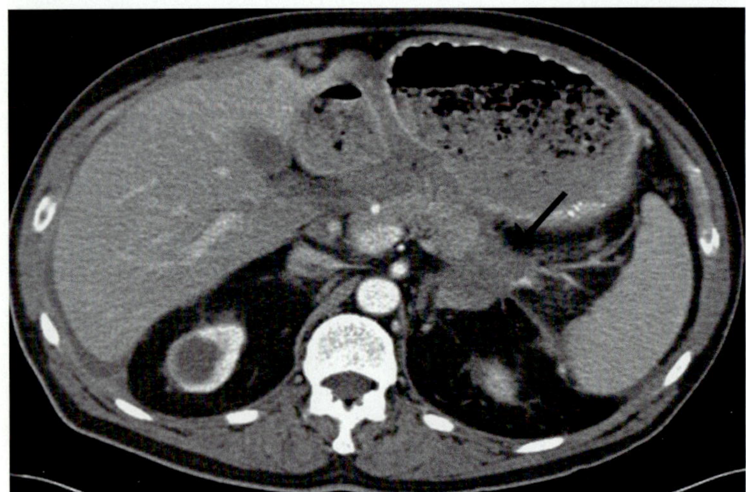

Figure 3.9 — Pancreas, Adenocarcinoma. This patient was a 70-year-old man with a history of superficial bladder cancer, who presented with abdominal pain. Axial contrast-enhanced CT shows an irregular mass with spiculation in the tail of the pancreas (arrow).

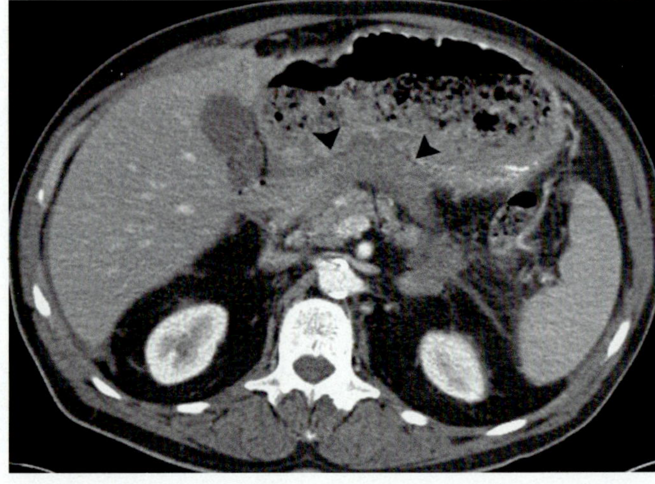

Figure 3.10 — Pancreas, Adenocarcinoma. Axial contrast-enhanced CT slightly more inferiorly shows an extensive soft tissue lesion involving the root of the mesentery (arrowheads). The mass abuts and likely involves the posterior aspect of the stomach. Pancreatic adenocarcinomas are typically ill defined and infiltrative, resulting in pancreatic duct dilation.

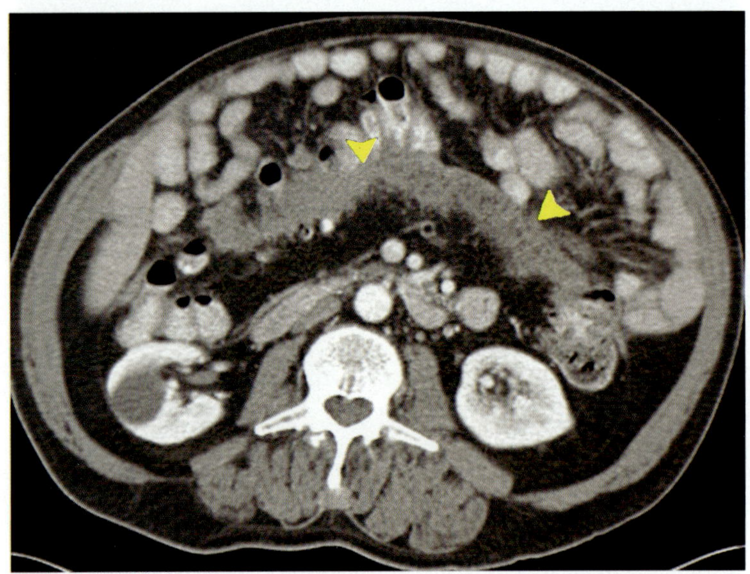

Figure 3.11 — Pancreas, Adenocarcinoma. There is extensive extension of the mass more inferiorly into the mesentery (arrowheads). This case is presumed to be pancreatic in origin with an atypical appearance extending into the root of the mesentery.

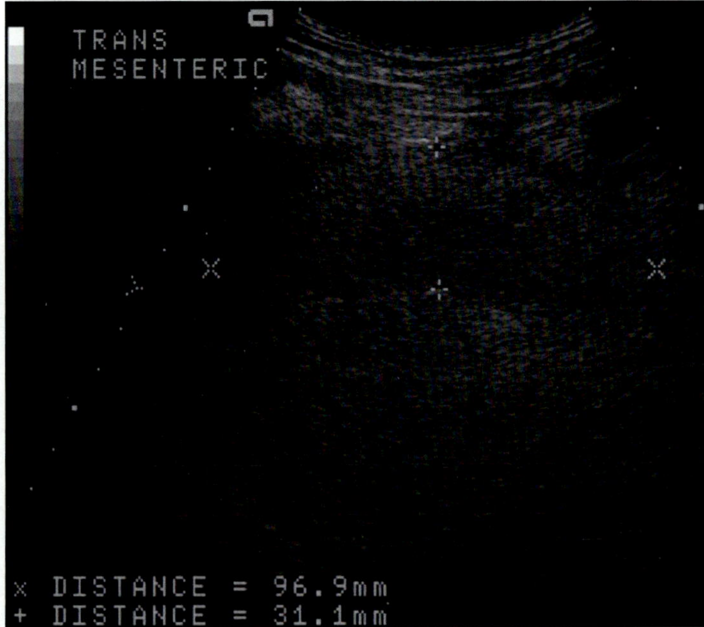

Figure 3.12 — Pancreas, Adenocarcinoma. Sonographic image shows the mesenteric mass which was targeted for biopsy. Pancreatic lesions are amenable to percutaneous or endoscopic ultrasound-guided FNA.

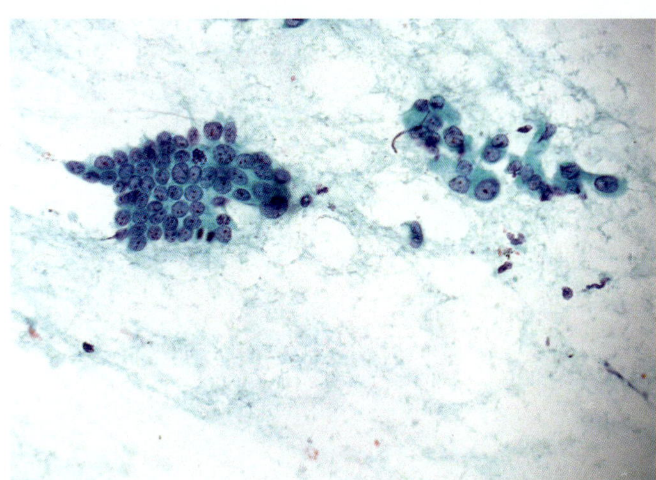

Figure 3.13 — Pancreas, Adenocarcinoma. Two fragments of adenocarcinoma are shown. The fragment on the left shows a sheet of tumor cells with slightly disrupted honeycomb architecture, while the fragment on the right shows a completely haphazard tumor cell arrangement. The malignant nuclei are enlarged and oval shaped with pale chromatin and small nucleoli. (Papanicolaou stain, high power)

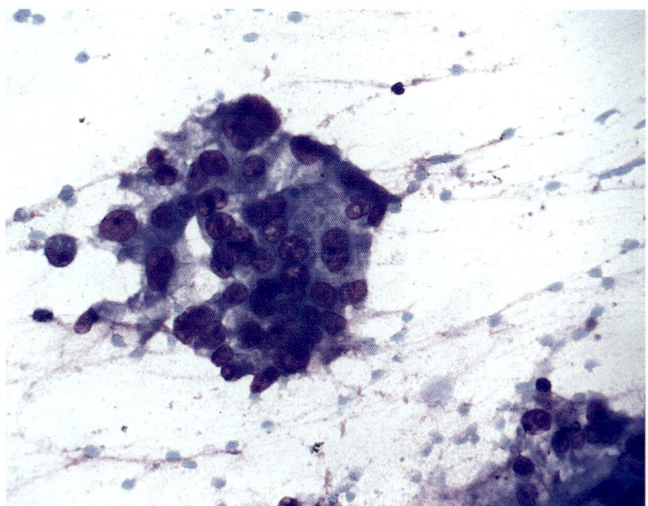

Figure 3.14 — Pancreas, Adenocarcinoma. These malignant cells are forming crude acinar structures consistent with glandular differentiation. The nuclei are enlarged with small nucleoli and show irregular contours with numerous divots, which some liken to an "Idaho potato." (Diff Quik stain, high power)

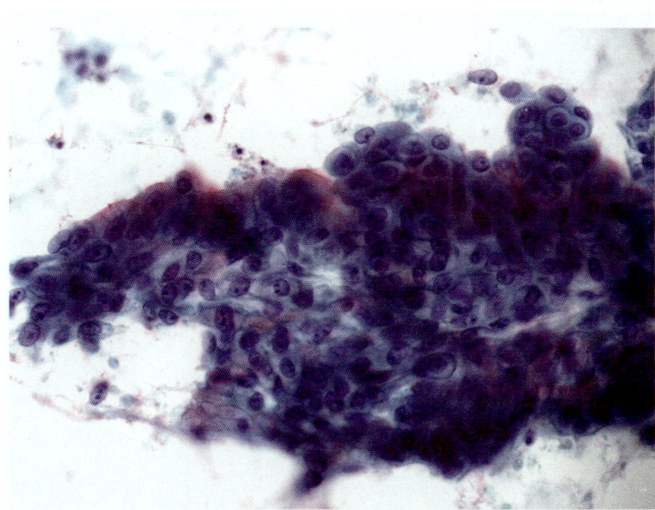

Figure 3.15 — Pancreas, Adenocarcinoma. This fragment of malignant epithelium shows complete disruption of the normal honeycomb architecture of ductal epithelium. The nuclei are slightly enlarged and there is slight anisonucleosis, consistent with a well-differentiated adenocarcinoma. (Papanicolaou stain, high power)

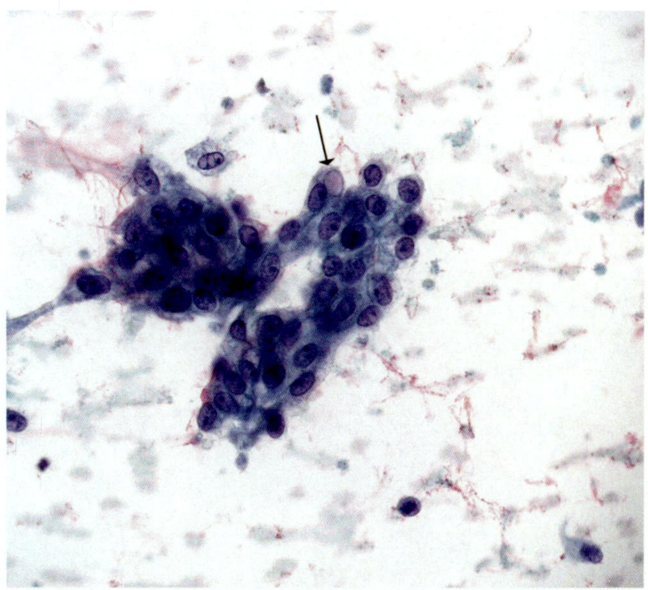

Figure 3.16 — Pancreas, Adenocarcinoma. A cohesive fragment of malignant epithelium is shown. One of the tumor cells shows an intracytoplasmic mucin droplet (arrow). FNAs of pancreatic adenocarcinoma often consist of a mixture of malignant epithelial fragments and single malignant cells (not shown). (Papanicolaou stain, high power)

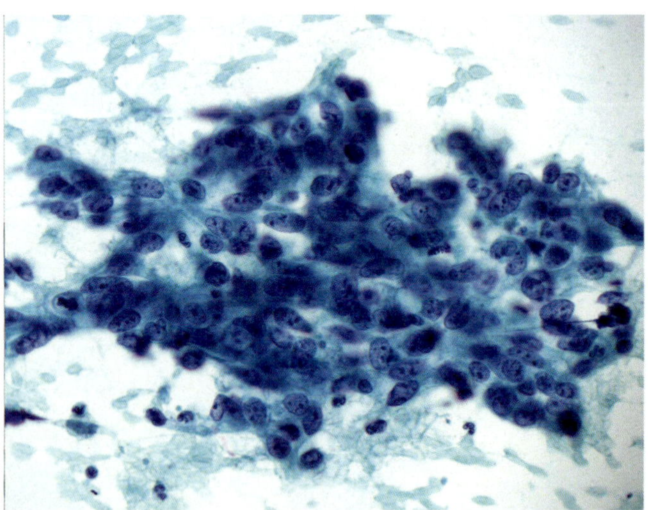

Figure 3.17 — Pancreas, Adenocarcinoma. This crowded sheet of malignant epithelial cells with moderate anisonucleosis and scattered mitotic figures is consistent with a moderately differentiated adenocarcinoma. One general rule of thumb is that nuclei should be four times the size of a normal ductal epithelial cell to make a diagnosis of adenocarcinoma. (Papanicolaou stain, high power)

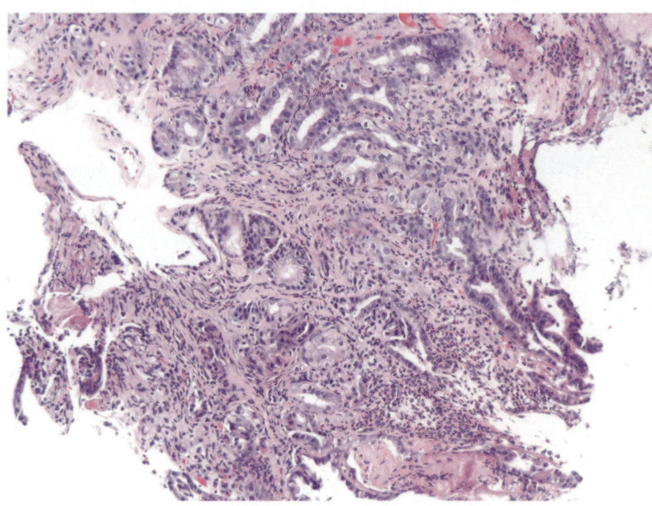

Figure 3.18 — Pancreas, Adenocarcinoma (Histology). Well to moderately differentiated pancreatic adenocarcinoma is shown with focally well-formed glands infiltrating a fibrotic stroma. Nuclei are crowded and stratified. There is moderate architectural disruption. (Hematoxylin and eosin stain, low power)

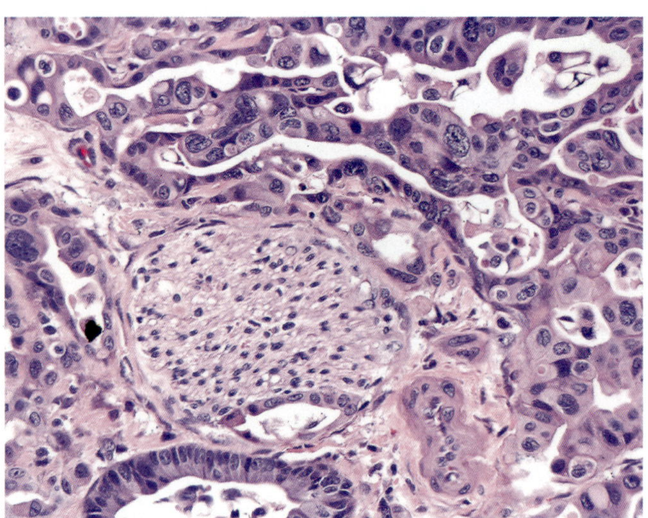

Figure 3.19 — Pancreas, Adenocarcinoma (Histology). Neoplastic glands show peri- and intraneural invasion. The glands are lined by epithelium which shows overt malignant features with pleomorphic large nuclei, small nucleoli, and architectural disruption. (Hematoxylin and eosin stain, high power)

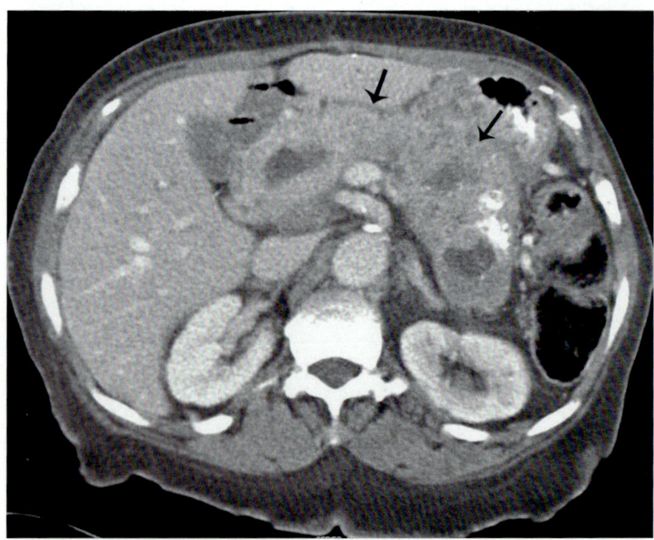

Figure 3.20 — Pancreas, Intraductal Papillary Mucinous Neoplasm. Axial contrast-enhanced CT in the venous phase shows enlargement of the pancreas (arrows) and several focal cystic areas in the pancreas. There are also coarse calcifications in the pancreatic parenchyma.

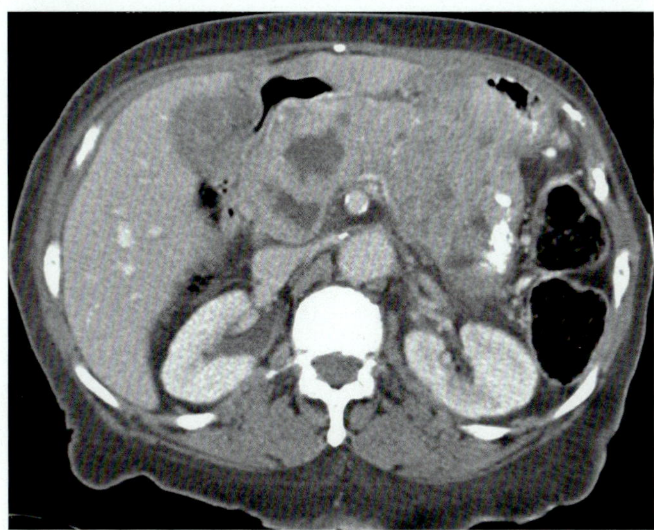

Figure 3.21 — Pancreas, Intraductal Papillary Mucinous Neoplasm. Axial contrast-enhanced CT in the venous phase slightly more inferiorly shows the entire pancreas is enlarged and contains several focal cystic areas.

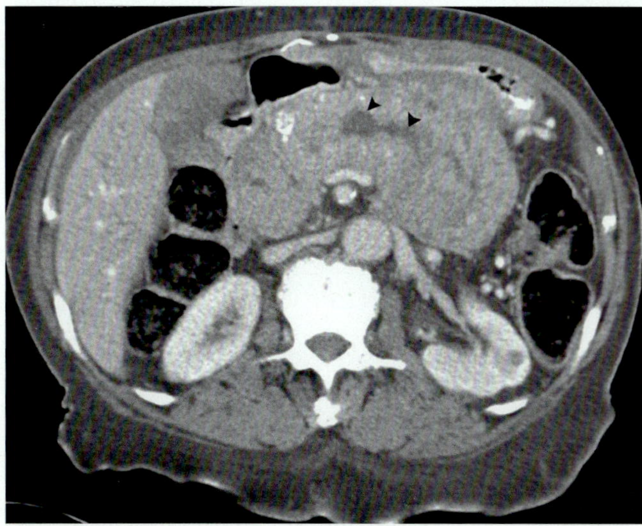

Figure 3.22 — Pancreas, Intraductal Papillary Mucinous Neoplasm. Axial contrast-enhanced CT in the venous phase shows, in addition, a dilated main pancreatic duct (arrowheads). Intraductal papillary mucinous neoplasms arise from the main pancreatic duct or side branches and result in dilation of the main pancreatic duct due to abundant mucin production.

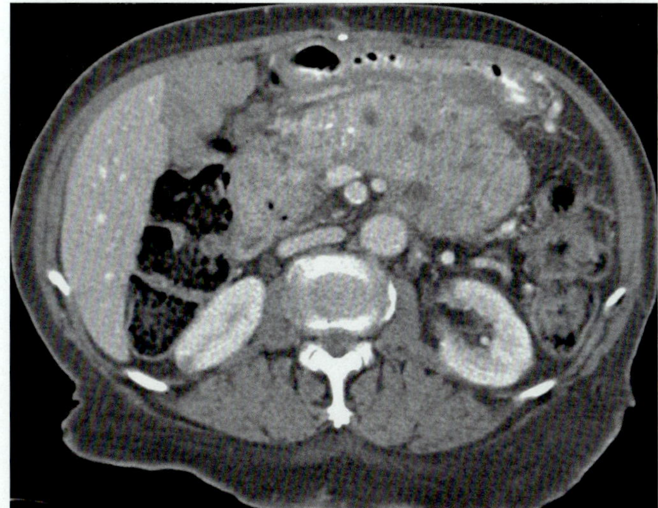

Figure 3.23 — Pancreas, Intraductal Papillary Mucinous Neoplasm. Axial contrast-enhanced CT in the venous phase more inferiorly shows the enlarged pancreas and several small cystic areas in the pancreas. These focal cystic areas in this patient likely represent dilated side branches. The presence of papillary projections, marked dilation of the main pancreatic duct, calcifications, or a soft tissue mass is suggestive of malignancy.

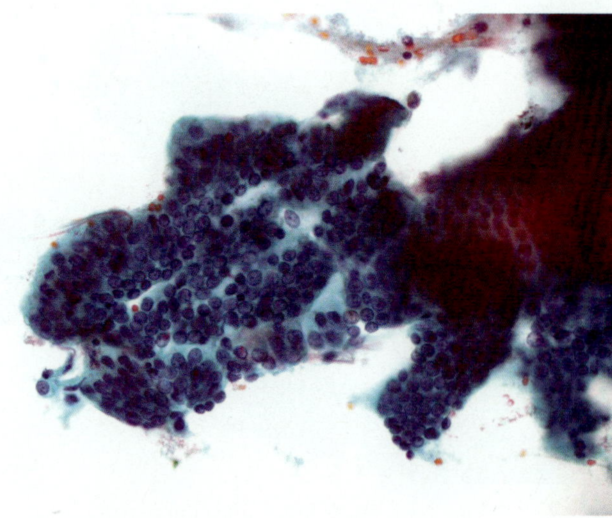

Figure 3.24 — Pancreas, Intraductal Papillary Mucinous Neoplasm. This fragment of mucinous epithelium shows an orderly arrangement of uniform columnar cells with only slight crowding. The mucinous cytoplasm of these cells is best appreciated in the top left portion of the field. (Papanicolaou stain, high power)

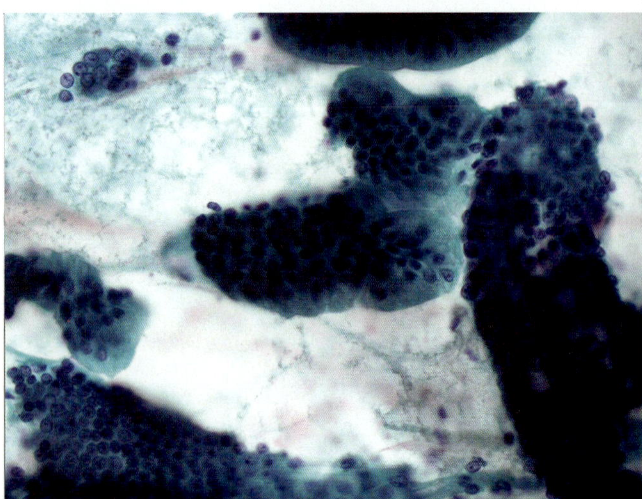

Figure 3.25 — Pancreas, Intraductal Papillary Mucinous Neoplasm. Papillary fragments of mucinous epithelium are shown composed of cells with ample pale cytoplasm and small, uniform nuclei. Dysplasia and adenocarcinoma may commonly arise in an intraductal papillary mucinous neoplasm; thus, careful examination of the epithelium at high power is essential to properly classify the lesion. (Papanicolaou stain, high power)

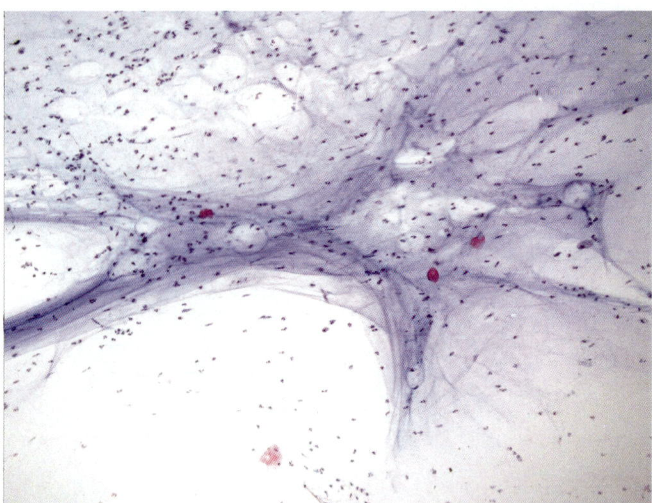

Figure 3.26 — Pancreas, Intraductal Papillary Mucinous Neoplasm. A background of thick "clean" mucin is suggestive of a neoplastic mucin-producing cyst. The mucin may not adhere well to the slide; thus, the gross appearance of the aspirate fluid should be noted for the pathologist to correlate with cytologic findings. This clean mucin should be distinguished from the thick, granular "dirty" mucin obtained as contamination from the gastrointestinal tract during endoscopic procedures. (Papanicolaou stain, medium power)

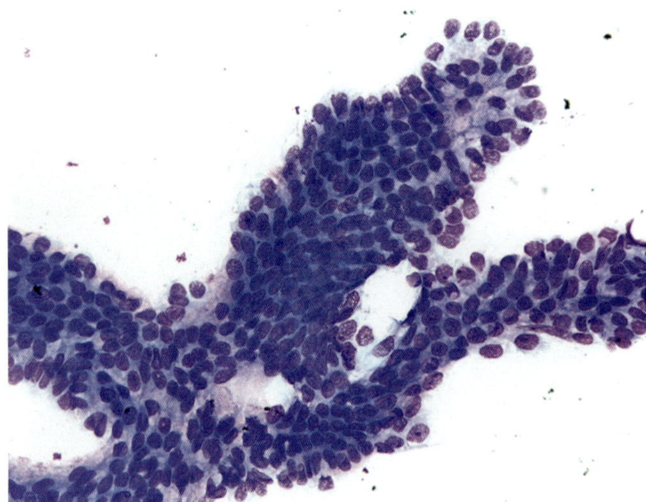

Figure 3.27 — Pancreas, Intraductal Papillary Mucinous Neoplasm. A papillary fragment of epithelium is shown with small, bland evenly spaced nuclei. An aliquot of the FNA specimen may be sent for chemistry analysis, which typically shows elevated CEA and normal amylase levels in an intraductal papillary mucinous neoplasm. (Diff Quik stain, medium power)

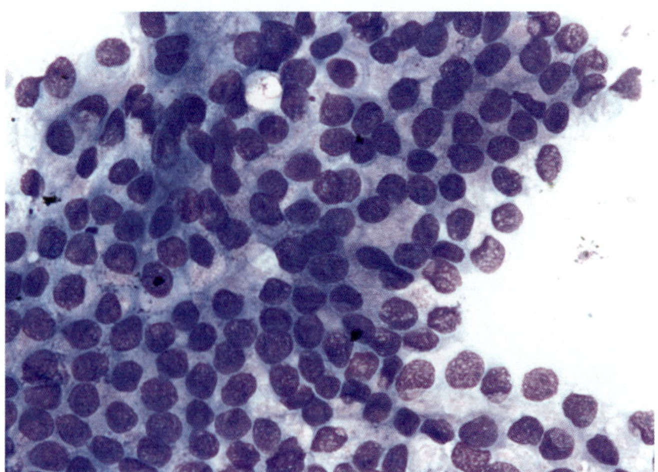

Figure 3.28 — Pancreas, Intraductal Papillary Mucinous Neoplasm. On high power, the cells show round- to oval-shaped nuclei with inconspicuous nucleoli. Intraductal papillary mucinous neoplasm is distinguished from a mucinous cystic neoplasm by the absence of ovarian-type stroma. (Diff Quik stain, medium power)

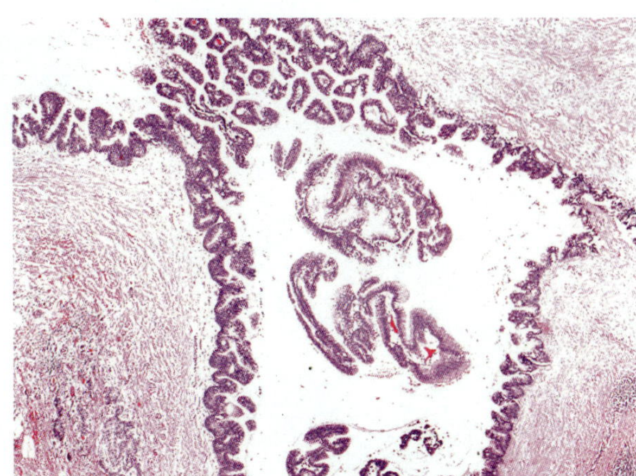

Figure 3.29 — Pancreas, Intraductal Papillary Mucinous Neoplasm (Histology). A papillary, mucin-producing epithelial neoplasm extending from the main pancreatic duct is shown. The current lesion is graded as having intermediate-grade dysplasia because it shows a degree of atypia similar to what would be seen in a tubular adenoma. (Hematoxylin and eosin stain, medium power)

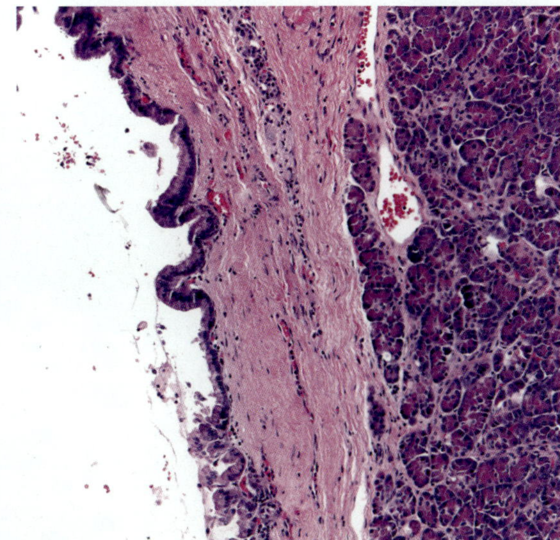

Figure 3.31 — Pancreas, Intraductal Papillary Mucinous Neoplasm (Histology). A proliferation of mucinous-type epithelium lines a pancreatic duct. This lesion shows no atypia. Benign pancreatic parenchyma is seen in the right portion of the field. Mucinous-type epithelium distinguishes these lesions from serous cystadenomas, and the absence of ovarian-type stroma differentiates it from a mucinous cystic neoplasm. (Hematoxylin and eosin stain, low power)

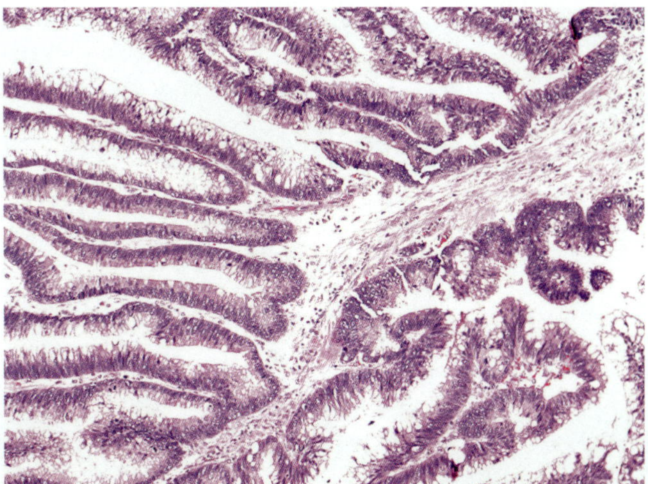

Figure 3.30 — Pancreas, Intraductal Papillary Mucinous Neoplasm (Histology). The neoplasm shows a papillary proliferation within the pancreatic duct system. These papillary projections have a focal cribriform architecture. The neoplasm involves a large duct and surrounding smaller ducts. The epithelium shows columnar cells with cytologic atypia analogous to that seen in colonic tubular adenoma. (Hematoxylin and eosin stain, high power)

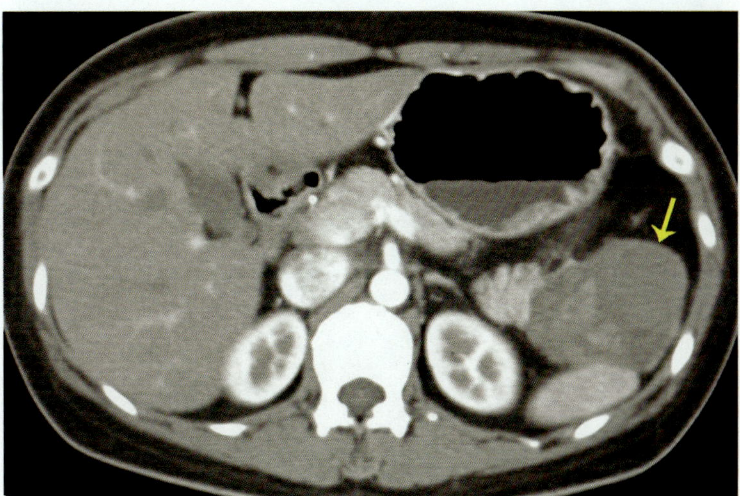

Figure 3.32 — Pancreas, Solid-Pseudopapillary Neoplasm. This 39-year-old woman presented with vague abdominal pain. Axial contrast-enhanced CT images in the arterial phases demonstrate a well-defined, 6.5-cm cystic mass in the tail of the pancreas (arrow). The mass contains heterogeneous areas of high density likely representing hemorrhage or a soft tissue component.

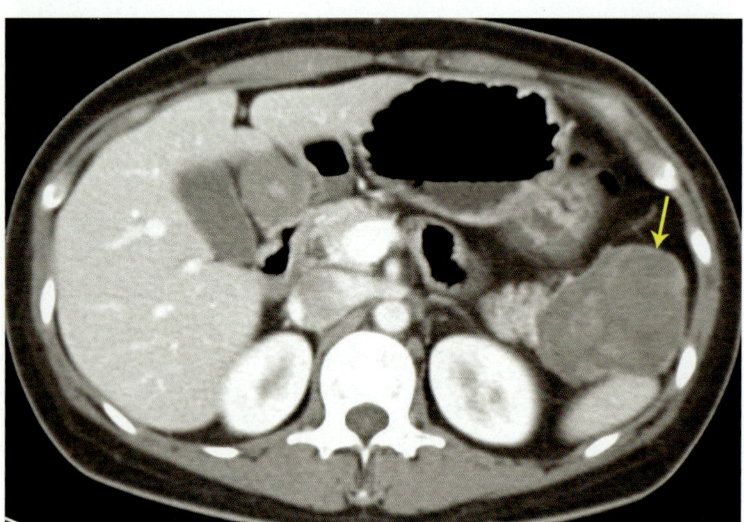

Figure 3.33 — Pancreas, Solid-Pseudopapillary Neoplasm. Axial contrast-enhanced CT in the venous phase confirms the heterogeneous appearance of the mass (arrow). Solid pseudopapillary epithelial neoplasms most commonly occur in young women and occur most often in the tail of the pancreas. Hemorrhage and necrosis are common.

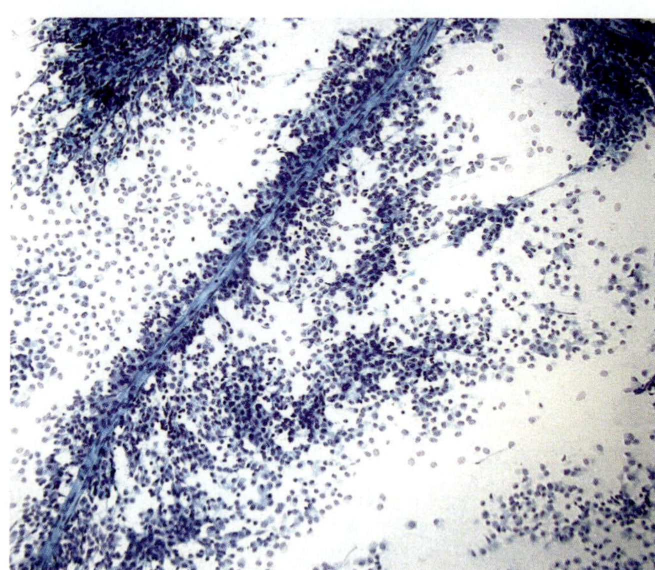

Figure 3.34 — Pancreas, Solid-Pseudopapillary Neoplasm. A fibrovascular core is seen traversing the field, surrounded by densely packed neoplastic cells. A population of single, dispersed tumor cells is present in the background. The main differential diagnostic consideration is a well-differentiated pancreatic neuroendocrine tumor. (Papanicolaou stain, low power)

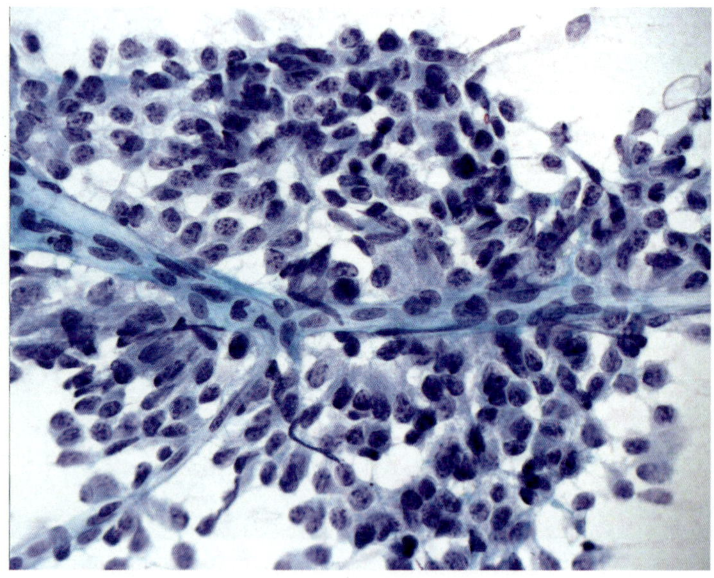

Figure 3.35 — Pancreas, Solid-Pseudopapillary Neoplasm. A small vessel is coursing through this fragment of neoplastic cells. The tumor cells have wispy cytoplasm and round to oval nuclei with pale, smooth to finely granular chromatin. Nucleoli are not commonly encountered. (Papanicolaou stain, medium power)

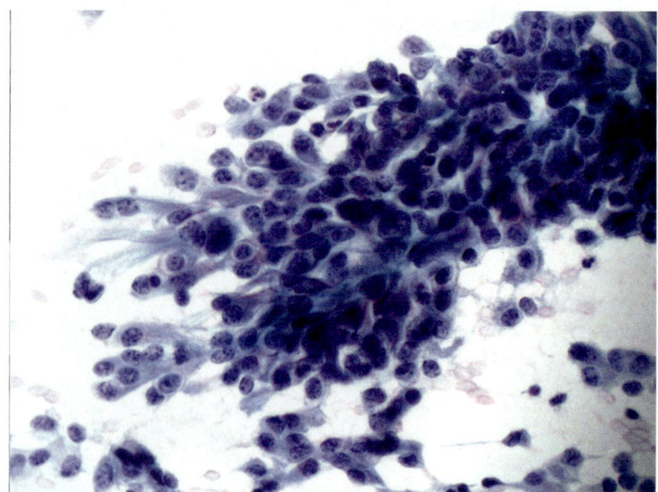

Figure 3.36 — Pancreas, Solid-Pseudopapillary Neoplasm. A densely cellular aggregate of neoplastic cells is shown. The cells have pale, wispy cytoplasm and ill-defined cell borders. An attempt should be made at the time of FNA to obtain material for cell block preparation as immunostains are often required to distinguish this lesion from a neuroendocrine tumor. (Papanicolaou stain, high power)

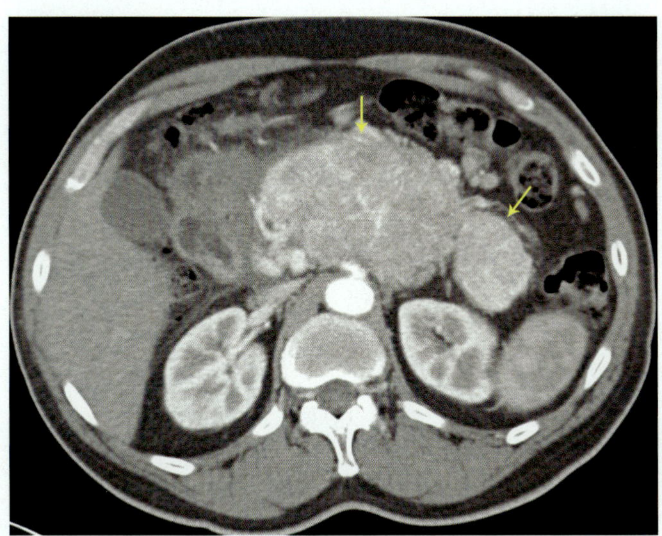

Figure 3.37 — Pancreas, Pancreatic Neuroendocrine Tumor. This 59-year-old man complained of vague abdominal pain for one month. Axial contrast-enhanced CT image in the arterial phase shows a large hypervascular mass involving the body and tail of the pancreas (arrows).

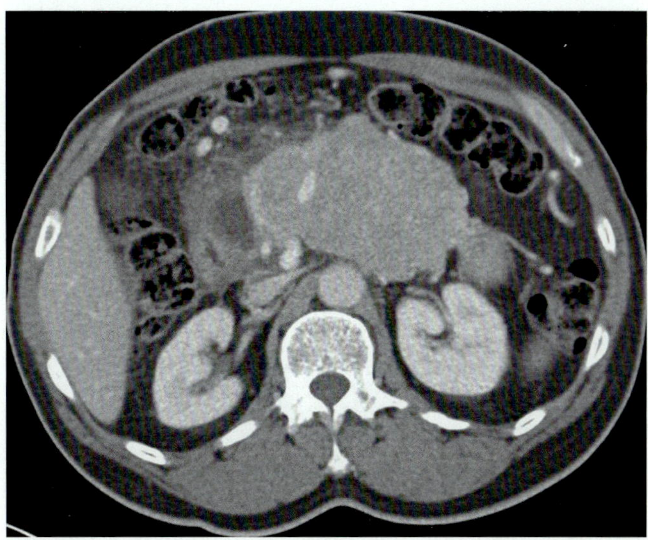

Figure 3.38 — Pancreas, Pancreatic Neuroendocrine Tumor. The mass shows homogeneous enhancement in the venous phase. Pancreatic neuroendocrine tumors are hypervascular after contrast enhancement. They are generally homogenous when small, but can become heterogeneous when large due to necrosis and hemorrhage. Vascular invasion and metastases are more common with larger lesions.

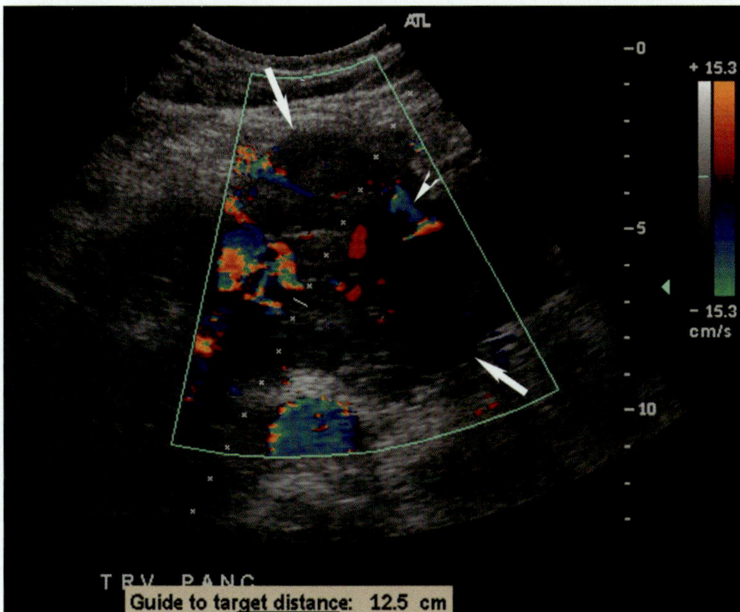

Figure 3.39 — Pancreas, Pancreatic Neuroendocrine Tumor. Sonographic image with color Doppler obtained during ultrasound-guided biopsy demonstrates a large hypoechoic mass in the pancreas (arrows) with marked internal vascularity.

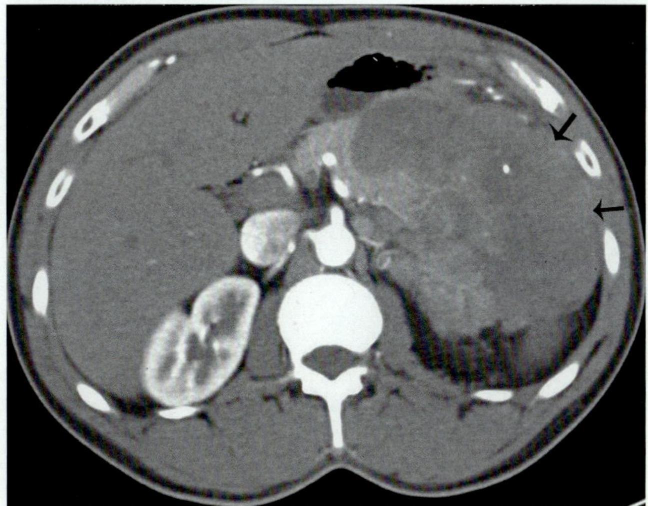

Figure 3.40 — Pancreas, Pancreatic Neuroendocrine Tumor. This 48-year-old man had a 2-year history of abdominal pain primarily in the left upper quadrant. Axial contrast-enhanced CT image in the arterial phase shows a large, 12.0-cm heterogeneous mass with areas of necrosis and calcification arising from the tail of the pancreas (arrows).

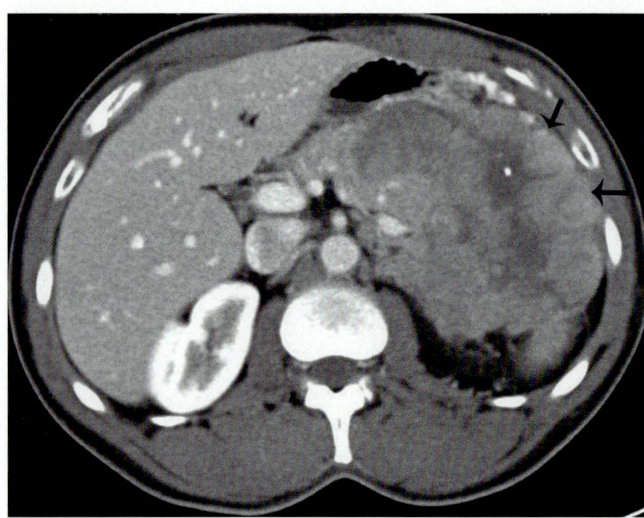

Figure 3.41 — Pancreas, Pancreatic Neuroendocrine Tumor. Axial contrast-enhanced CT image in the venous phase at the same level shows a prominent enhancing soft tissue component and necrosis within the mass (arrows). Pancreatic neuroendocrine tumors can become heterogeneous when large, as in this case, due to necrosis and hemorrhage. Vascular invasion and metastases are more common with larger lesions.

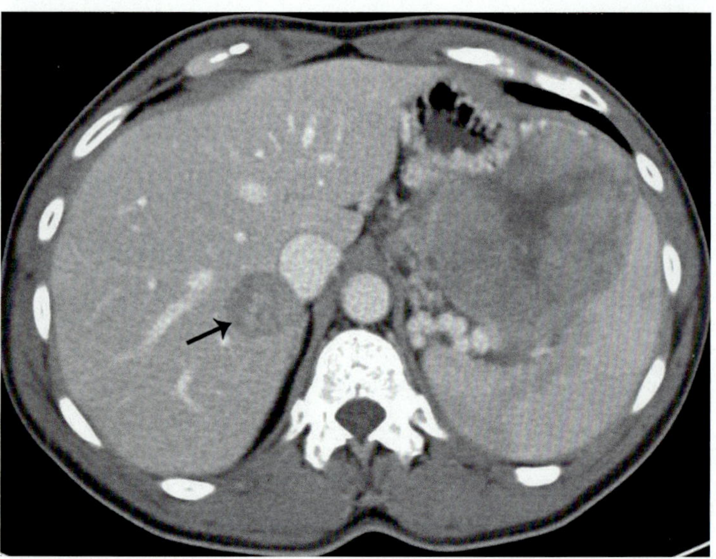

Figure 3.42 — Pancreas, Pancreatic Neuroendocrine Tumor. Axial contrast-enhanced CT in the venous phase shows a small heterogeneous mass in the right lobe of the liver which is suspicious for a metastasis (arrow). Metastases from neuroendocrine tumors are commonly hypervascular.

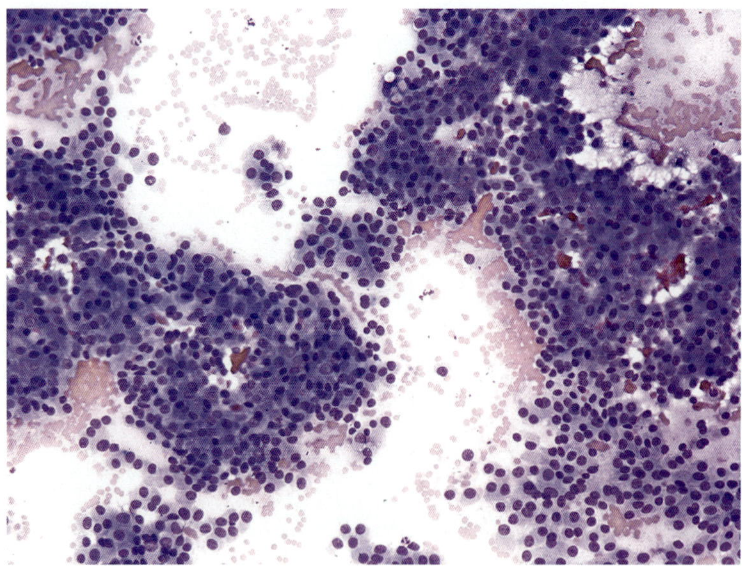

Figure 3.43 — Pancreas, Pancreatic Neuroendocrine Tumor. Sheets of neoplastic cells with uniform, round nuclei and ample granular cytoplasm are characteristic of a well-differentiated neuroendocrine tumor. Few scattered single cells are present, and bare nuclei may be encountered. (Diff Quik stain, medium power)

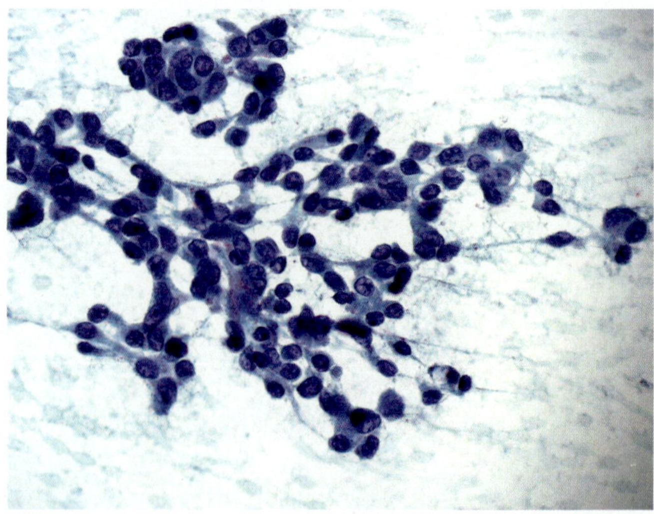

Figure 3.44 — Pancreas, Pancreatic Neuroendocrine Tumor. Loosely cohesive neoplastic cells with round to oval nuclei are present. The cytoplasm demonstrates granularity attributable to neurosecretory granules. The presence of necrosis and mitotic figures should be noted, as they relate to tumor prognosis. (Papanicolaou stain, medium power)

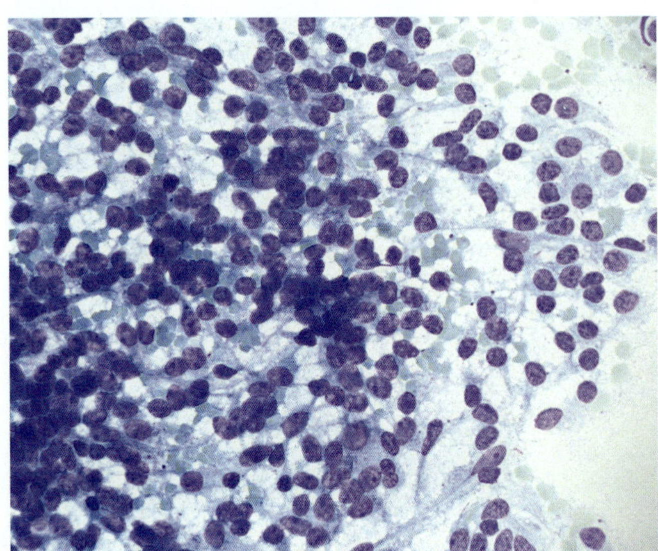

Figure 3.45 — Pancreas, Pancreatic Neuroendocrine Tumor. A dispersed population of uniform, round to oval neoplastic cells is shown. The chromatin is evenly dispersed with rare small nucleoli. Pancreatic neuroendocrine tumors often arise in the setting of MEN1 and may be multiple in those patients. (Diff Quik stain, medium power)

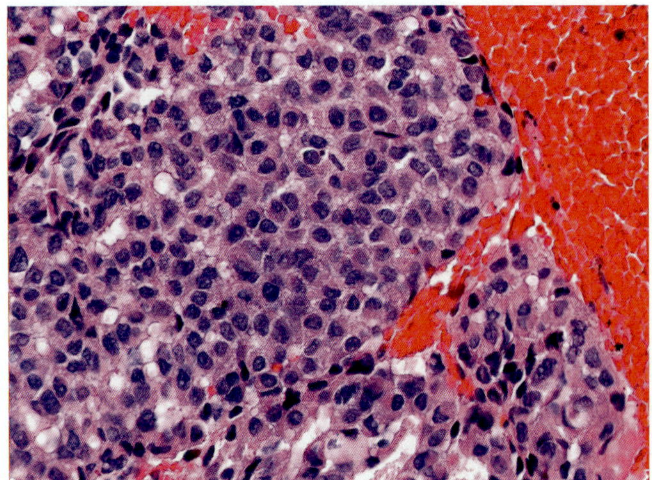

Figure 3.46 — Pancreas, Pancreatic Neuroendocrine Tumor (Cell Block). The neoplasm is composed of a uniform population of cells with low nuclear-to-cytoplasmic ratios and round nuclei with minimal pleomorphism. Chromatin is uniformly distributed. Nucleoli are not evident, although they may be present in neuroendocrine tumors, raising the differential diagnosis of acinar cell carcinoma. (Hematoxylin and eosin stain, high power)

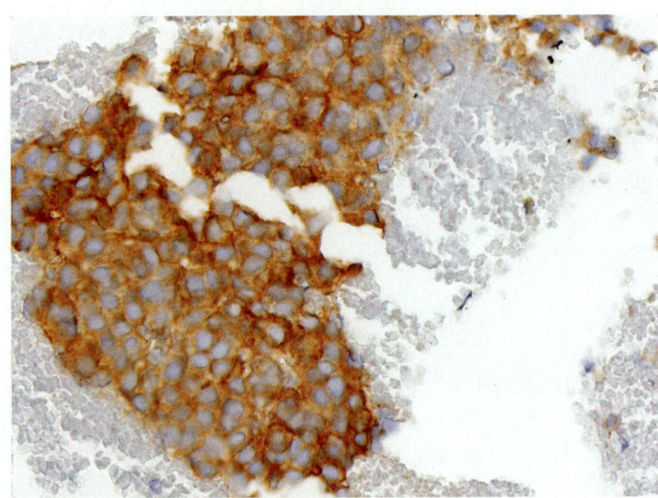

Figure 3.47 — Pancreas, Pancreatic Neuroendocrine Tumor (Cell Block). The tumor is positive for CD56 immunostain, reflecting neuroendocrine differentiation. Synaptophysin and chromogranin stains were also positive. PAX8 is also positive in neuroendocrine tumors of pancreatic origin. (CD56 immunostain, high power)

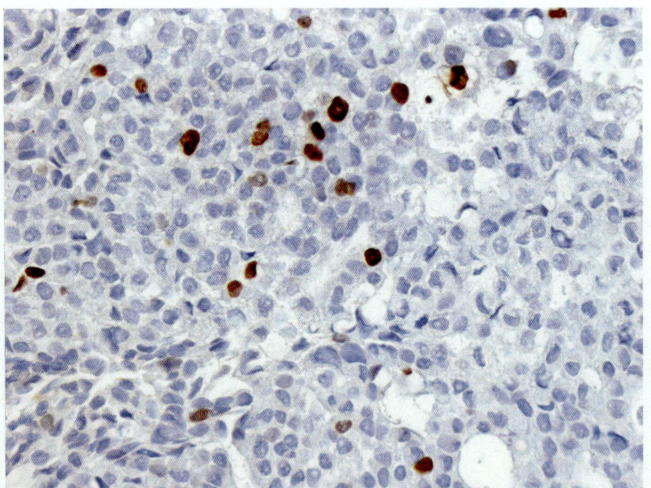

Figure 3.48 — Pancreas, Pancreatic Neuroendocrine Tumor (Cell Block). The proliferative rate of this tumor is quite low (less than 2%), as highlighted by this Ki67 immunostain. A low mitotic rate is needed to classify these lesions as well-differentiated pancreatic neuroendocrine tumors (PanNETs). (Ki67 immunostain, high power)

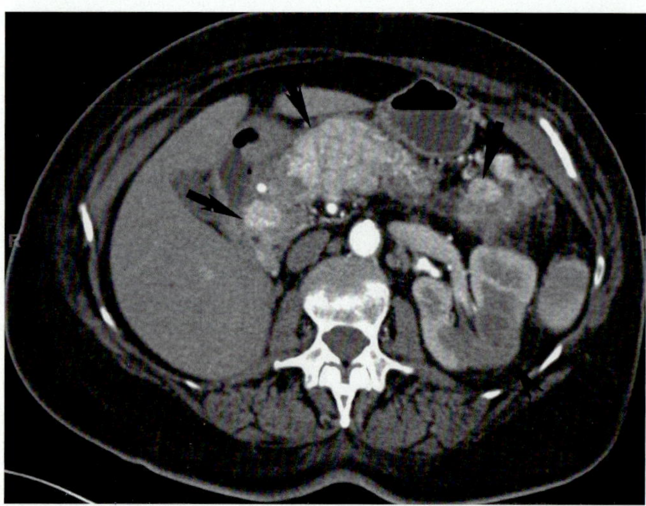

Figure 3.49 — Pancreas, Metastatic Renal Cell Carcinoma. This 70-year-old woman had a history of a right nephrectomy for renal cell carcinoma and was in a car accident prompting a trauma CT. Axial contrast-enhanced CT image in the arterial phase shows multiple hypervascular, arterially enhancing masses in the pancreas (arrowhead). Note the ill-defined hypodense area in the left kidney arrowhead which likely represents infection or inflammation as it decreased in size on subsequent studies (not shown).

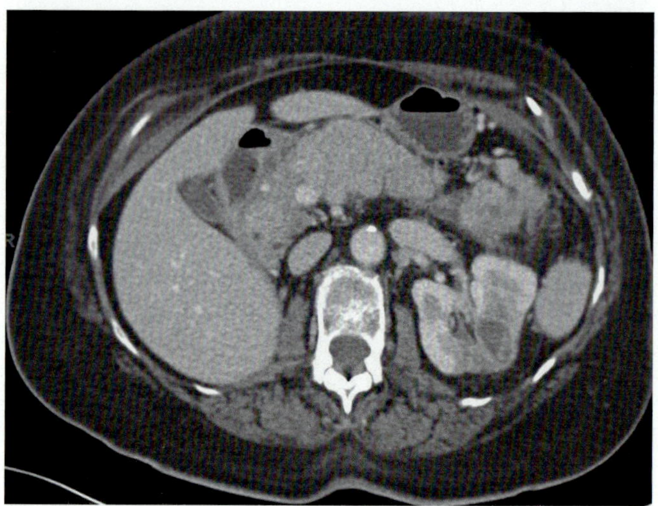

Figure 3.50 — Pancreas, Metastatic Renal Cell Carcinoma. The multiple masses in the pancreas de-enhance in the venous phase. Metastases to the pancreas occur with hematogeneous spread of lung, renal, breast, and colon cancers and melanoma. Depending on the primary tumor, pancreatic metastases can be hypovascular or as in this case, hypervascular (renal cell carcinoma, sarcoma).

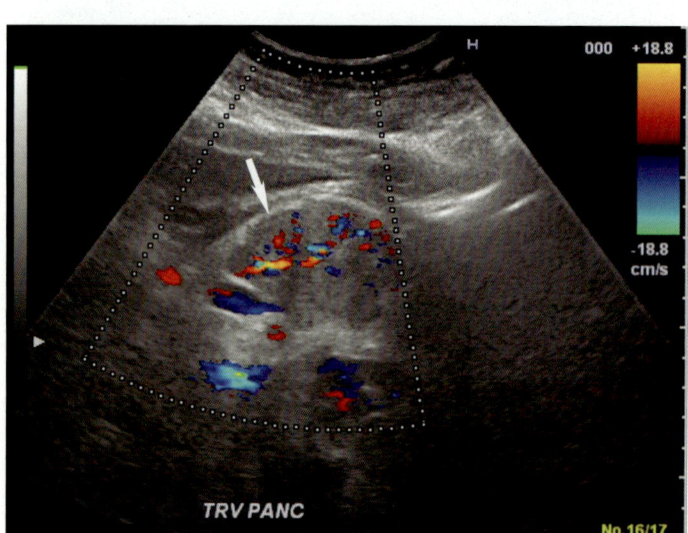

Figure 3.51 — Pancreas, Metastatic Renal Cell Carcinoma. Sonographic image confirms hypervascular masses in the pancreas. Renal cell carcinoma metastases to the pancreas can mimic islet cell tumors as both are hypervascular.

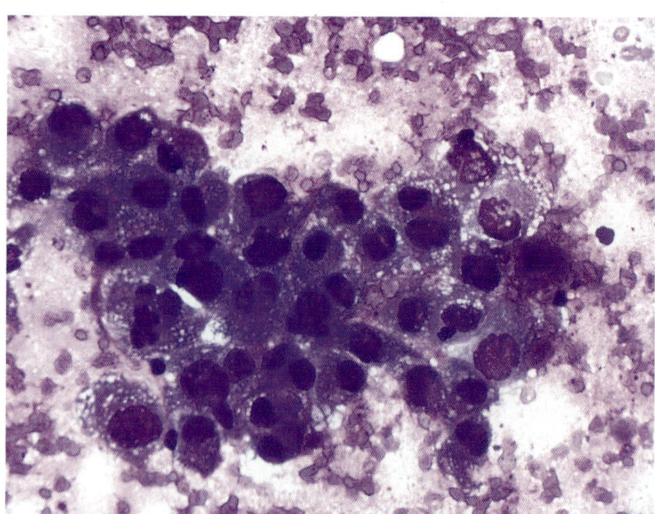

Figure 3.52 — Pancreas, Metastatic Renal Cell Carcinoma. Abundant vacuolated cytoplasm is evident in these neoplastic cells. The nuclei are enlarged and hyperchromatic, but the nuclear-to-cytoplasmic ratio is still relatively low. An acinar cell carcinoma would be considered in the differential diagnosis. (Diff Quik stain, high power)

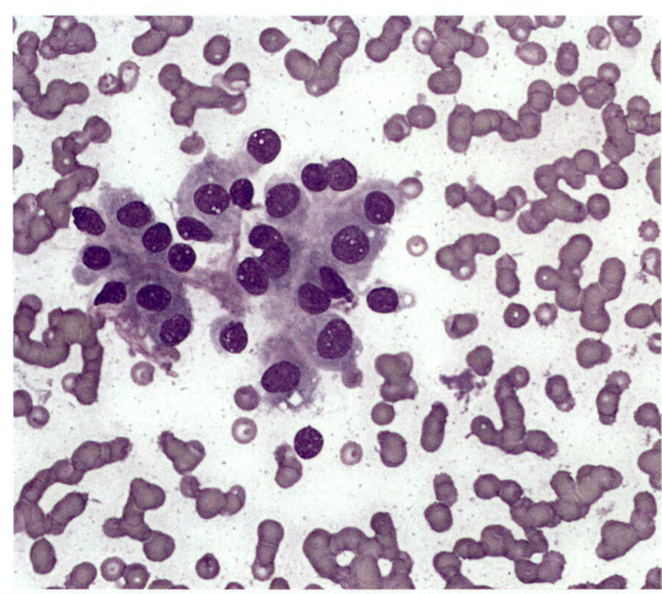

Figure 3.53 — Pancreas, Metastatic Renal Cell Carcinoma. These neoplastic cells have a polygonal shape with abundant cytoplasm and round nuclei. Both acinar cell carcinoma and a neuroendocrine tumor are in the differential. (Diff Quik stain, high power)

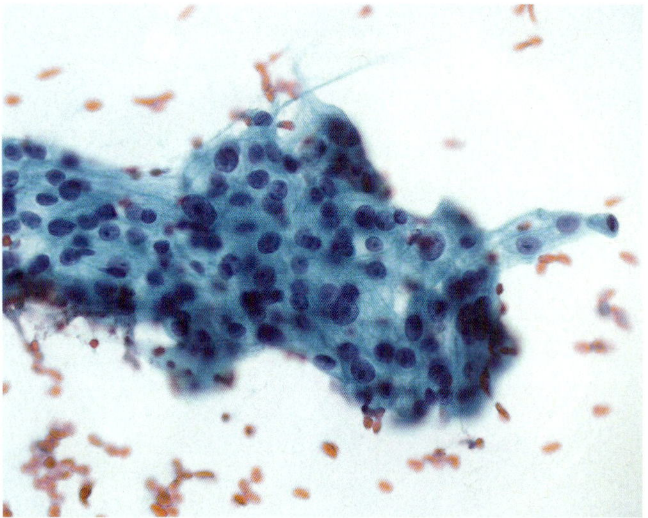

Figure 3.54 — Pancreas, Metastatic Renal Cell Carcinoma. Abundant delicate cytoplasm surrounds round to oval nuclei with prominent nucleoli. As per usual, a thorough patient history is essential to diagnosis, as a pancreatic metastasis long removed in time from a primary renal cell carcinoma is not uncommon. (Papanicolaou stain, high power)

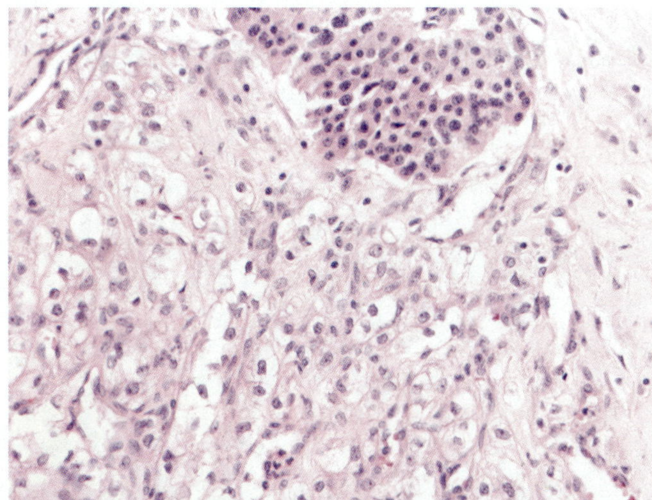

Figure 3.55 — Pancreas, Metastatic Renal Cell Carcinoma (Histology). A richly vascular, clear cell epithelial tumor with large polygonal cells with large nuclei and macronucleoli is seen surrounding an intact pancreatic islet. Confirmatory immunostains can be easily performed in cases where no definite history of a primary renal cell carcinoma is available. (Hematoxylin and eosin stain, medium power)

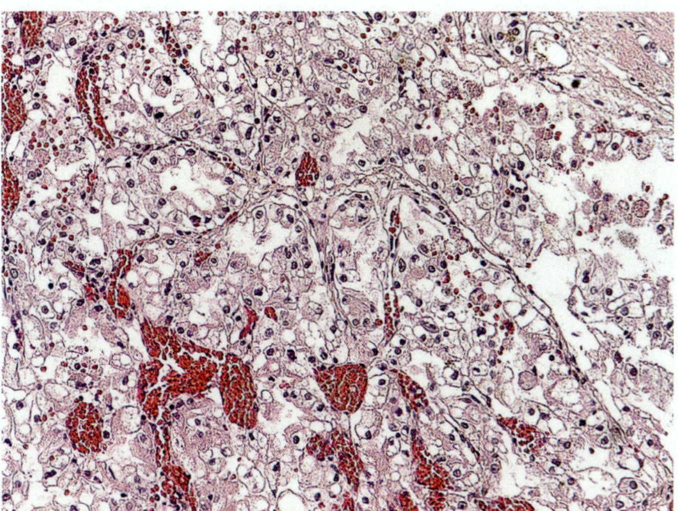

Figure 3.56 — Pancreas, Metastatic Renal Cell Carcinoma. The neoplastic cells are large and polygonal. The cell membranes are distinct and surround abundant clear cytoplasm. The nuclei are round to oval and small with minimal variation in size and inconspicuous nucleoli. (Hematoxylin and eosin stain, medium power)

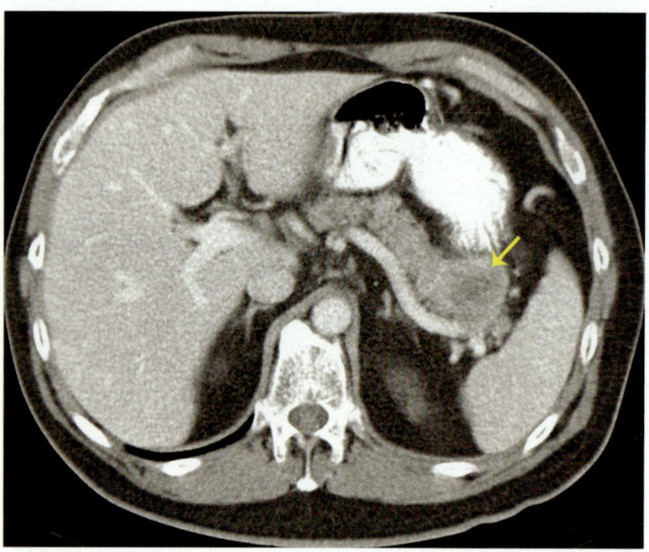

Figure 3.57 — Pancreas, Metastatic Merkel Cell Carcinoma. This 61-year-old man presented with abdominal pain. Axial contrast-enhanced CT shows a mass with central necrosis in the pancreatic tail (arrow).

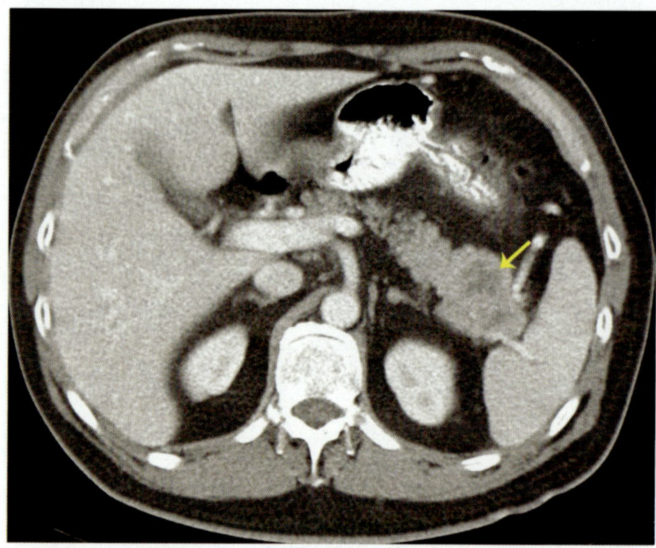

Figure 3.58 — Pancreas, Metastatic Merkel Cell Carcinoma. Axial contrast-enhanced CT slightly more inferiorly shows the focal mass in the pancreatic tail with central necrosis (arrow). Depending on the primary tumor, pancreatic metastases can be hypovascular, as in this case, and may mimic pancreatic adenocarcinoma.

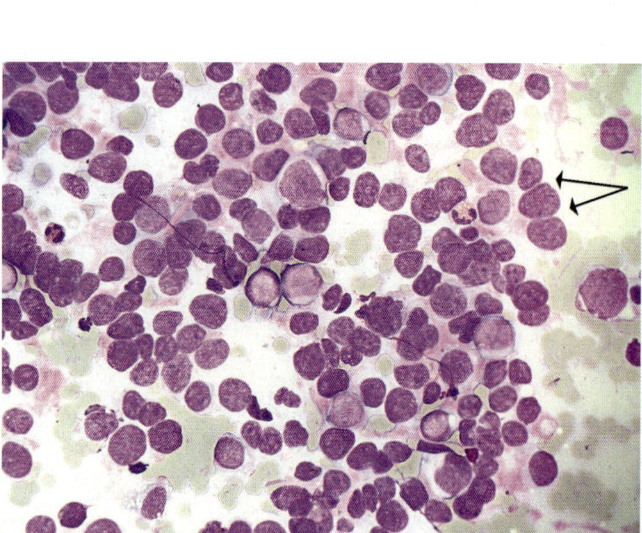

Figure 3.59 — Pancreas, Metastatic Merkel Cell Carcinoma. A dispersed population of neoplastic cells is present. The differential diagnosis includes a hematopoietic neoplasm, metastatic small cell carcinoma, and a metastatic Merkel cell carcinoma. Focal nuclear molding (arrows) is suggestive of neuroendocrine differentiation, but confirmatory immunostains are warranted. (Diff Quik stain, high power)

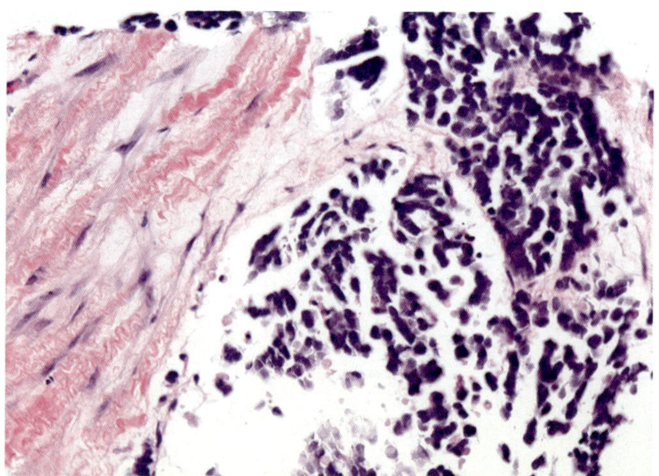

Figure 3.60 — Pancreas, Metastatic Merkel Cell Carcinoma (Core Biopsy). A metastatic Merkel cell carcinoma is indistinguishable cytologically from a small cell carcinoma, as both show small cells with scant cytoplasm, neuroendocrine nuclear features, and frequent crush artifact. This small core biopsy provided adequate material on which to perform immunostains. (Hematoxylin and eosin stain, high power)

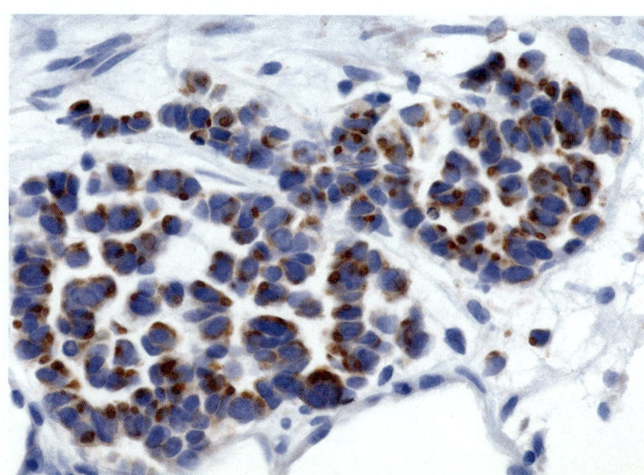

Figure 3.61 — Pancreas, Metastatic Merkel Cell Carcinoma (Core Biopsy). A CK20 immunostain shows the characteristic perinuclear dot-like positivity for Merkel cell carcinoma. A TTF-1 stain was negative, which also supports Merkel cell carcinoma over small cell carcinoma. (Cytokeratin 20, high power)

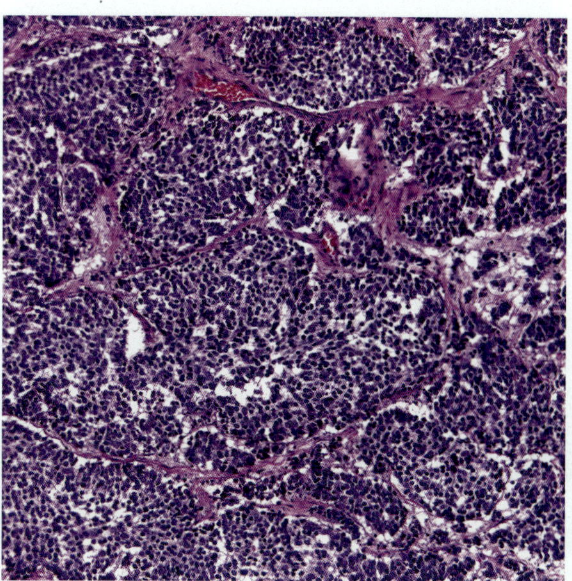

Figure 3.62 — Pancreas, Metastatic Merkel Cell Carcinoma (Histology). The metastatic neoplasm is composed of small blue cells with scant cytoplasm and a high nuclear-to-cytoplasmic ratio. Note the round nuclei with fine chromatin. Nucleoli are absent or inconspicuous. Mitotic activity is typically brisk. (Hematoxylin and eosin stain, low power)

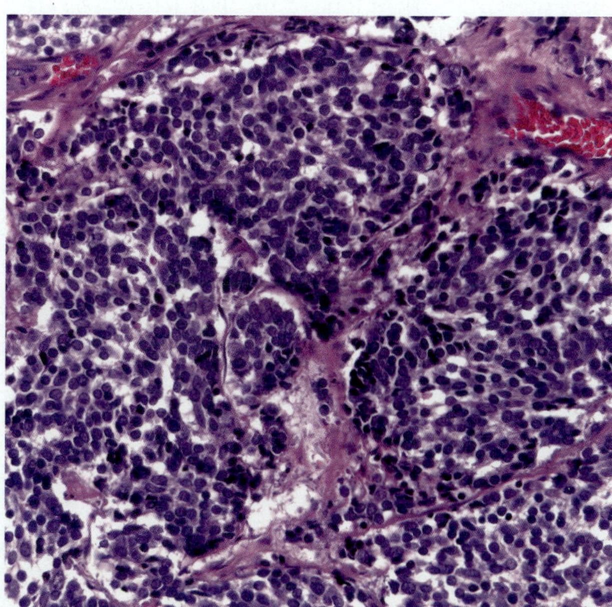

Figure 3.63 — Pancreas, Metastatic Merkel Cell Carcinoma (Histology). The normal pancreatic parenchyma is replaced by small round blue cells. The neoplastic nuclei have a "ground glass" appearance with "dusty" chromatin. The tumor is associated with necrosis and mitotic figures are easily identified. Nuclear molding is not seen. (Hematoxylin and eosin stain, medium power)

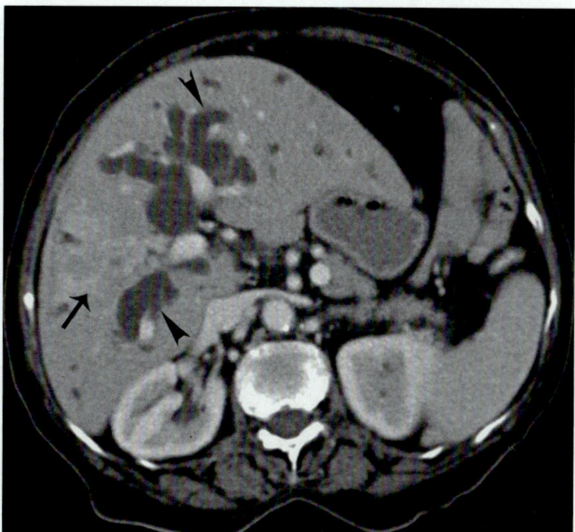

Figure 3.64 — Liver, Cholangiocarcinoma. A 78-year-old woman presented with jaundice, right upper quadrant pain, and elevated bilirubin. Axial contrast-enhanced CT image demonstrates an infiltrative mass in the right hepatic lobe (arrowheads). There is moderate dilatation of the right and left biliary ducts arrowheads.

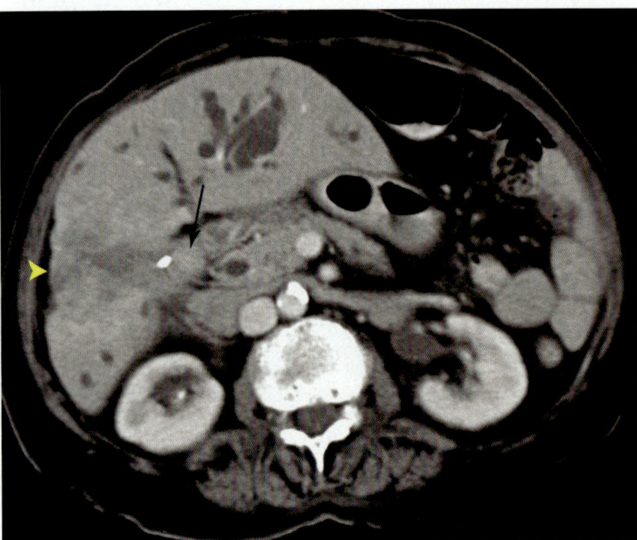

Figure 3.65 — Liver, Cholangiocarcinoma. Note retraction of the liver capsule (arrowhead), which is characteristic of a cholangiocarcinoma. The mass extends inferiorly to the porta hepatis (arrow) resulting in marked intrahepatic biliary duct dilation in both the right and left hepatic lobes.

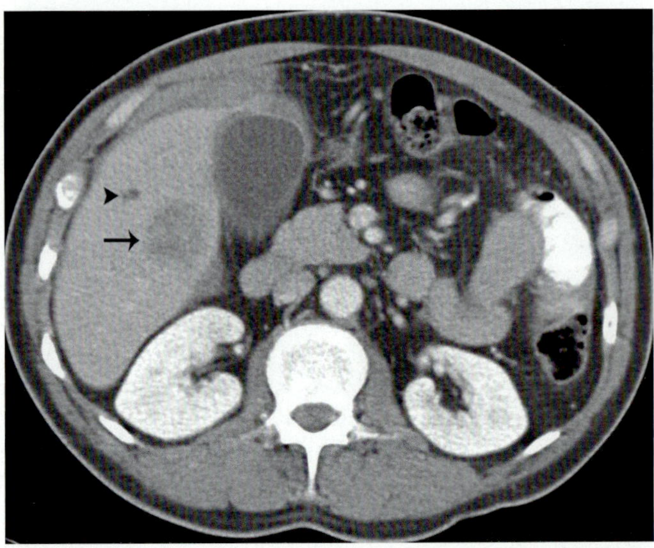

Figure 3.66 — Liver, Cholangiocarcinoma. This 49-year-old man with a history of Crohn's disease and primary sclerosing cholangitis was found to have a mass in the right lobe of the liver. Axial contrast-enhanced CT image demonstrates an ill-defined hypoechoic mass in the right lobe of the liver (arrow). There is mild biliary duct dilation in the right hepatic lobe (arrowhead). Cholangiocarcinomas frequently cause focal dilatation of intrahepatic ducts distal to the tumor.

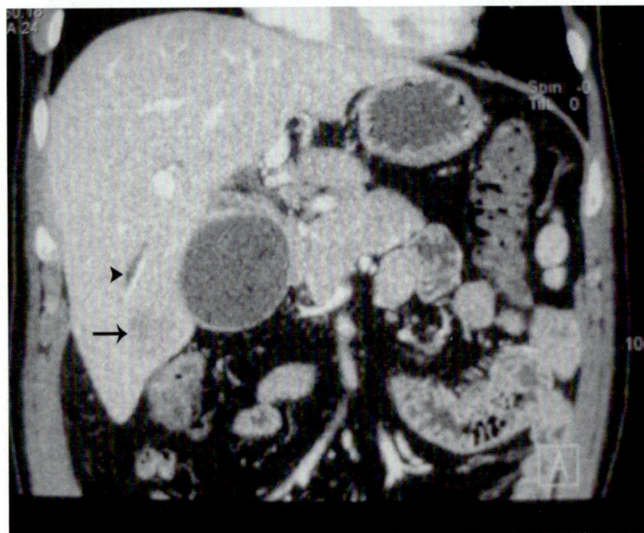

Figure 3.67 — Liver, Cholangiocarcinoma. Coronal contrast-enhanced CT image confirms an ill-defined hypoechoic mass in the right lobe of the liver (arrow). There is mild biliary duct dilation in the right hepatic lobe (arrowhead).

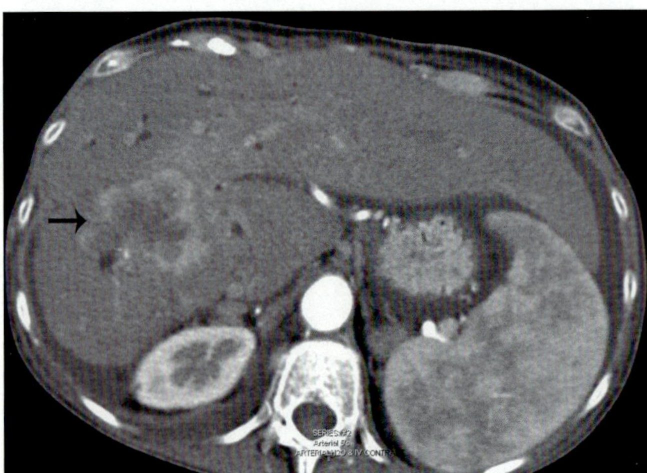

Figure 3.68 — Liver, Cholangiocarcinoma. This 62-year-old woman was noted to have elevated liver function tests, prompting further work-up. Axial contrast-enhanced CT image of the liver in the arterial phase demonstrates an infiltrative mass with peripheral enhancement located centrally in the right hepatic lobe (arrow).

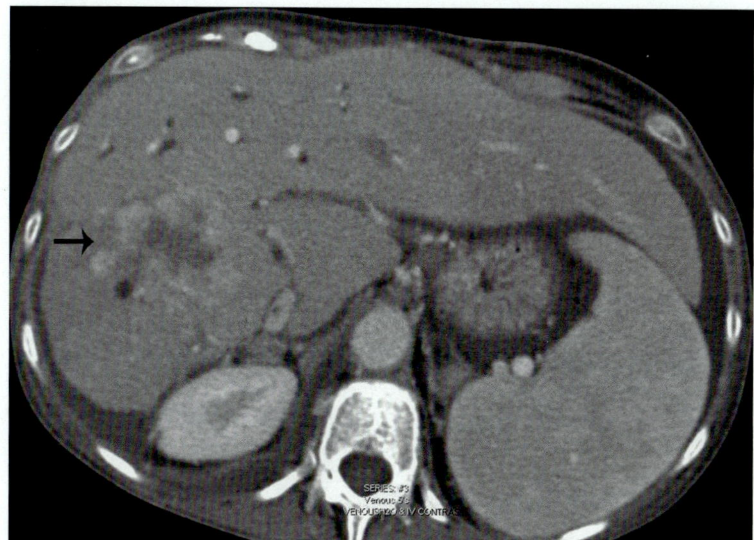

Figure 3.69 — Liver, Cholangiocarcinoma. The mass enhances in the venous phase (arrow). Cholangiocarcinoma may arise in the setting of primary sclerosing cholangitis, as in this patient.

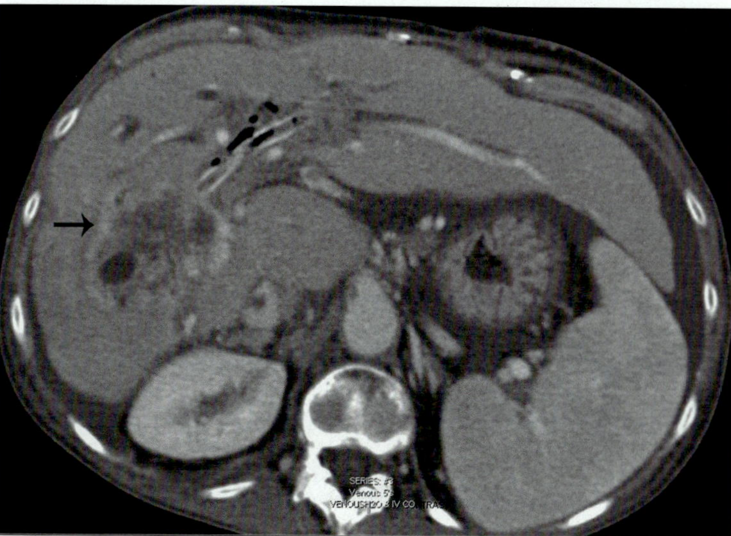

Figure 3.70 — Liver, Cholangiocarcinoma. There is mild intrahepatic biliary duct dilation and biliary drains are also seen. Centrally located cholangiocarcinomas (arrow) often result in dilation of distal intrahepatic bile ducts.

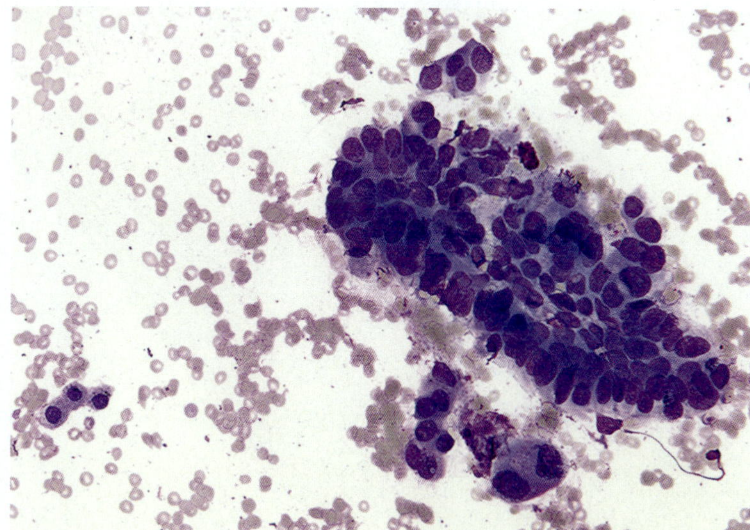

Figure 3.71 — Liver, Cholangiocarcinoma. The epithelial fragment shown demonstrates a glandular configuration. The nuclei are moderately enlarged and crowded, consistent with a well-differentiated adenocarcinoma. A few benign hepatocytes are present in the lower left portion of the field for size comparison. (Diff Quik stain, medium power)

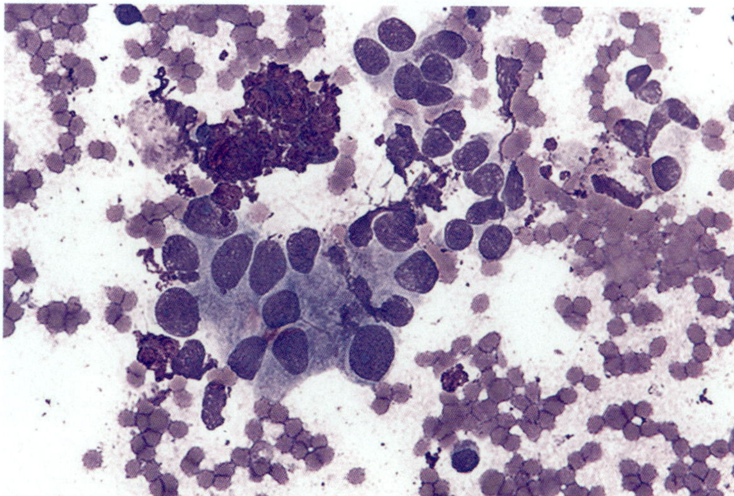

Figure 3.72 — Liver, Cholangiocarcinoma. The glandular nature of the tumor is demonstrated here as two acinar structures are present adjacent to one another. Cholangiocarcinoma cannot be distinguished morphologically or immunohistochemically from a metastatic adenocarcinoma from the pancreas or extrahepatic biliary tree; thus, clinical and radiographic correlation is essential. (Diff Quik stain, high power)

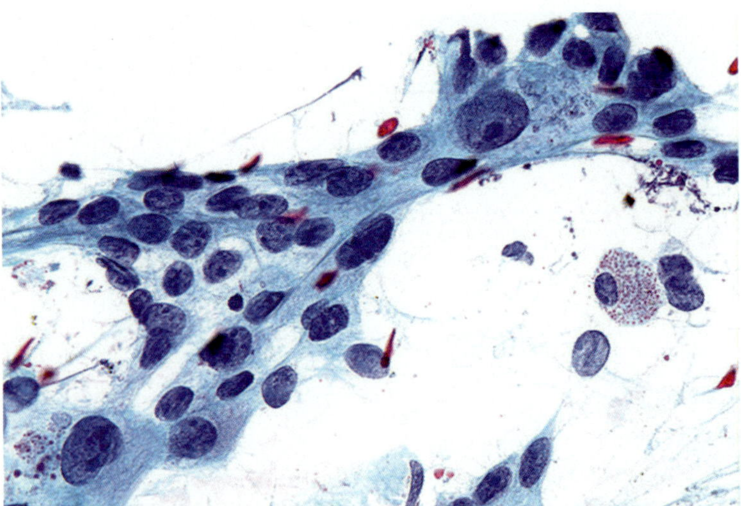

Figure 3.73 — Liver, Cholangiocarcinoma. These malignant epithelial cells show anisonucleosis and irregular nuclear contours. The nuclei are hyperchromatic and have nucleoli ranging from small to prominent. A single hepatocyte with granular cytoplasm is present in the background. (Papanicolaou stain, high power)

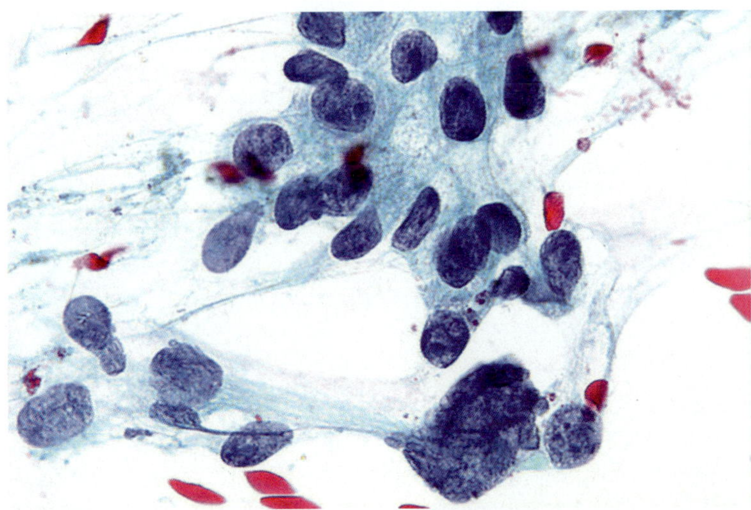

Figure 3.74 — Liver, Cholangiocarcinoma. Marked nuclear atypia is demonstrated. Metastatic adenocarcinoma to the liver is far more common than primary cholangiocarcinoma and may occur in the absence of a clinical history of prior malignancy. (Papanicolaou stain, high power)

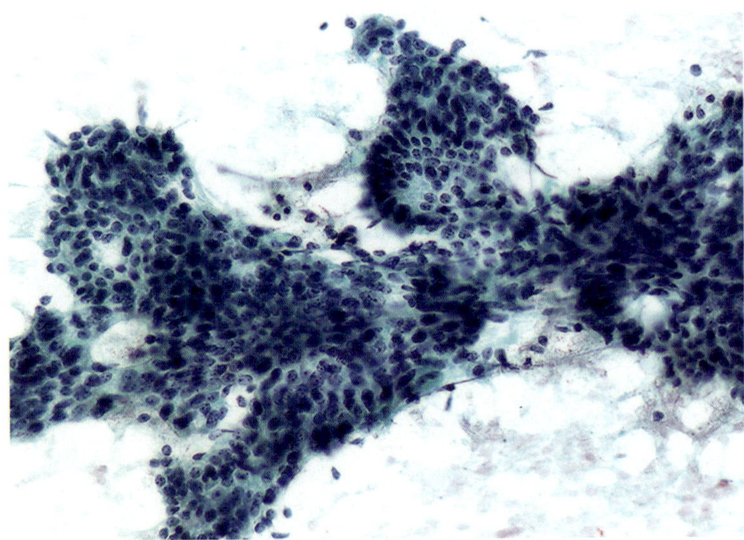

Figure 3.75 — Liver, Cholangiocarcinoma. This tumor is well differentiated and displays a predominantly flat, sheet-like pattern with focal glandular formations. The tumor cells show focal nuclear stratification and have round to oval mildly pleomorphic nuclei with small nucleoli. (Papanicolaou stain, low power)

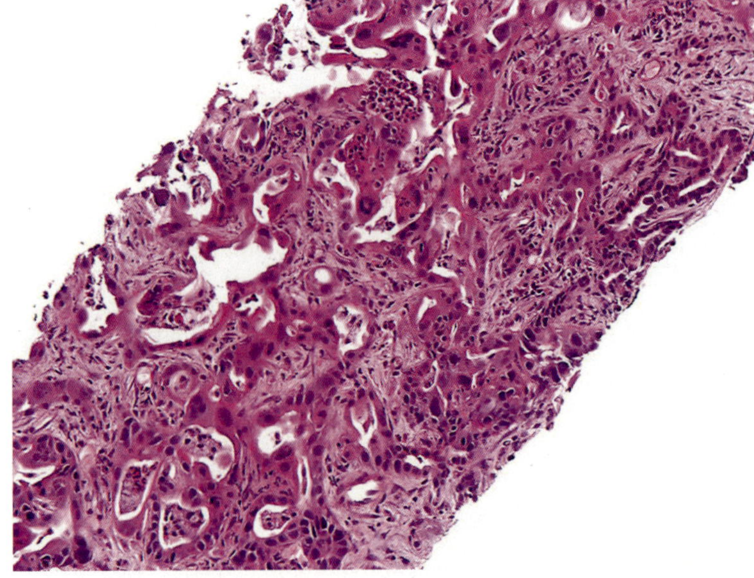

Figure 3.76 — Liver, Cholangiocarcinoma (Core Biopsy). A moderately to poorly differentiated adenocarcinoma is shown with extensive cytological atypia. The neoplastic cells have pleomorphic nuclei and the infiltrating glands are seen embedded in a fibrous stroma. (Hematoxylin and eosin stain, low power)

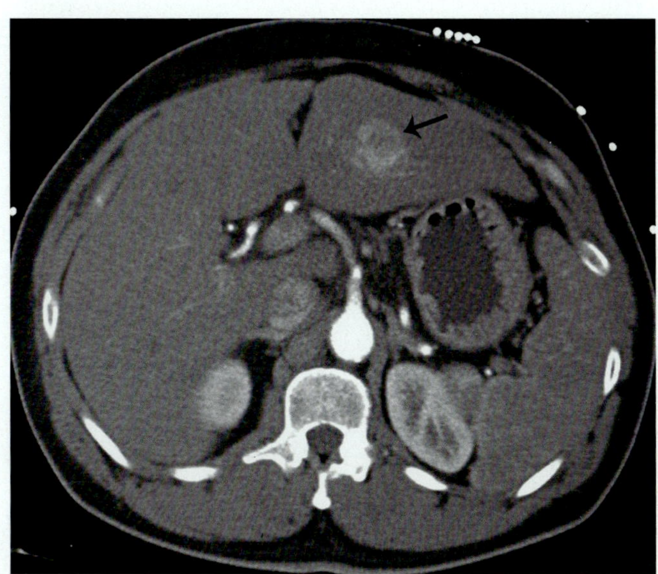

Figure 3.77 — Liver, Hepatocellular Carcinoma. This 57-year-old man complained of epigastric pain. Contrast-enhanced CT axial image in the arterial phase shows a slightly heterogeneous, hypervascular lesion in the left lobe of the liver (arrow).

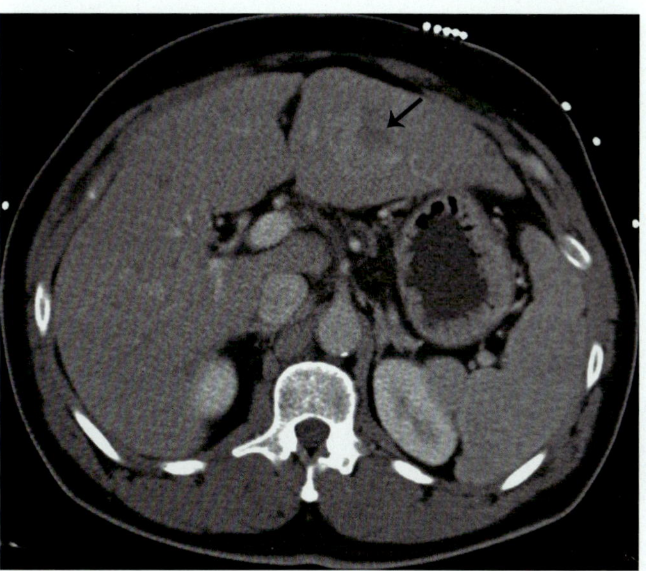

Figure 3.78 — Liver, Hepatocellular Carcinoma. In this contrast-enhanced CT, the lesion demonstrates washout of contrast in the venous phase (arrow), characteristic of hepatocellular carcinoma.

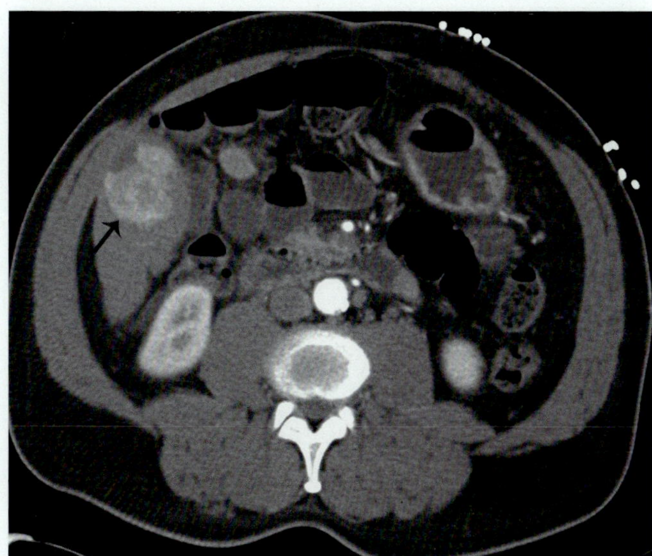

Figure 3.79 — Liver, Hepatocellular Carcinoma. This contrast-enhanced CT, arterial phase, shows that an additional heterogeneous, hypervascular lesion is present in the inferior right lobe of the liver (arrow).

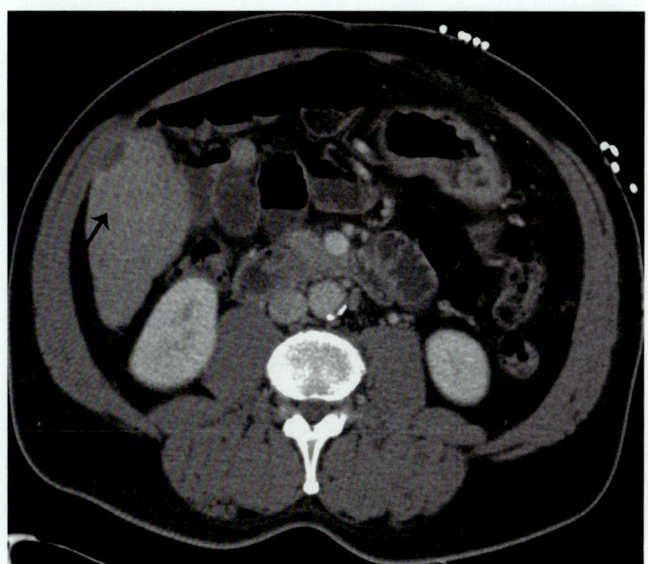

Figure 3.80 — Liver, Hepatocellular Carcinoma. Contrast-enhanced CT in the venous phase shows this mass also washes out in the venous phase (arrow) and blends in with the liver parenchyma.

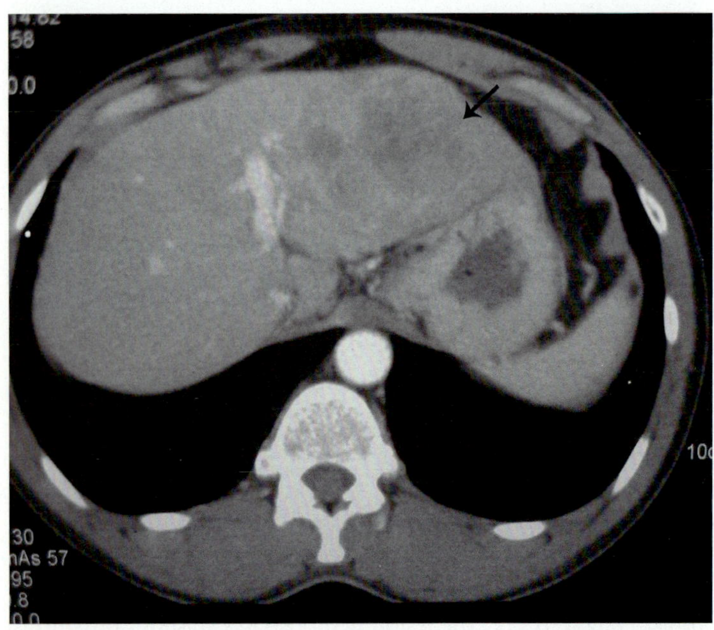

Figure 3.81 — Liver, Hepatocellular Carcinoma. This 41-year-old man complained of abdominal pain and distension. Axial contrast-enhanced CT image shows a large, heterogeneous mass in the left lobe of the liver with mild peripheral enhancement (arrow).

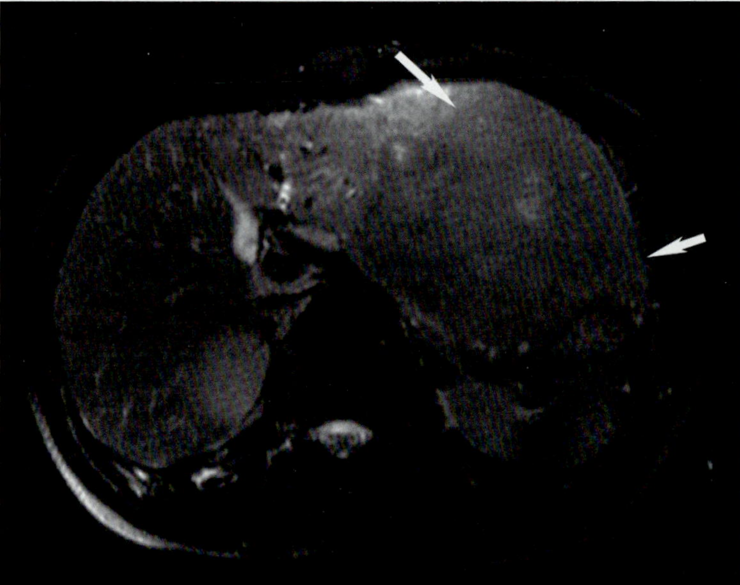

Figure 3.82 — Liver, Hepatocellular Carcinoma. Axial T2-weighted MR image with fat saturation shows the large mass replacing and enlarging the left lobe of the liver (arrows).

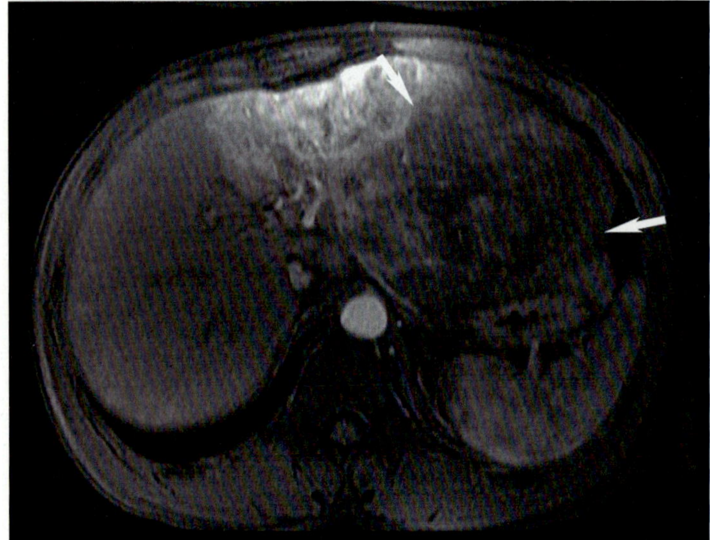

Figure 3.83 — Liver, Hepatocellular Carcinoma. Axial post-contrast T1-weighted MR image in the arterial phase shows a large, heterogeneous, mildly hypervascular mass in the left lobe of the liver (arrows).

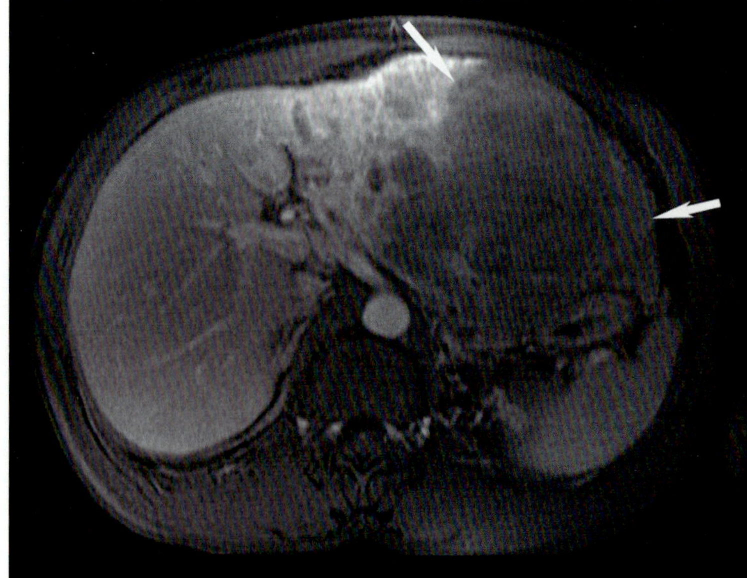

Figure 3.84 — Liver, Hepatocellular Carcinoma. Axial post-contrast T1-weighted MR image is shown in the venous phase. The mass shows some washout in this phase (arrows).

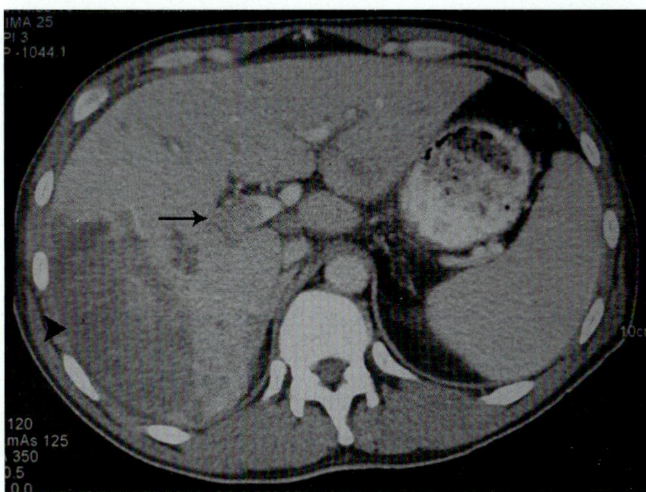

Figure 3.85 — Liver, Hepatocellular Carcinoma. A 51-year-old man with a history of hepatitis B presented with fever, cough, elevated liver functions tests, and an alpha-fetoprotein level of 23,000. Axial contrast-enhanced CT image shows a large, low-density, infiltrative area within the right lobe of the liver (arrowhead). Note the tumor thrombus in the right portal vein (arrow).

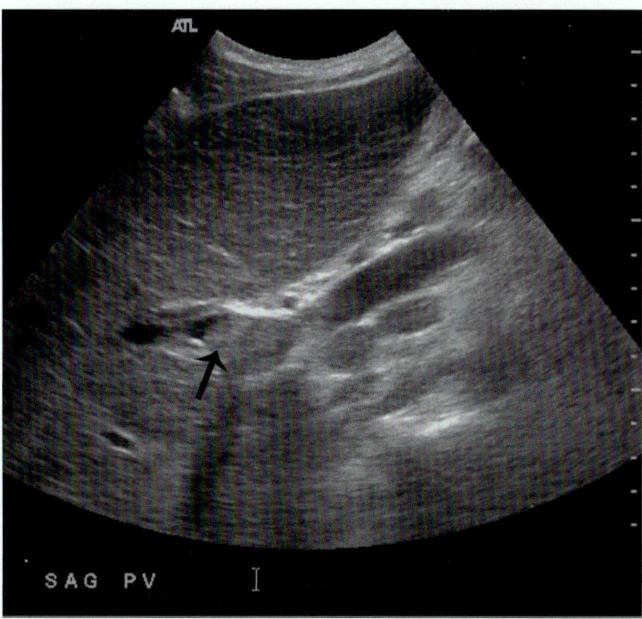

Figure 3.86 — Liver, Hepatocellular Carcinoma. Sonographic image confirms expansion of the portal vein with echogenic tumor thrombus (arrow).

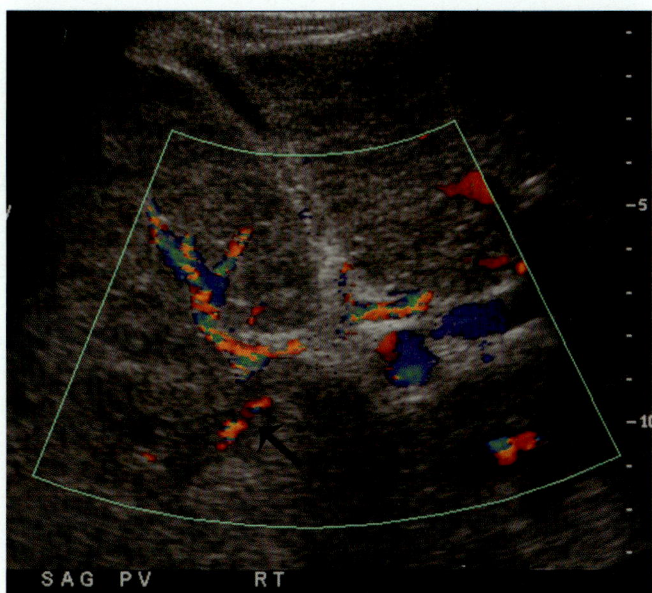

Figure 3.87 — Liver, Hepatocellular Carcinoma. Color Doppler image confirms internal vascularity in the right portal vein tumor thrombus (arrow).

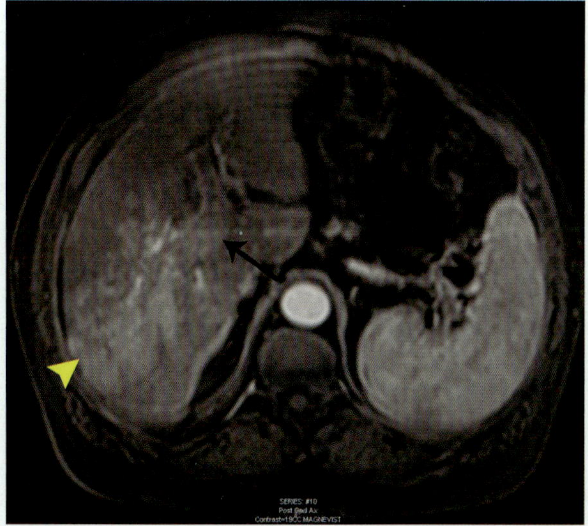

Figure 3.88 — Liver, Hepatocellular Carcinoma. This 70-year-old man with HIV, hepatitis C, and cirrhosis presented to the ED with vertigo and fever. Axial T1 fat-saturated post-contrast MR in the arterial phase shows a hypervascular mass in the right lobe of the liver (arrowhead). There is enhancing tumor thrombus in the right portal vein extending into the main portal vein (arrow). The liver is nodular, compatible with cirrhosis.

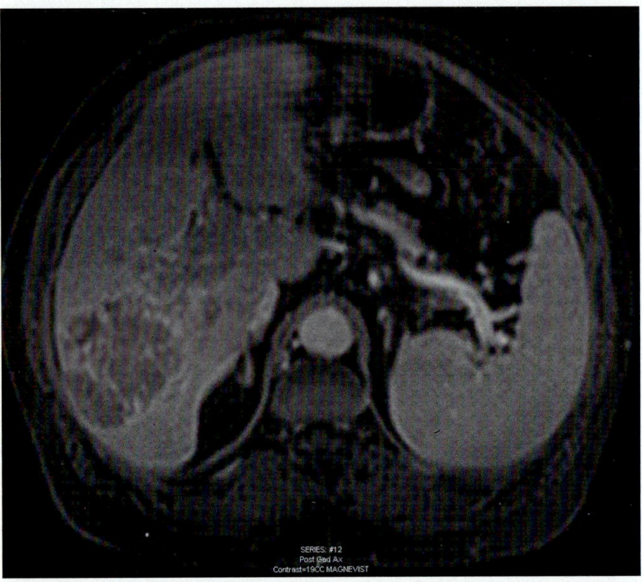

Figure 3.89 — Liver, Hepatocellular Carcinoma. Axial T1 fat-saturated post-contrast MR in the venous phase shows the mass washes out in this phase. This enhancement pattern is suggestive of hepatocellular carcinoma.

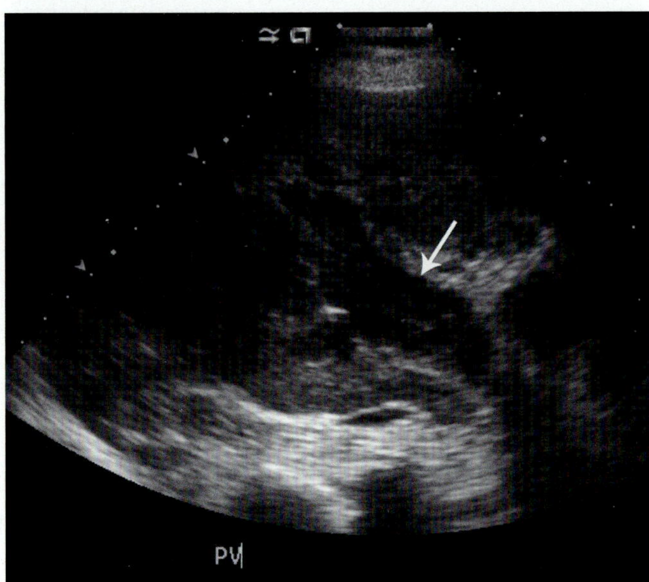

Figure 3.90 — Liver, Hepatocellular Carcinoma. Sonographic image confirms enlargement of the portal vein with hypoechoic tumor thrombus (arrow). Tumor invasion into the portal vein is highly suggestive of hepatocellular carcinoma.

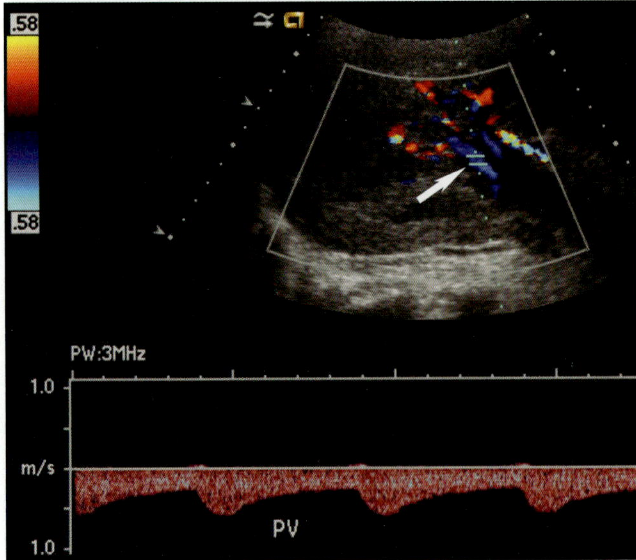

Figure 3.91 — Liver, Hepatocellular Carcinoma. Spectral color Doppler shows arterial-type flow away from the liver within thrombosed portal vein (arrow) characteristic of tumor thrombus.

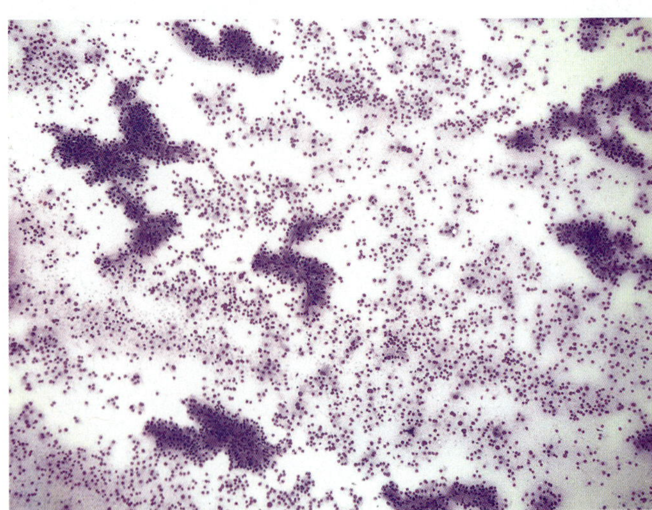

Figure 3.92 — Liver, Hepatocellular Carcinoma. The high cellularity of this aspirate is evident at low power. There is a mixture of fragments and numerous single cells, characteristic of moderately differentiated hepatocellular carcinoma. (Diff Quik stain, low power)

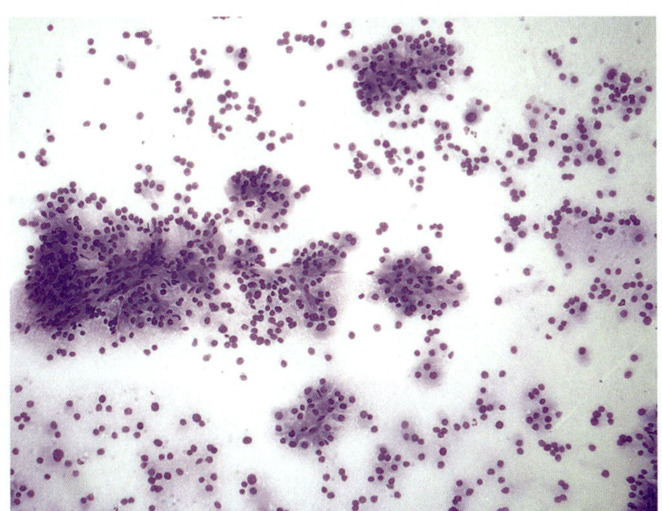

Figure 3.93 — Liver, Hepatocellular Carcinoma. On higher power, it is apparent that the cells have abundant cytoplasm and relatively uniform round nuclei. Numerous small blood vessels, characteristic of hepatocellular carcinoma, are seen coursing through the tissue fragments. (Diff Quik stain, medium power)

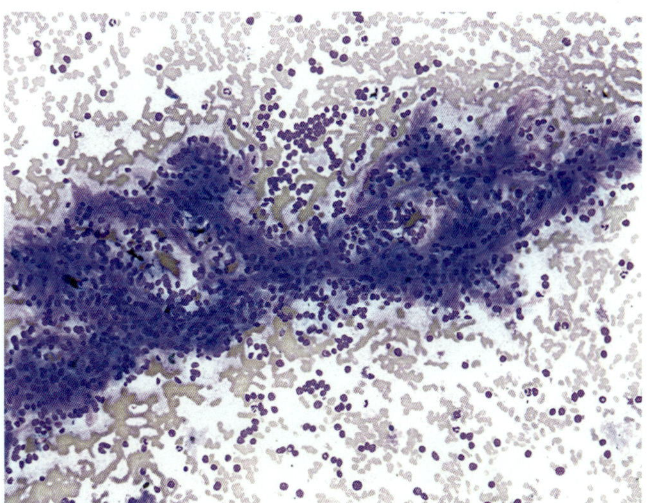

Figure 3.94 — Liver, Hepatocellular Carcinoma. The prominent vascular network is demonstrated. Abundant neoplastic hepatocytes are seen surrounding the small vessels. In addition, numerous bare tumor nuclei are present in the background. (Diff Quik stain, medium power)

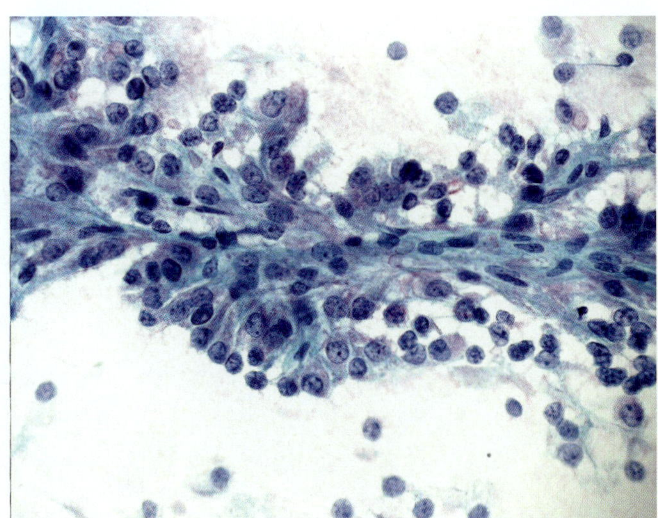

Figure 3.95 — Liver, Hepatocellular Carcinoma. These neoplastic cells show ample granular cytoplasm and fairly uniform round nuclei. Nucleoli are not noted in this case, but may be prominent. Perivascular nesting by neoplastic cells is characteristic. (Papanicolaou stain, high power)

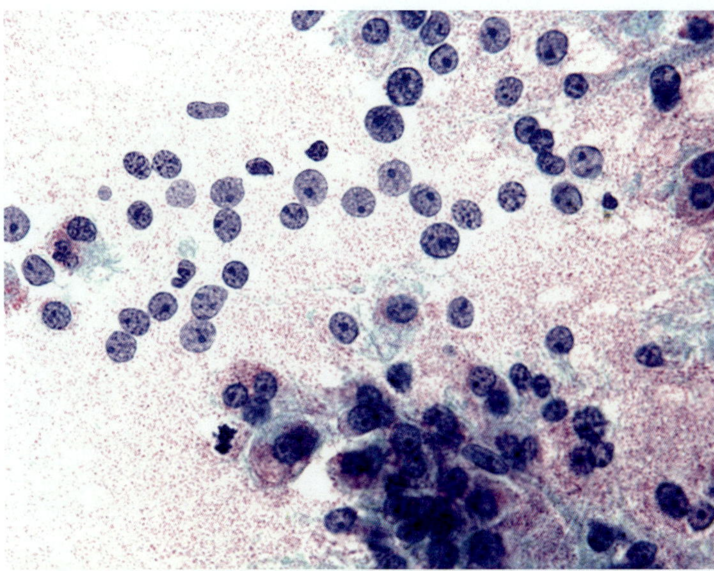

Figure 3.96 — Liver, Hepatocellular Carcinoma. Bare malignant nuclei are shown, some with nucleoli. The background shows granular debris which represents the remnants of the tumor cell cytoplasm. (Papanicolaou stain, high power)

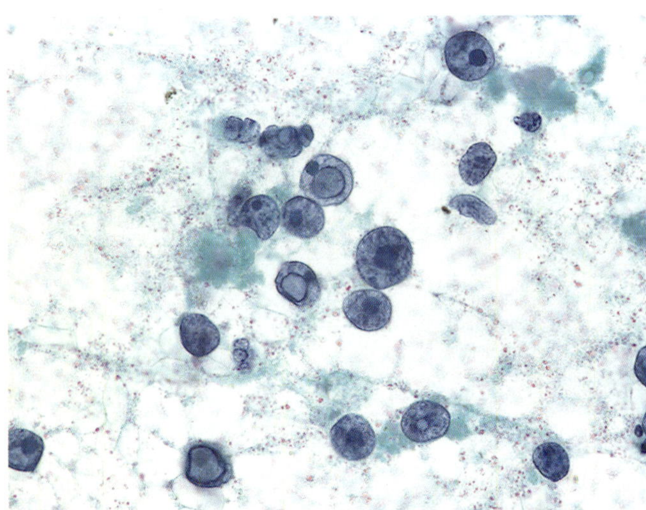

Figure 3.97 — Liver, Hepatocellular Carcinoma. Intranuclear inclusions are present in several malignant nuclei, a common, though nonspecific, finding in hepatocellular carcinoma. Differential diagnostic considerations should include other tumors with intranuclear inclusions, particularly malignant melanoma. (Papanicolaou stain, high power)

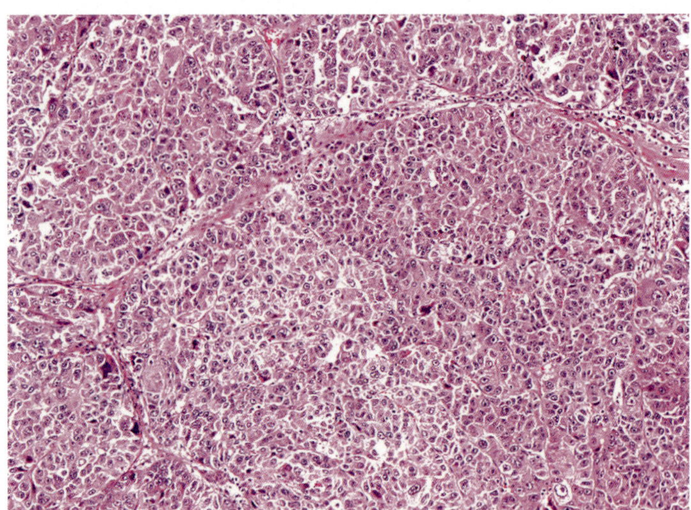

Figure 3.98 — Liver, Hepatocellular Carcinoma (Histology). This well-differentiated tumor has a predominant solid and trabecular growth pattern. The nests of tumor cells are surrounded by sinusoidal vessels. Immunohistochemical staining with AFP and HepPar-1 can be helpful in confirming the hepatic origin in a poorly differentiated lesion. (Hematoxylin and eosin stain, low power)

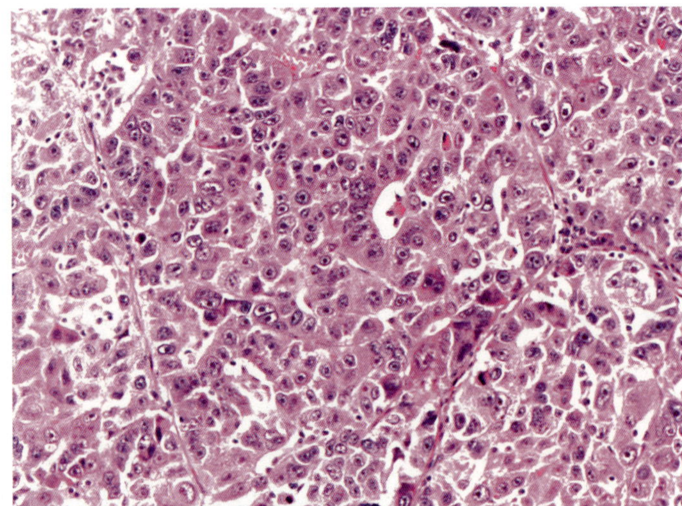

Figure 3.99 — Liver, Hepatocellular Carcinoma (Histology). The tumor consists of thickened trabeculae of hepatocytes. The trabeculae predominantly have five or more cells in thickness. The neoplastic cells have abundant eosinophilic cytoplasm with round to oval nuclei and prominent nucleoli. (Hematoxylin and eosin stain, medium power)

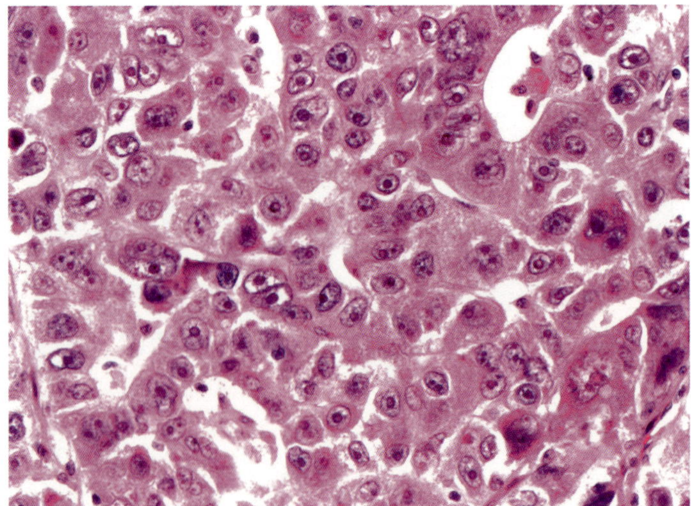

Figure 3.100 — Liver, Hepatocellular Carcinoma (Histology). The neoplastic cells show hepatocytic differentiation, but are atypical. The cells have an increased nucleus-to-cytoplasm ratio, anisonucleosis, and prominent macronucleoli. (Hematoxylin and eosin stain, high power)

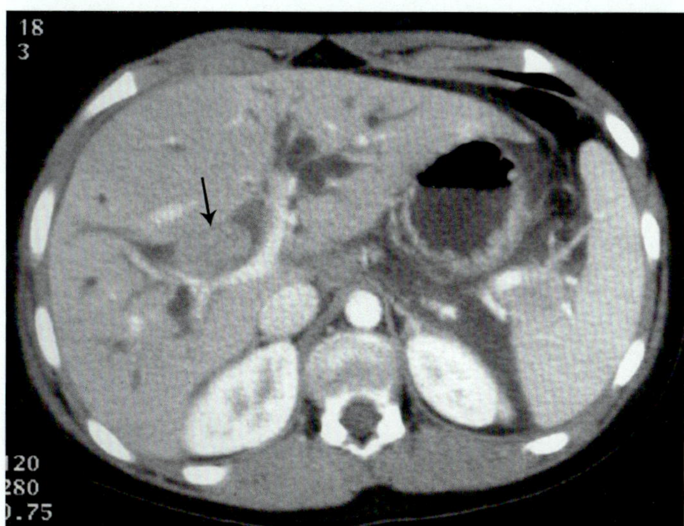

Figure 3.101 — Liver, Hepatocellular Carcinoma, Fibrolamellar Variant. This 13-year-old boy had right upper quadrant pain with elevated alkaline phosphatase and bilirubin levels. Axial contrast-enhanced CT shows a well-defined soft tissue mass in the central bile duct (arrow) and marked intrahepatic biliary duct dilation.

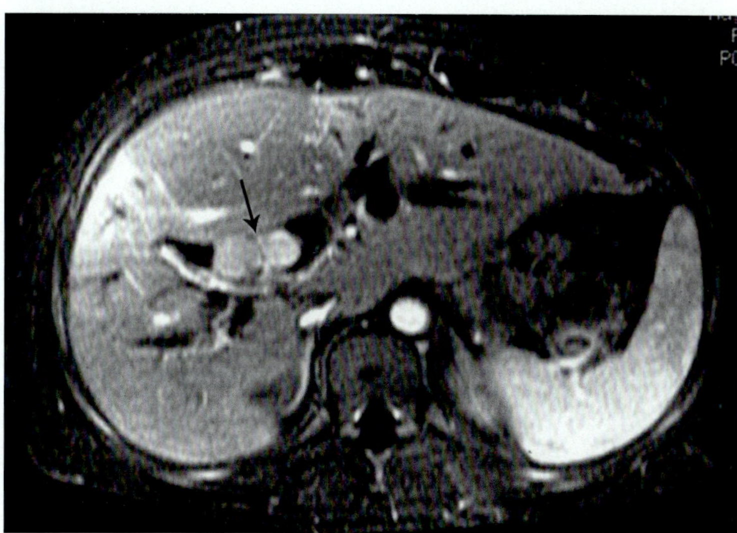

Figure 3.102 — Liver, Hepatocellular Carcinoma, Fibrolamellar Variant. Axial contrast-enhanced MR confirms the presence of an enhancing soft tissue mass in the central bile duct (arrow).

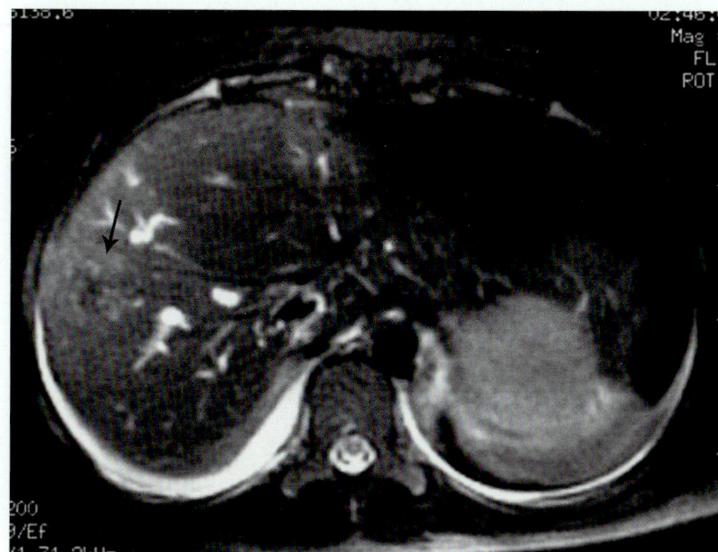

Figure 3.103 — Liver, Hepatocellular Carcinoma, Fibrolamellar Variant. Axial T2-weighted MR image more superiorly in the same patient demonstrates a subtle heterogeneous mass present in segment 8 of the right lobe of the liver (arrow).

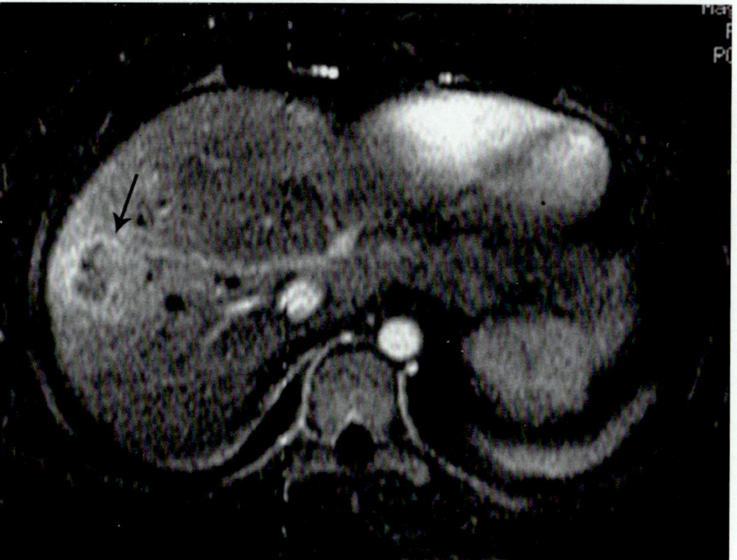

Figure 3.104 — Liver, Hepatocellular Carcinoma, Fibrolamellar Variant. Axial contrast-enhanced MR is shown. The mass shows mild peripheral enhancement post-contrast, suspicious for tumor (arrow). This mass was found to represent fibrolamellar hepatocellular carcinoma.

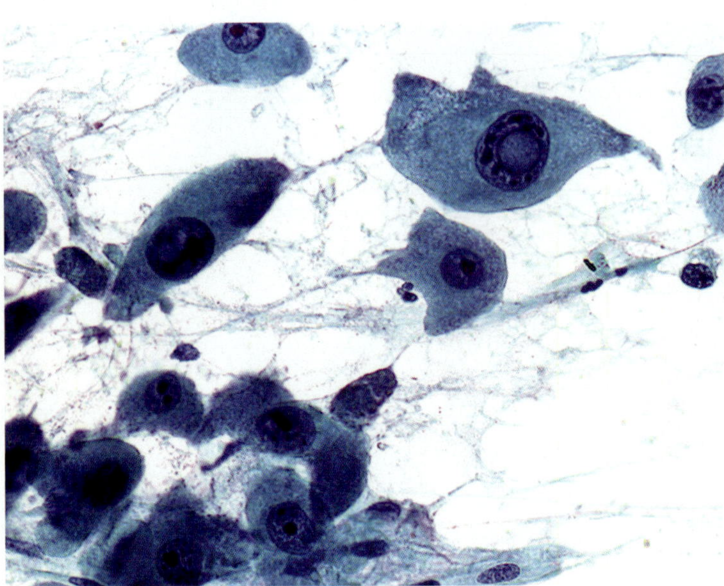

Figure 3.105 — Liver, Hepatocellular Carcinoma, Fibrolamellar Variant. Markedly pleomorphic single tumor cells are seen with increased nuclear-to-cytoplasmic ratios and macronucleoli. An intranuclear inclusion is present (top right), characteristic (but not diagnostic) of hepatocellular carcinoma. (Papanicolaou stain, high power)

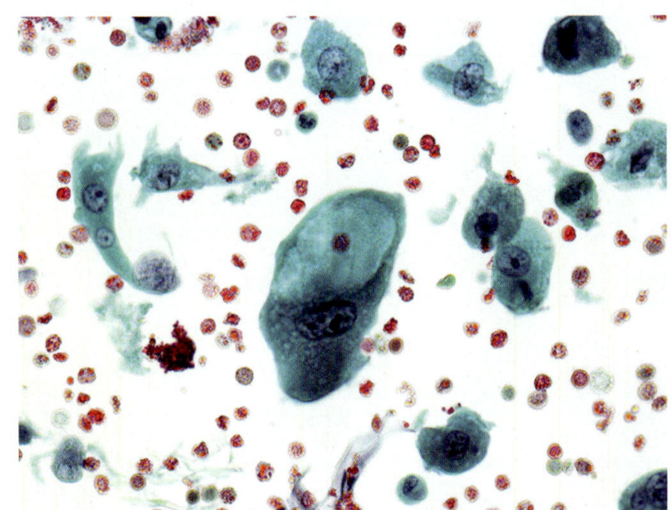

Figure 3.106 — Liver, Hepatocellular Carcinoma, Fibrolamellar Variant. A cytoplasmic clearing, termed a "pale body" is seen in the center of the field, surrounded by other malignant hepatocytes. Strands of fibrous tissue also may be prominent in aspirates of fibrolamellar variant of hepatocellular carcinoma (not shown). (Papanicolaou stain, high power)

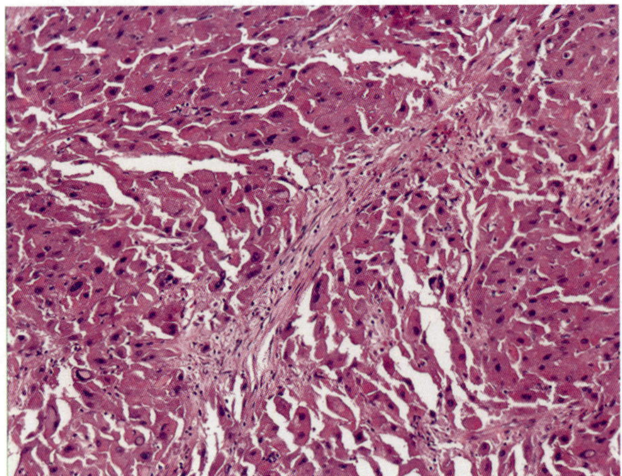

Figure 3.107 — Liver, Hepatocellular Carcinoma, Fibrolamellar Variant (Histology). The fibrolamellar variant of hepatocellular carcinoma is seen predominantly in young patients without cirrhosis. The tumor has a characteristic growth pattern with nests of malignant hepatocytes with "oncocytic-type" cytoplasm, separated by a fine lamellar fibrosis. (Hematoxylin and eosin stain, low power)

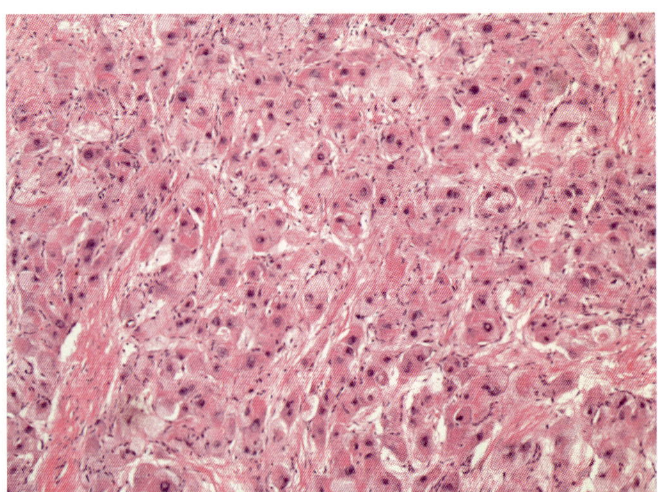

Figure 3.108 — Liver, Hepatocellular Carcinoma, Fibrolamellar Variant (Histology). The neoplastic cells have a polygonal shape and abundant eosinophilic cytoplasm. The nuclei are round to oval with prominent nucleoli. Note the fibrosis which is arranged in a lamellar, or layered, manner around the neoplastic cells. (Hematoxylin and eosin stain, medium power)

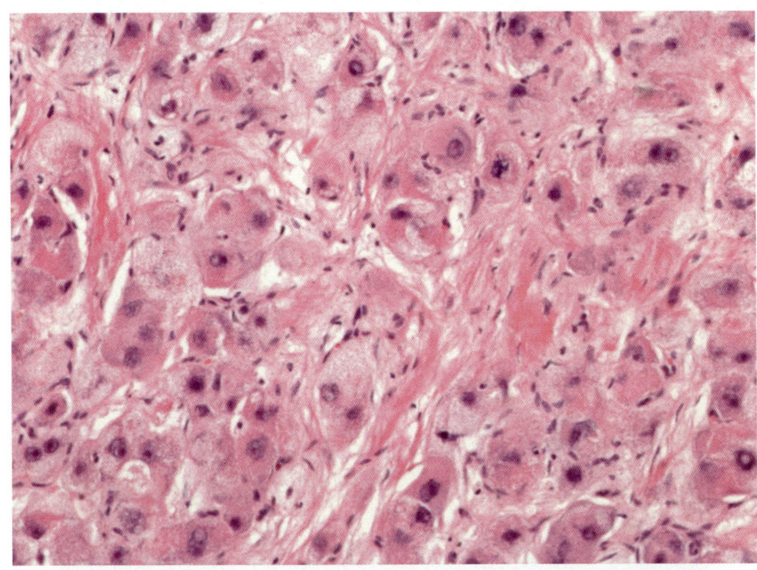

Figure 3.109 — Liver, Hepatocellular Carcinoma, Fibrolamellar Variant (Histology). These malignant hepatocytes show increased nuclear-to-cytoplasmic ratios and irregular nuclear contours with occasional prominent nucleoli (7 o'clock) in a background of lamellar fibrosis. (Hematoxylin and eosin stain, high power)

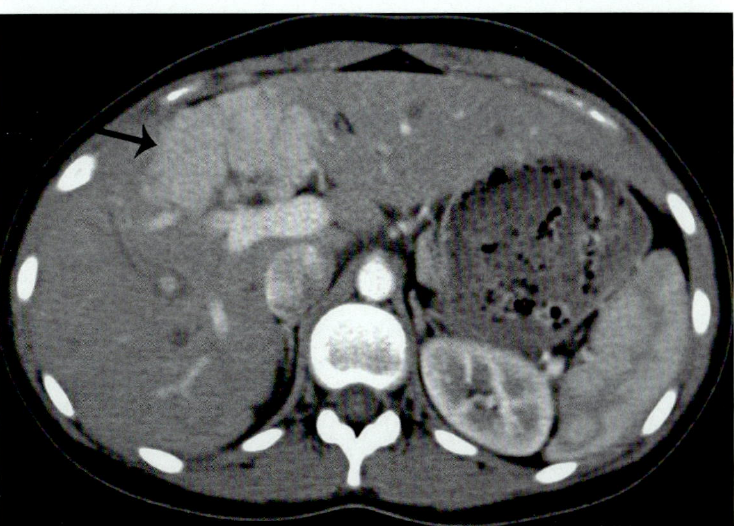

Figure 3.110 — Liver, Focal Nodular Hyperplasia. A 16-year-old girl presented with mild right hip pain and a subsequent CT showed an incidental liver mass requiring further work up. Axial contrast-enhanced CT image in the arterial phase shows a mass in segment 4 of the liver (arrow) which homogeneously enhances in the arterial phase.

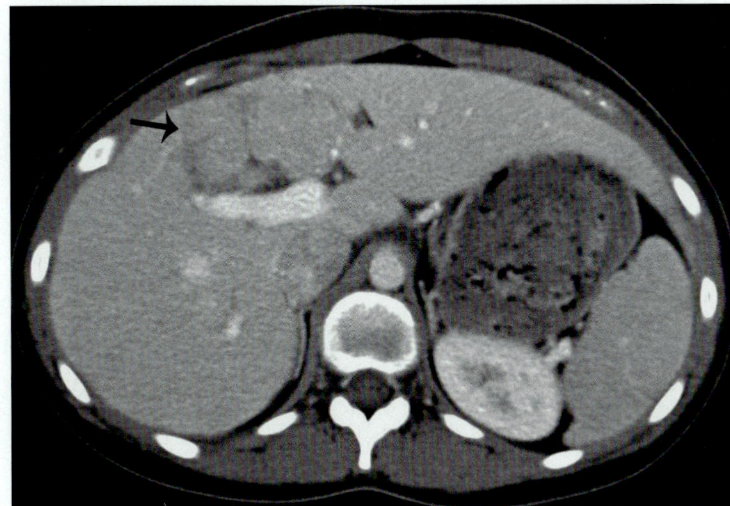

Figure 3.111 — Liver, Focal Nodular Hyperplasia. Axial contrast-enhanced CT image in the venous phase shows the mass becomes nearly isodense to the liver in this phase (arrow).

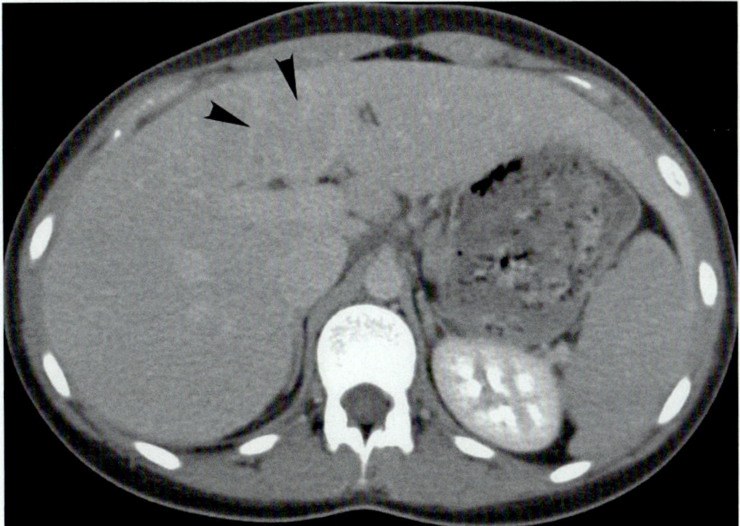

Figure 3.112 — Liver, Focal Nodular Hyperplasia. Axial contrast-enhanced CT image in the delayed phase is shown. There is a central scar and several septations arrowheads which enhance late in the delayed phase. This is characteristic of a focal nodular hyperplasia.

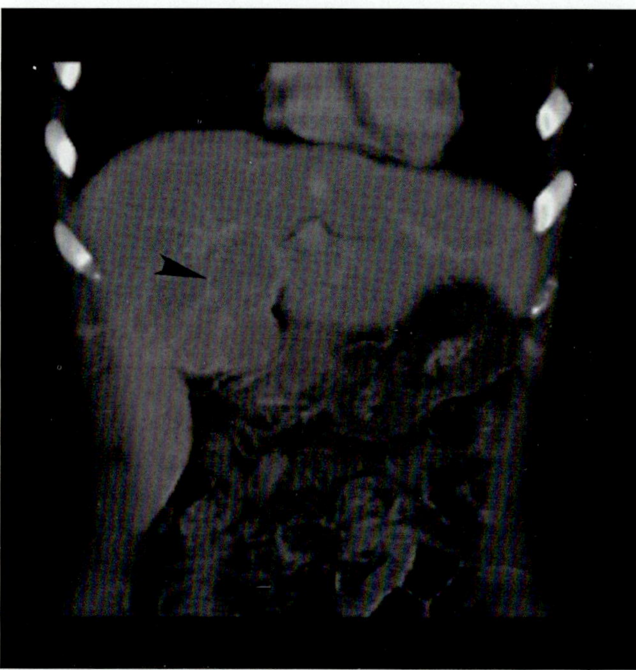

Figure 3.113 — Liver, Focal Nodular Hyperplasia. Coronal contrast-enhanced CT in the delayed phase confirms the delayed enhancement of the central scar (arrowhead) as well as the presence of several septations.

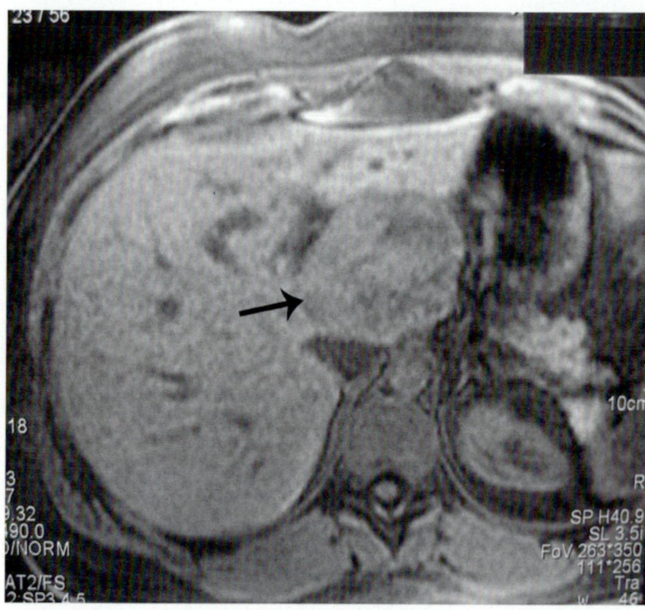

Figure 3.114 — Liver, Focal Nodular Hyperplasia. This 22-year-old woman presented with abdominal pain. Axial T1-weighted MR without intravenous contrast shows a mass in the caudate lobe (arrow) which is mildly T1 hypointense.

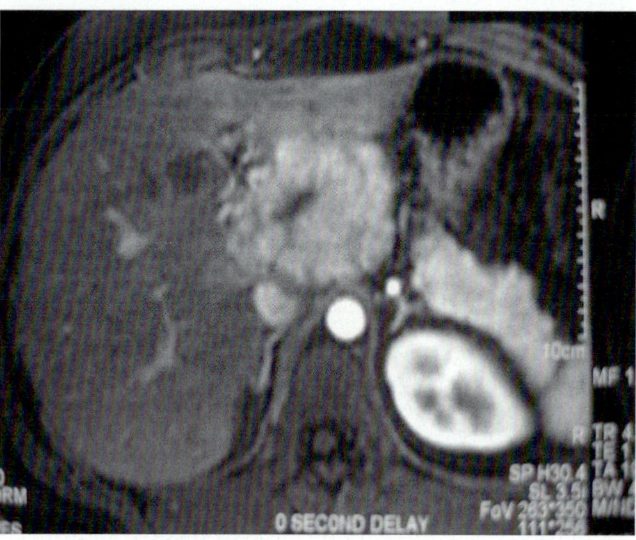

Figure 3.115 — Liver, Focal Nodular Hyperplasia. Axial T1-weighted MR with contrast in the arterial phase shows the mass enhances homogeneously.

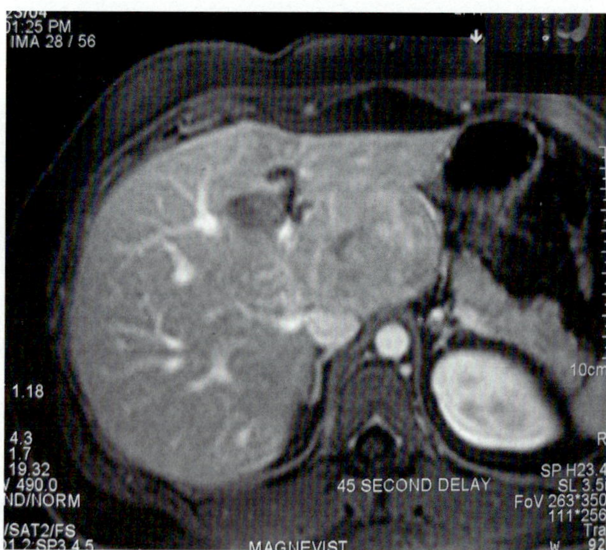

Figure 3.116 — Liver, Focal Nodular Hyperplasia. Axial T1-weighted MR with contrast in the venous phase demonstrates that the mass becomes isointense to the liver in the venous phase and is no longer visible. This enhancement pattern is characteristic of focal nodular hyperplasia.

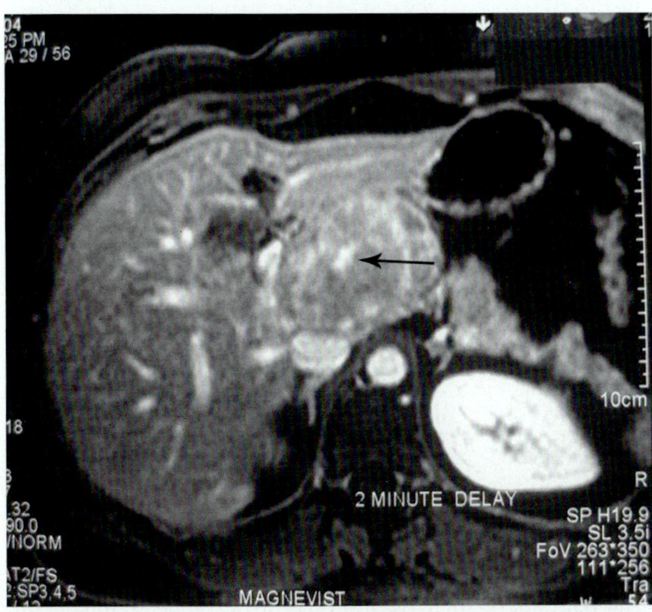

Figure 3.117 — Liver, Focal Nodular Hyperplasia. The central scar (arrow) enhances late in the delayed phase which is also characteristic of focal nodular hyperplasia.

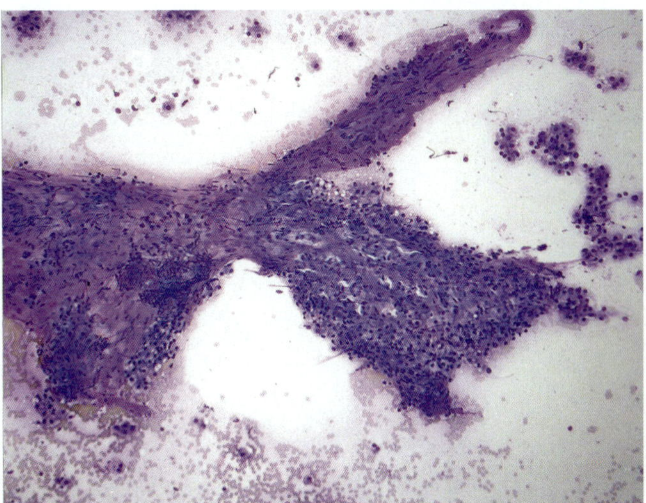

Figure 3.118 — Liver, Focal Nodular Hyperplasia. A large tissue fragment is present consisting of fibrous tissue (upper and left portions) and a population of hepatocytes (right lower portion). This mixture of cells is consistent with focal nodular hyperplasia, but is not specific. (Diff Quik stain, medium power)

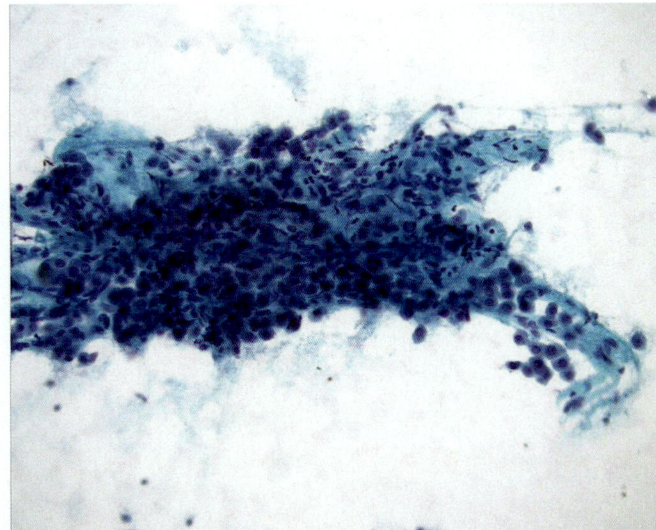

Figure 3.119 — Liver, Focal Nodular Hyperplasia. Fibrous tissue is intimately admixed with benign-appearing hepatocytes. Cirrhosis may also have a similar cytologic appearance; thus, the clinical and radiographic impression is important in ascertaining the diagnosis. (Papanicolaou stain, high power)

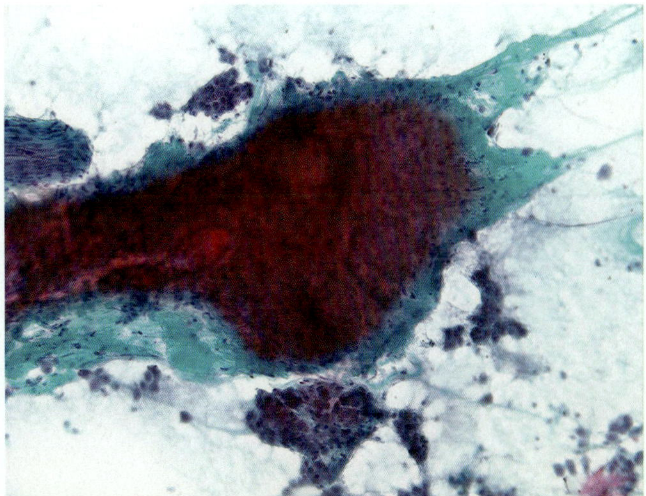

Figure 3.120 — Liver, Focal Nodular Hyperplasia. A large fragment of fibrous tissue surrounded by small groups of benign-appearing hepatocytes. The cytomorphology is totally nonspecific and a diagnosis of focal nodular hyperplasia can only be rendered after careful clinico–radiologic correlation. (Papanicolaou stain, low power)

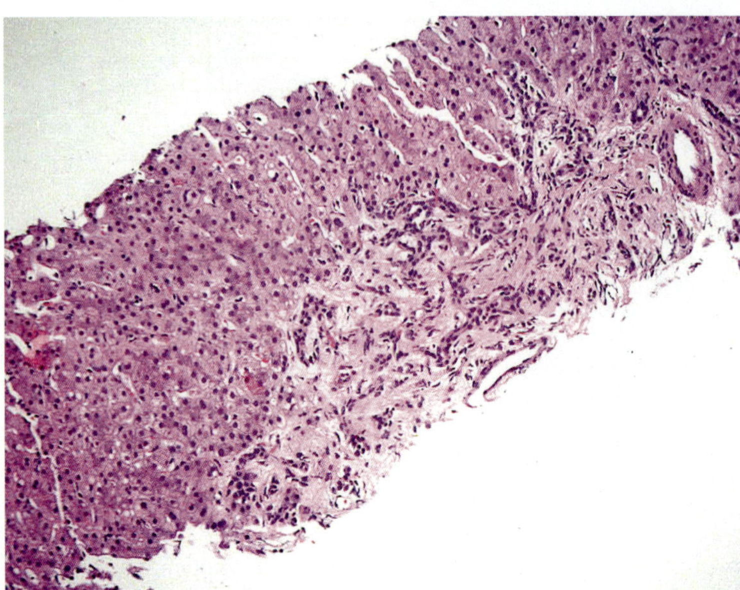

Figure 3.121 — Liver, Focal Nodular Hyperplasia. If possible, core biopsy should be obtained to aid in the diagnosis. Areas of fibrous tissue with bile ductular proliferation are surrounded by benign hepatocytes consistent with focal nodular hyperplasia. (Hematoxylin and eosin stain, medium power)

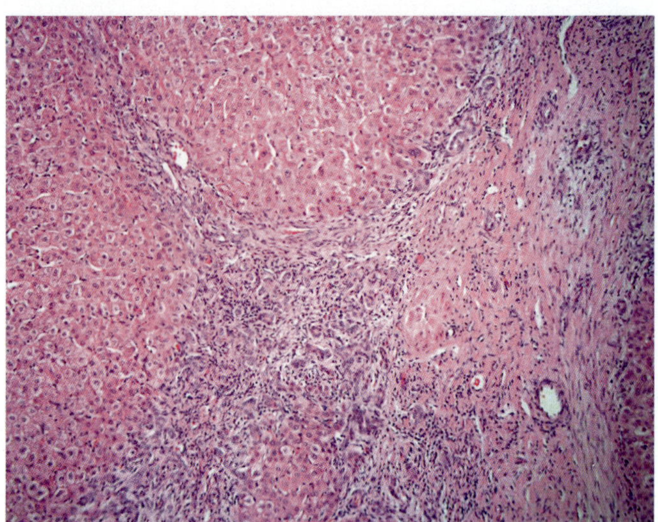

Figure 3.122 — Liver, Focal Nodular Hyperplasia (Histology). Focal nodular hyperplasia is a lesion that occurs predominantly in young patients in their twenties to thirties. The characteristic pathological features are the presence of bridging fibrosis and nodular hyperplasia, showing a "focal cirrhosis" pattern. (Hematoxylin and eosin stain, low power)

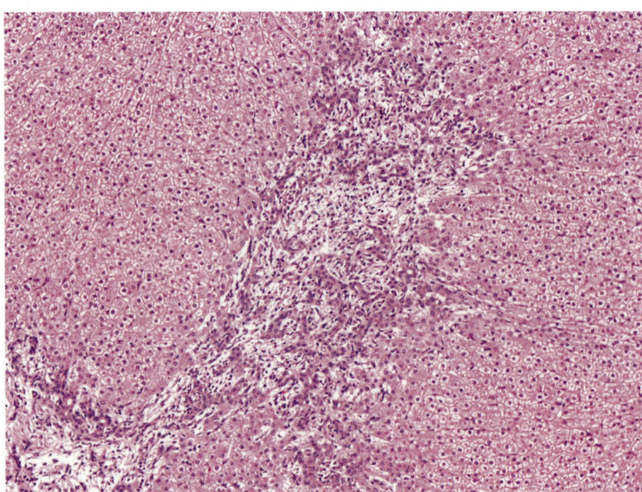

Figure 3.123 — Liver, Focal Nodular Hyperplasia (Histology). Hyperplastic nodules of hepatocytes are separated by dense fibrotic bands that contain inflammatory cells, thick-walled arteries, and bile ductules. It should be noted that all of the normal components of a liver lobule are present. (Hematoxylin and eosin stain, medium power)

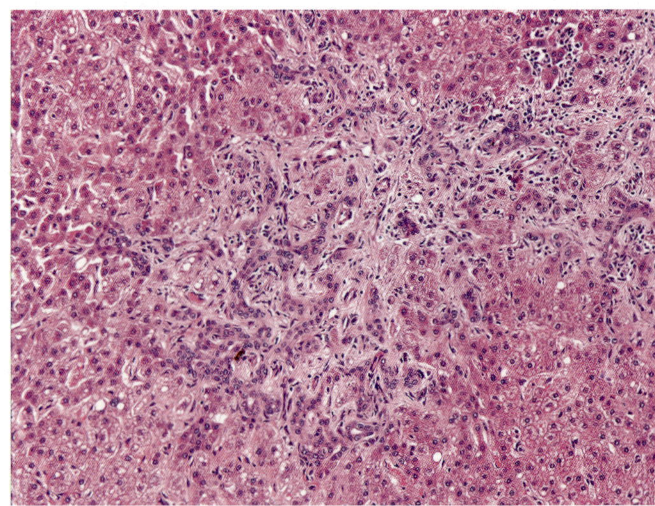

Figure 3.124 — Liver, Focal Nodular Hyperplasia (Histology). Proliferation of bile ductules in the portal triads is occasionally seen as a reactive phenomenon. Most tumors (80%) have the three classic features of abnormal architecture, bile ductular proliferation, and malformed vessels. (Hematoxylin and eosin stain, high power)

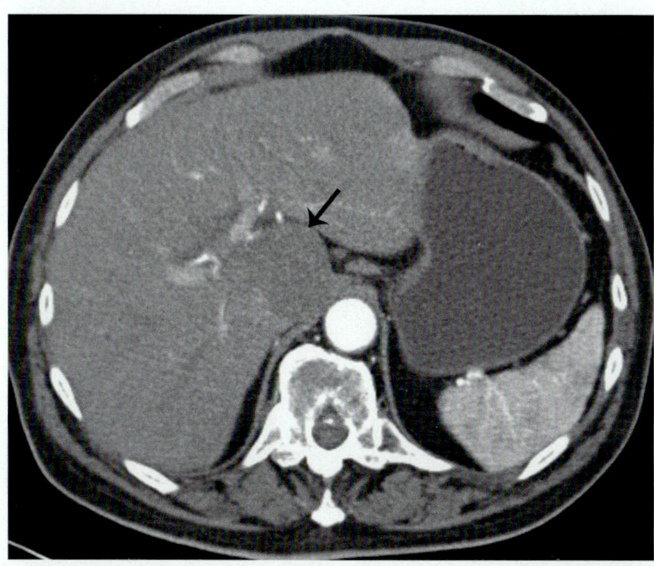

Figure 3.125 — Liver, Hemangioma. This 77-year-old woman had a history of hepatitis C and unintentional weight loss. Axial contrast-enhanced CT image in the arterial phase shows a hypovascular mass (arrow) in the caudate lobe. The mass mildly compresses the IVC.

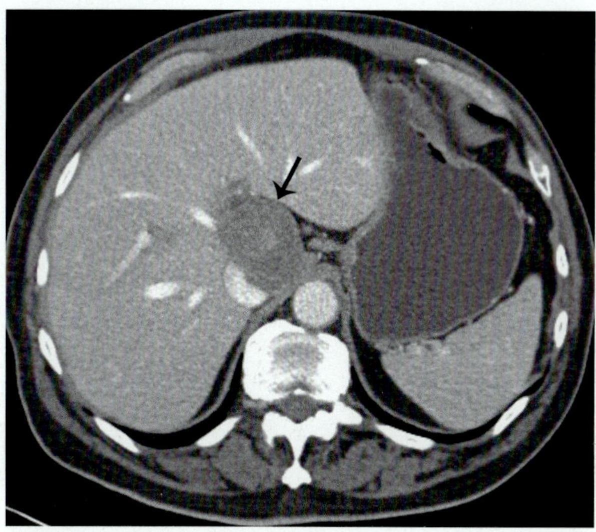

Figure 3.126 — Liver, Hemangioma. Axial contrast-enhanced CT image in the venous phase demonstrates that the mass remains hypovascular in this phase (arrow). This lesion does not show the typical imaging features of a hemangioma which usually demonstrates peripheral, discontinuous, nodular enhancement with gradual, delayed fill-in of contrast. Biopsy was therefore requested.

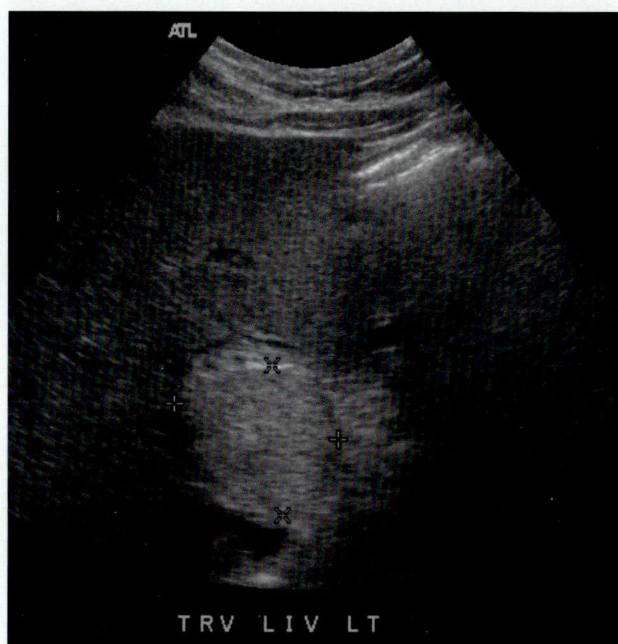

Figure 3.127 — Liver, Hemangioma. Sonographic image confirms an echogenic caudate lobe mass (calipers). Hemangiomas are commonly echogenic.

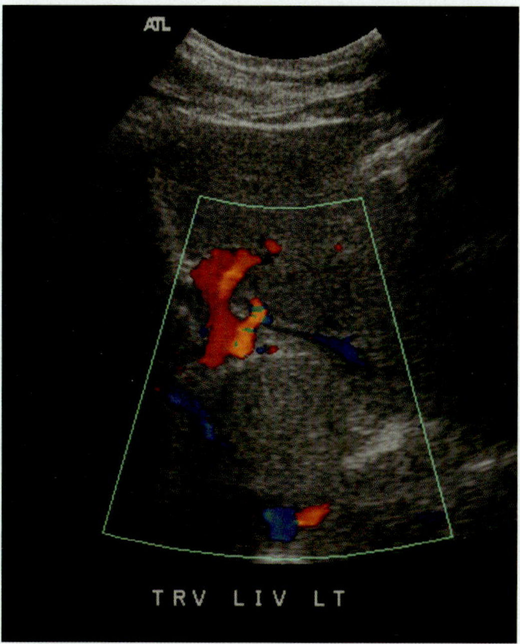

Figure 3.128 — Liver, Hemangioma. There is no internal vascularity with color Doppler. This mass was found to be a sclerotic hemangioma.

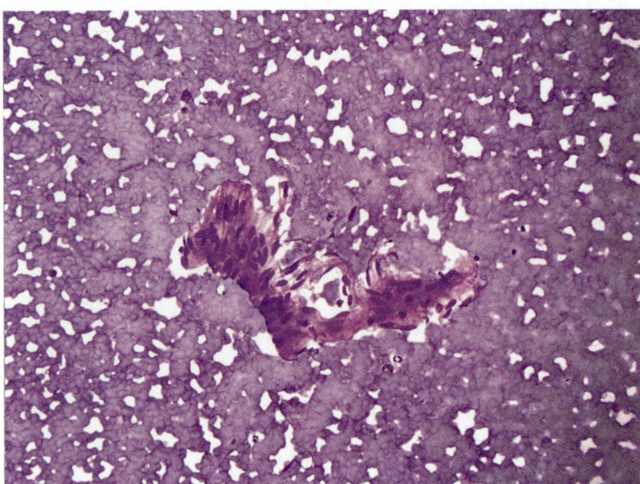

Figure 3.129 — Liver, Hemangioma. Aspirate smears from hemangioma are often sparsely cellular and consist predominantly of blood, so-called unyielding FNAs. There is a single fragment of fibrous tissue shown here with small spindle cells without atypia. (Diff Quik stain, medium power)

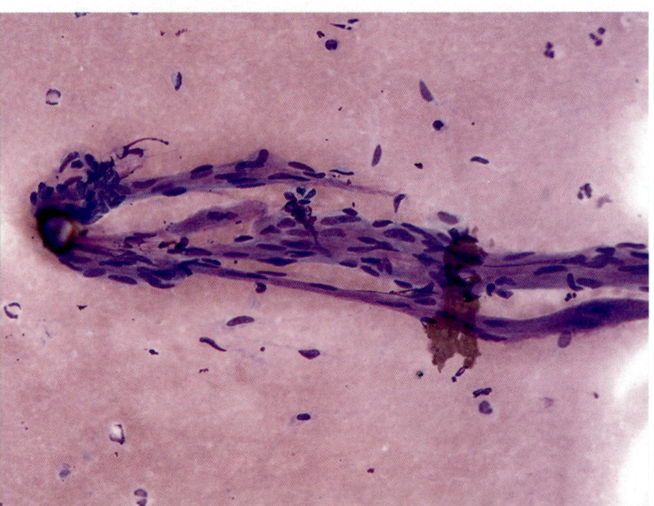

Figure 3.130 — Liver, Hemangioma. Bundles of mesenchymal-type cells with elongated fusiform nuclei are seen in a hemorrhagic background. These cells represent the supporting stromal (fibrous) tissue of hepatic hemangioma and are not diagnostic of this lesion. (Diff Quik stain, medium power)

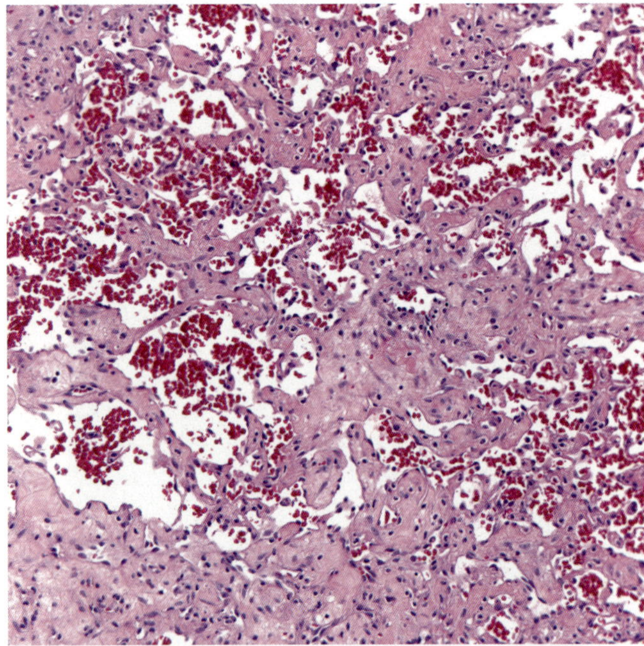

Figure 3.131 — Liver, Hemangioma (Histology). Hemangioma is the most frequent benign tumor of the liver. The neoplasm consists of variably sized blood vessels lined by endothelial cells. These interconnected spaces are separated by fibrous tissue. (Hematoxylin and eosin stain, low power)

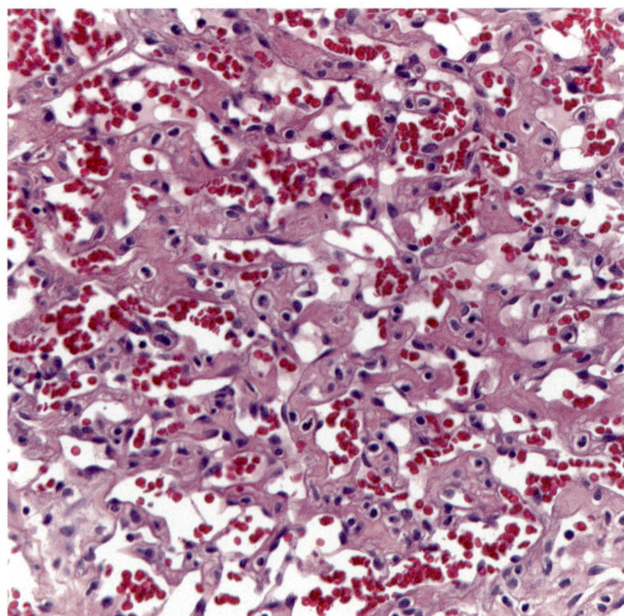

Figure 3.132 — Liver, Hemangioma (Histology). Hemangiomas are often solitary, but multiple lesions may be present in both the right and left lobes of the liver. Note the vascular channels with endothelial lining. There is no atypia or mitotic activity. These tumors can be less than 1 cm or grow up to 20 cm in size. (Hematoxylin and eosin stain, medium power)

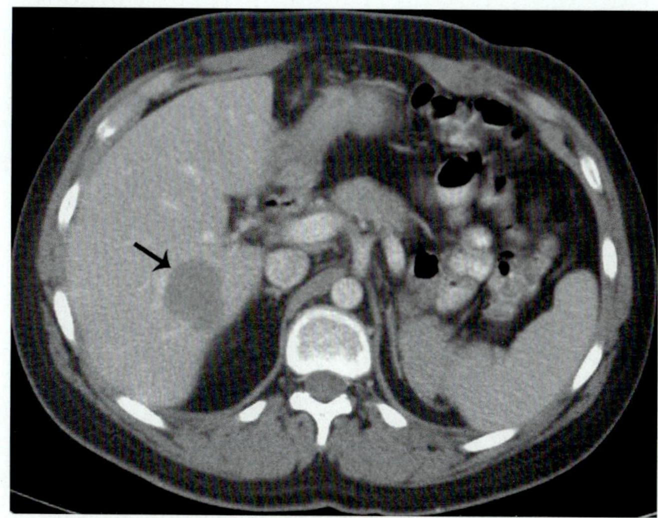

Figure 3.133 — Liver, Post-transplant Lymphoproliferative Disorder. This 21-year-old man was status post heart transplant and had elevated liver function tests. Axial contrast-enhanced CT shows a 4-cm hypodense mass in the right lobe of the liver (arrow).

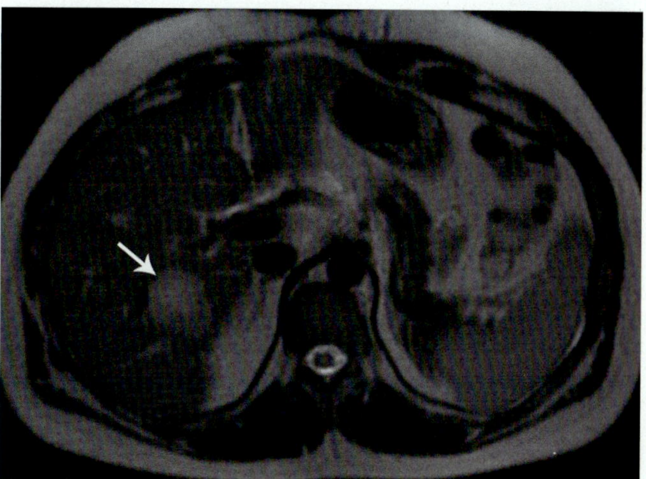

Figure 3.134 — Liver, Post-transplant Lymphoproliferative Disorder. Axial MR is shown. T2-weighted image confirms a T2 hyperintense mass (arrow).

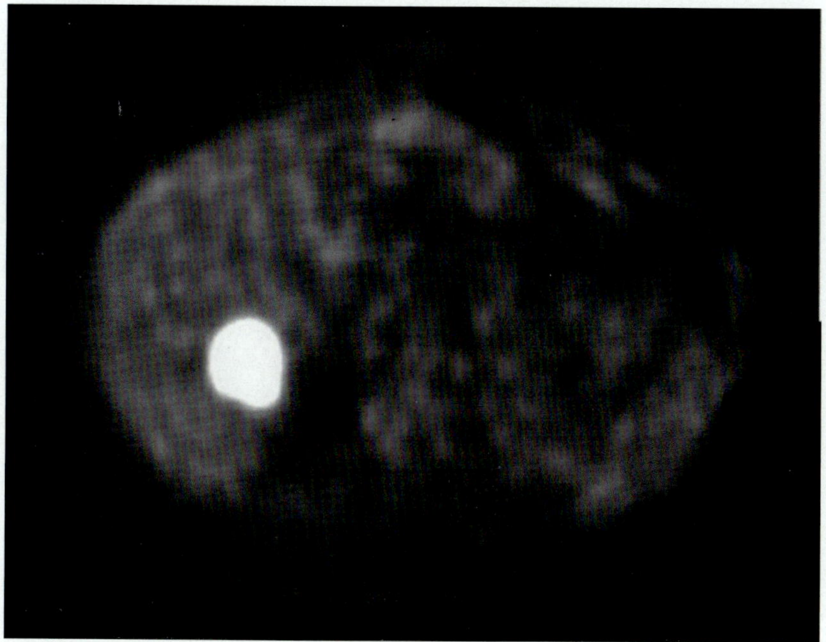

Figure 3.135 — Liver, Post-transplant Lymphoproliferative Disorder. PET scan demonstrates that the mass is markedly FDG avid.

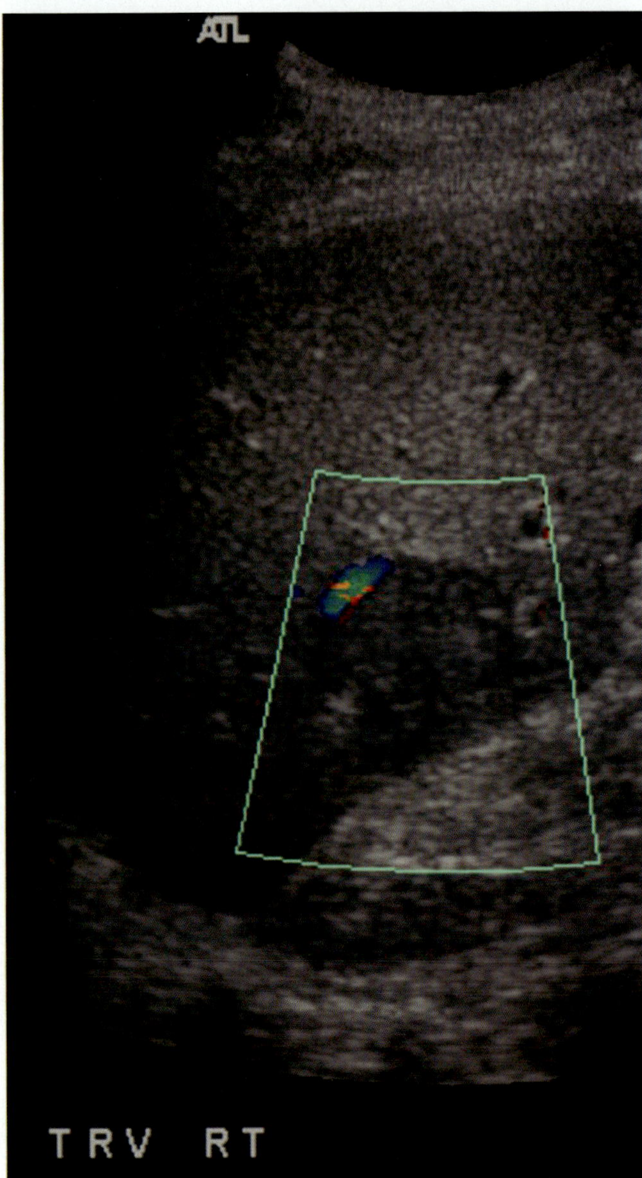

Figure 3.136 — Liver, Post-transplant Lymphoproliferative Disorder. Sonographic image with color Doppler confirms a hypoechoic mass in the right lobe of the liver. The appearance is nonspecific.

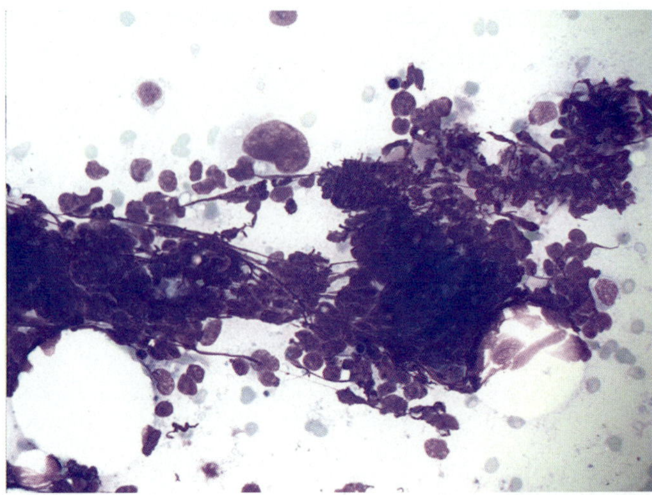

Figure 3.137 — Liver, Post-transplant Lymphoproliferative Disorder. It is difficult to distinguish cellular morphology in these two groups of crushed cells. Single cells surrounding the groups show marked nuclear atypia and scant cytoplasm. Crush artifact is characteristic of lymphoid cells, but is not a specific finding. (Diff Quik stain, high power)

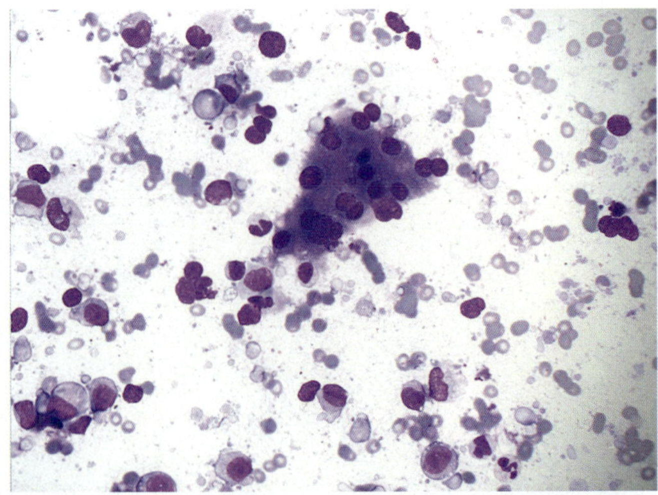

Figure 3.138 — Liver, Post-transplant Lymphoproliferative Disorder. A fragment of benign hepatocytes is surrounded by scattered single cells with large, irregular nuclei and a moderate amount of basophilic cytoplasm suggestive of a hematopoietic neoplasm. The specimen was sent for flow cytometry, which showed a clonal population of B-lymphocytes. (Diff Quik stain, high power)

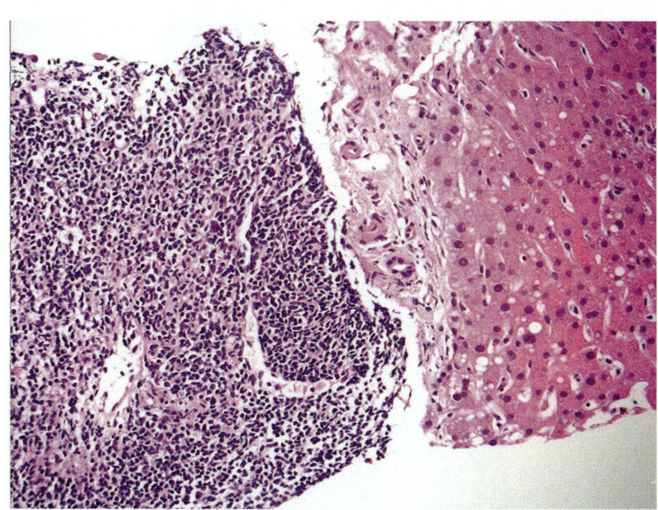

Figure 3.139 — Liver, Post-transplant Lymphoproliferative Disorder (Core Biopsy). On core biopsy, an atypical lymphoid proliferation is juxtaposed with normal hepatic tissue (right side of field). Post-transplant lymphoproliferative disorder is most often a clonal proliferation of lymphoid or plasma cells resulting from immunosuppression following solid organ or bone marrow transplant. (Hematoxylin and eosin stain, medium power)

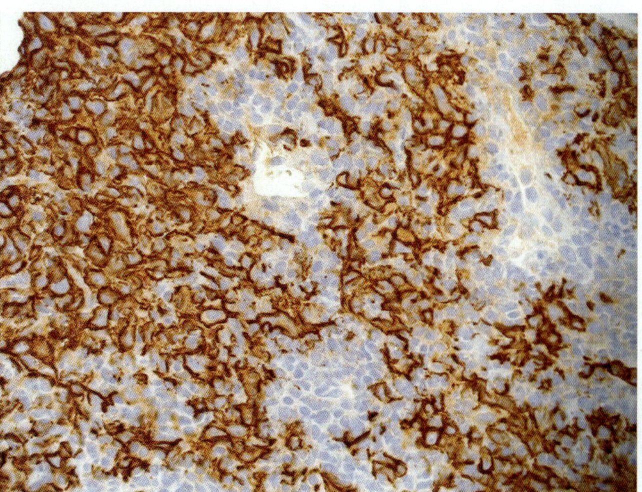

Figure 3.140 — Liver, Post-transplant Lymphoproliferative Disorder (Core Biopsy). A CD20 immunostain highlights the predominant B-cell population. Post-transplant lymphoproliferative disorder often occurs in the first year post-transplant when the patient's immunosuppression is at its highest. (CD20 immunostain, high power)

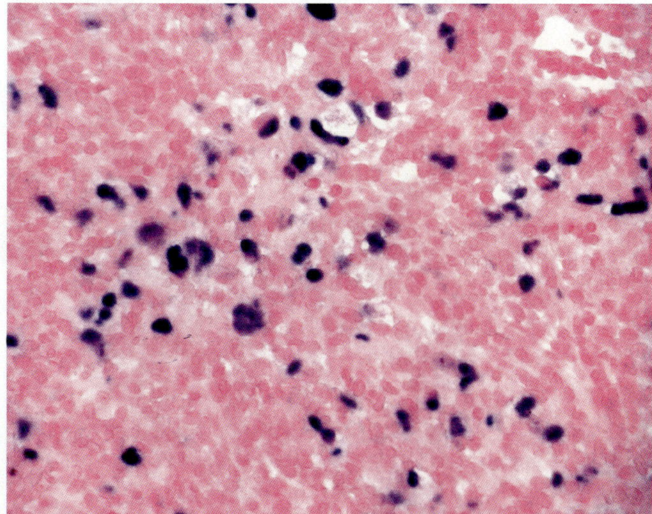

Figure 3.141 — Liver, Post-transplant Lymphoproliferative Disorder (Core Biopsy). EBV *in situ* hybridization shows numerous positive nuclei (dark blue). Post-transplant lymphoproliferative disorder is more common in pediatric transplant patients because they are often EBV naïve at the time of transplant and subsequently become infected. (EBV *in situ* hybridization, high power)

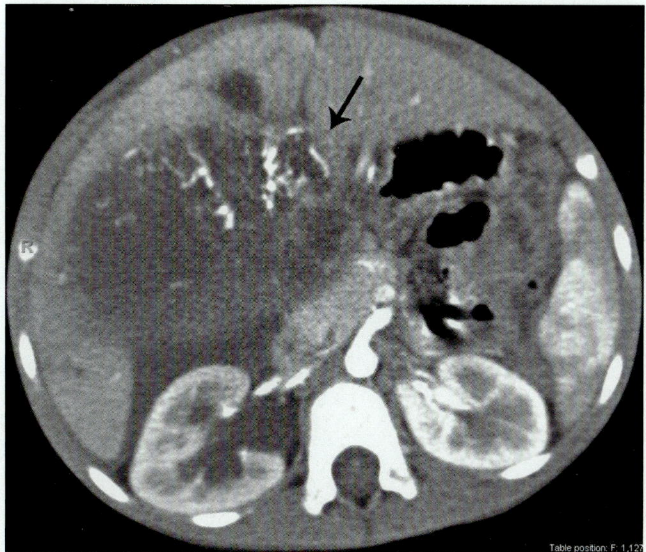

Figure 3.142 — Liver, Undifferentiated (Embryonal) Sarcoma. This 6-year-old boy presented with flu-like symptoms, abdominal distention, and failure to thrive. Axial contrast-enhanced CT of the upper abdomen in the arterial phase shows a large mass extending inferiorly from the liver (arrow). There is prominent internal vascularity.

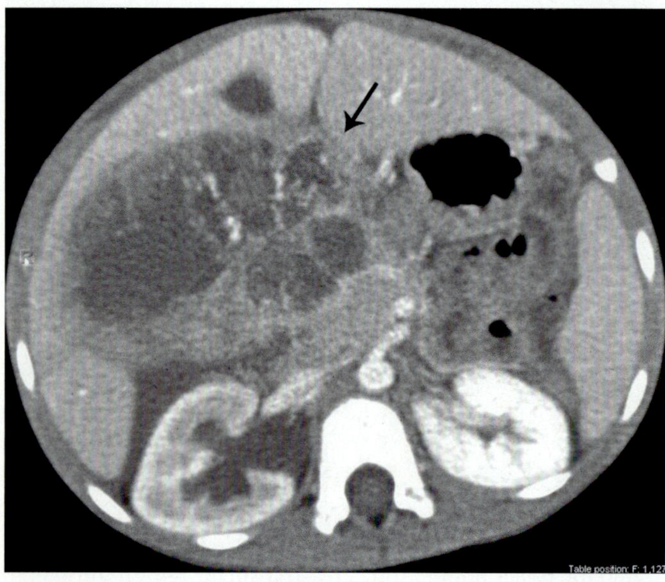

Figure 3.143 — Liver, Undifferentiated (Embryonal) Sarcoma. Axial contrast-enhanced CT in the venous phase shows the mass (arrow) contains enhancing soft tissue components and internal necrosis or cystic change. These tumors typically occur in children between ages 6 and 10 years. Serum AFP is typically normal.

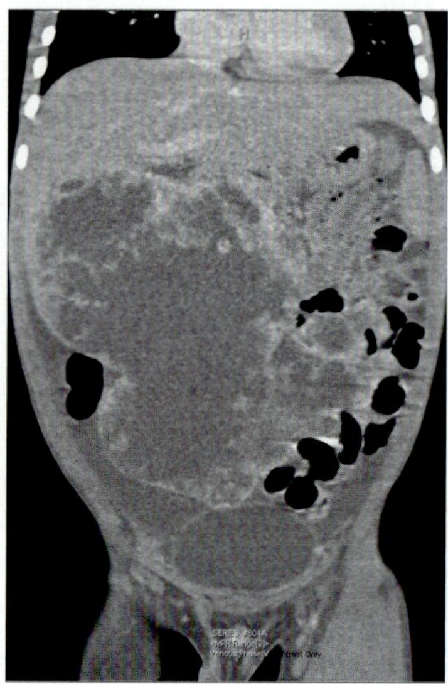

Figure 3.144 — Liver, Undifferentiated (Embryonal) Sarcoma. Coronal contrast-enhanced CT shows the craniocaudal extent of the mass. Undifferentiated sarcomas are rare tumors and are frequently cystic, as in this case; however, they can contain solid components, usually at the periphery. There is small amount of ascites in the abdomen.

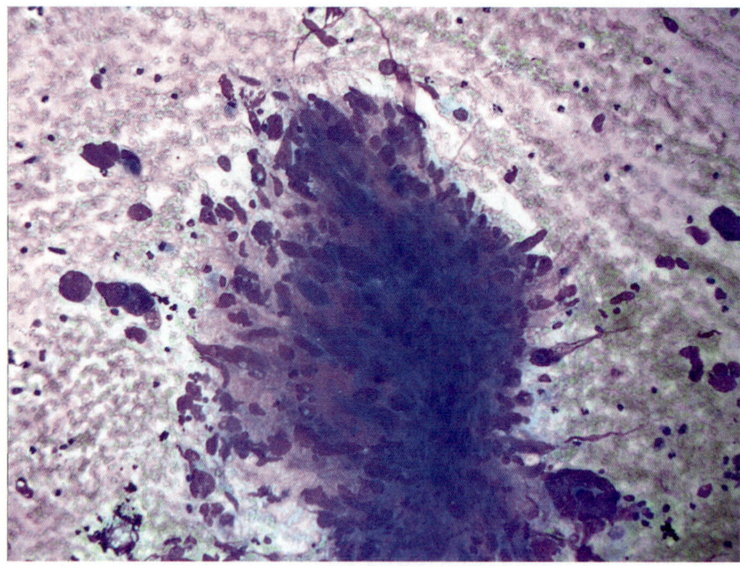

Figure 3.145 — Liver, Undifferentiated (Embryonal) Sarcoma. A cohesive group of spindle-shaped cells with ill-defined cell borders shows anisonucleosis with focal marked nuclear enlargement. These features suggest a sarcoma. (Diff Quik stain, high power)

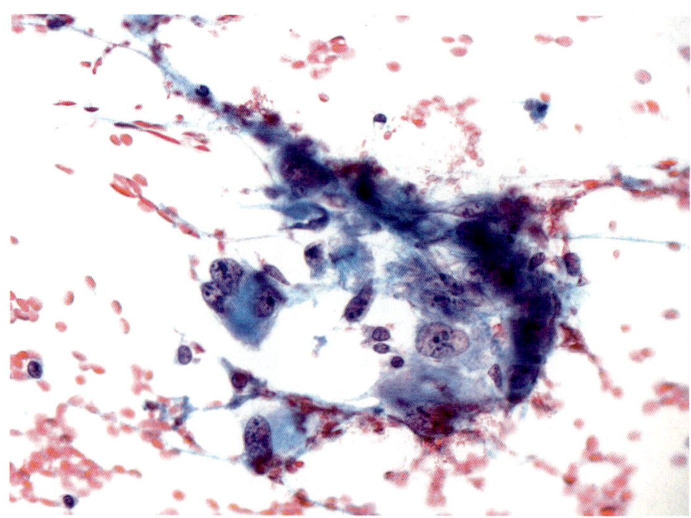

Figure 3.146 — Liver, Undifferentiated (Embryonal) Sarcoma. Markedly enlarged atypical nuclei with variably prominent nucleoli are demonstrated. The differential diagnosis includes sarcomatoid hepatocellular carcinoma and embryonal rhabdomyosarcoma. (Papanicolaou stain, high power)

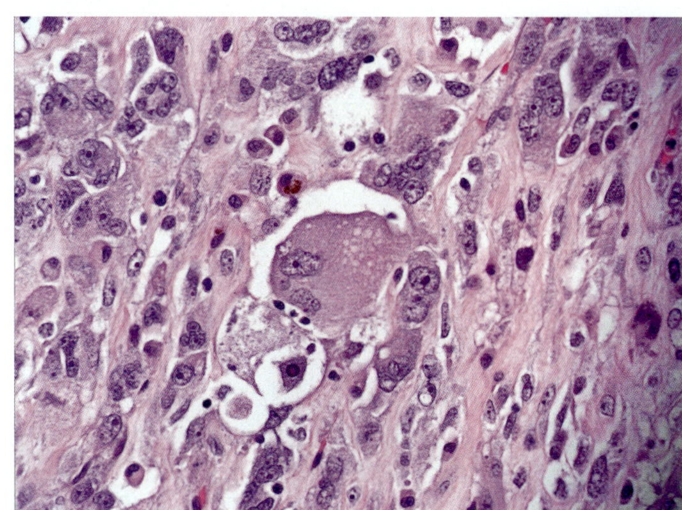

Figure 3.147 — Liver, Undifferentiated (Embryonal) Sarcoma (Histology). The resection specimen shows a cellular lesion with marked anisonucleosis and cellular pleomorphism. Occasional giant tumor cells are present showing voluminous cytoplasm. (Hematoxylin and eosin stain, high power)

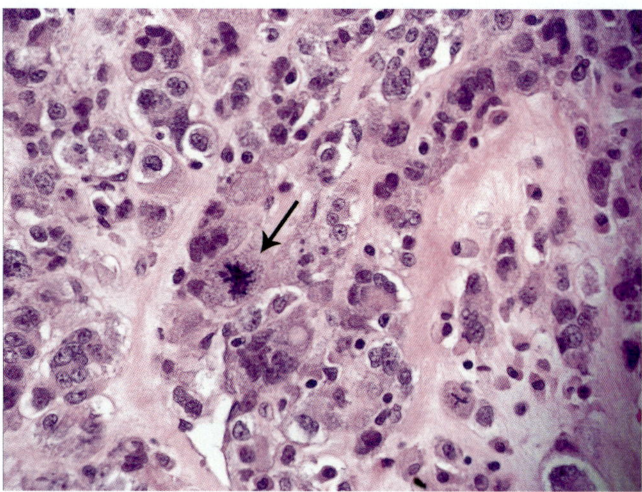

Figure 3.148 — Liver, Undifferentiated (Embryonal) Sarcoma (Histology). An atypical mitotic figure, a feature of malignancy, is present (arrow). Densely packed tumor cells show irregular, hyperchromatic nuclei and occasional multinucleation. (Hematoxylin and eosin stain, high power)

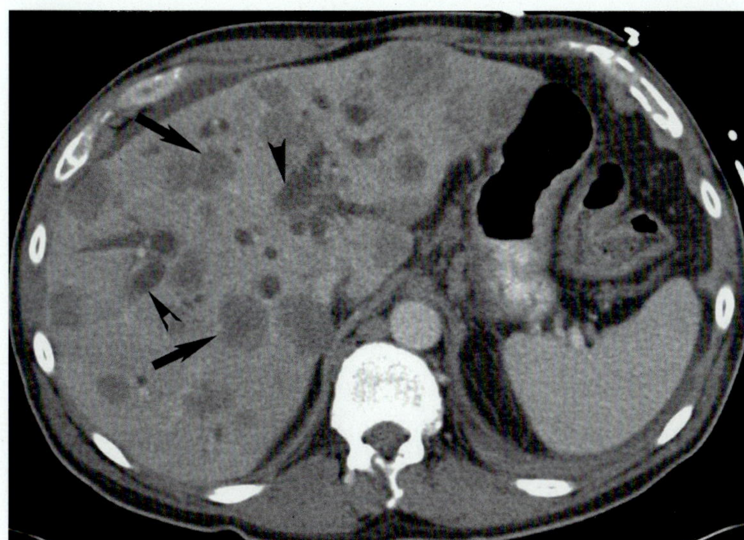

Figure 3.149 — Liver, Metastatic Colonic Adenocarcinoma. This 60-year-old-man was recently diagnosed with an extensive carcinoma of unknown primary, presumably colorectal cancer. Axial contrast-enhanced CT image of the abdomen in the venous phase shows numerous low-density liver masses (arrows). There is associated biliary ductal dilatation (arrowheads).

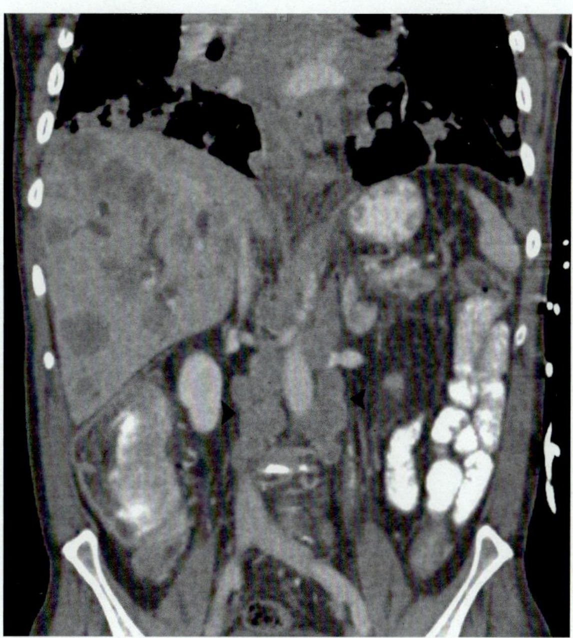

Figure 3.150 — Liver, Metastatic Colonic Adenocarcinoma. Coronal contrast-enhanced CT image of the abdomen confirms multiple low-density liver masses. There is also retroperitoneal adenopathy (arrowheads). Most hepatic metastases are multiple and hypovascular.

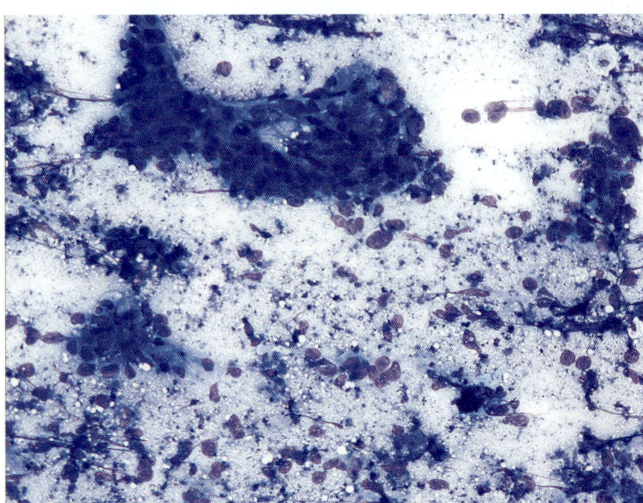

Figure 3.151 — Liver, Metastatic Colonic Adenocarcinoma. Fragments of malignant glandular epithelium are shown in a background of granular necrotic debris characteristic of colonic adenocarcinoma. (Diff Quik stain, medium power)

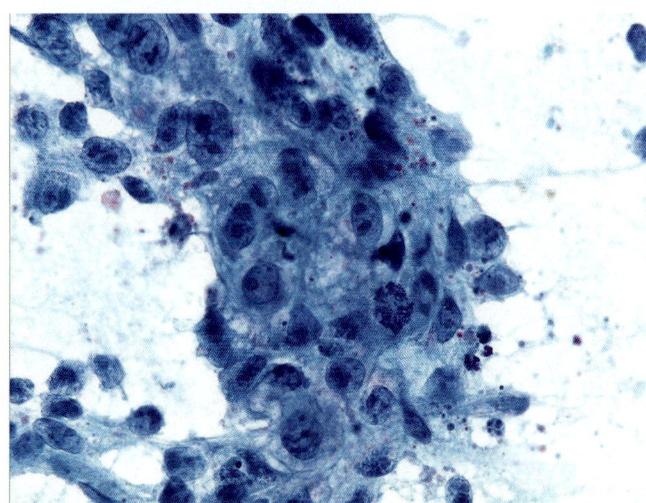

Figure 3.152 — Liver, Metastatic Colonic Adenocarcinoma. Tumor cells show anisonucleosis with prominent nucleoli. A mitotic figure is present and there are fragments of cellular debris scattered about. Cell block or core biopsy material is helpful in determining a primary site for a metastatic adenocarcinoma. Colonic adenocarcinoma is immunoreactive for CK20 and CDX2. (Papanicolaou stain, high power)

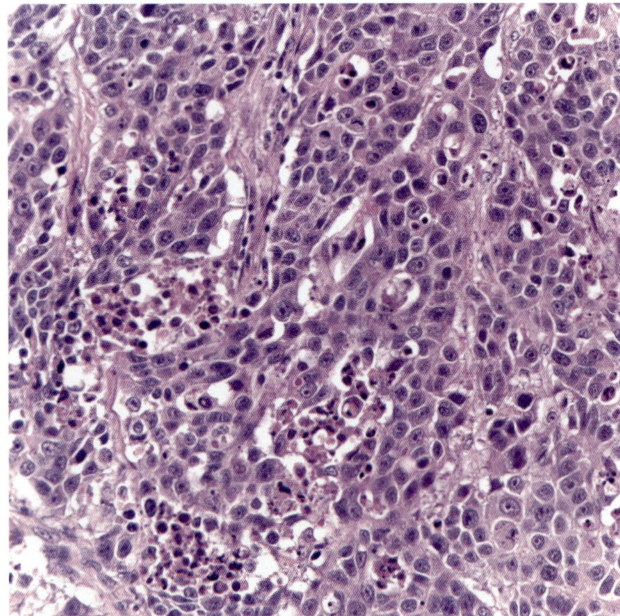

Figure 3.153 — Liver, Metastatic Colonic Adenocarcinoma (Histology). Poorly differentiated adenocarcinoma originating from the colon is illustrated. Solid sheets of neoplastic glands are composed of cells with round- to oval-shaped nuclei and prominent nuclei. Focal necrosis is evident. (Hematoxylin and eosin stain, medium power)

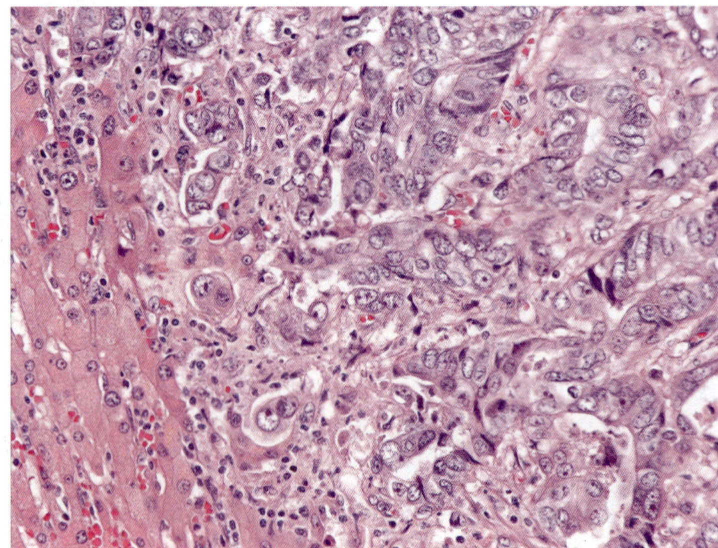

Figure 3.154 — Liver, Metastatic Colonic Adenocarcinoma (Histology). These malignant glands show nuclear pleomorphism, stratification, and occasional nucleoli. Abundant necrosis is typically present. Neoplastic cells are positive for CK20 and CDX2. (Hematoxylin and eosin stain, high power)

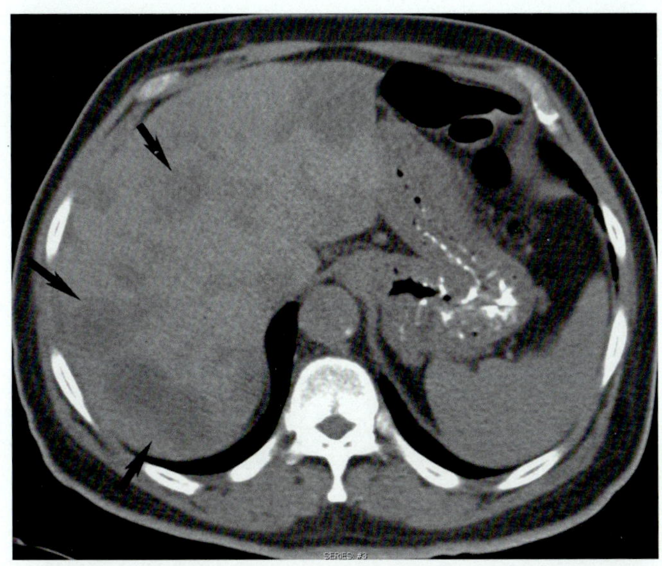

Figure 3.155 — Liver, Metastatic Pancreatic Adenocarcinoma. A 57-year-old man complained of abdominal pain. Axial noncontrast CT shows multiple ill-defined hypodense liver lesions (arrows).

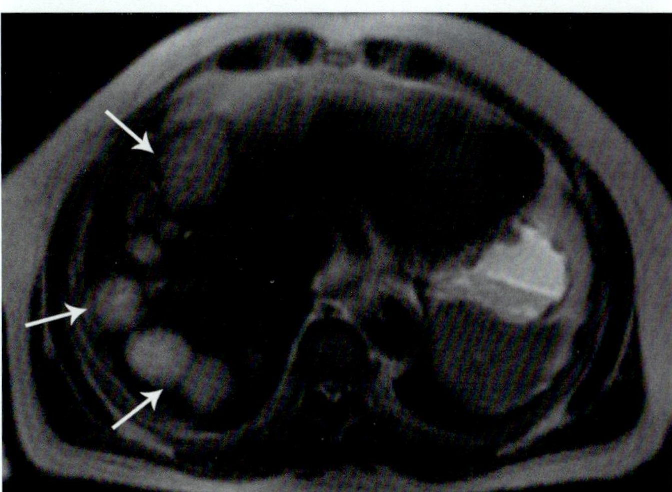

Figure 3.156 — Liver, Metastatic Pancreatic Adenocarcinoma. Axial T2-weighted MR shows the lesions are hyperintense on this sequence (arrows).

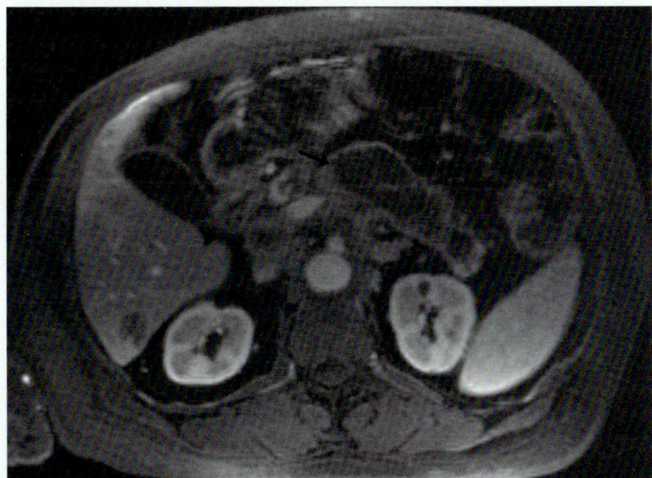

Figure 3.157 — Liver, Metastatic Pancreatic Adenocarcinoma. Axial T1 fat-saturated post-contrast MR image in the arterial phase in the same patient also shows there is marked dilation of the pancreatic duct with an abrupt cut-off in the proximal pancreatic body (arrow) highly suspicious for a pancreatic adenocarcinoma. Hepatic metastases from pancreatic adenocarcinoma are commonly hypovascular.

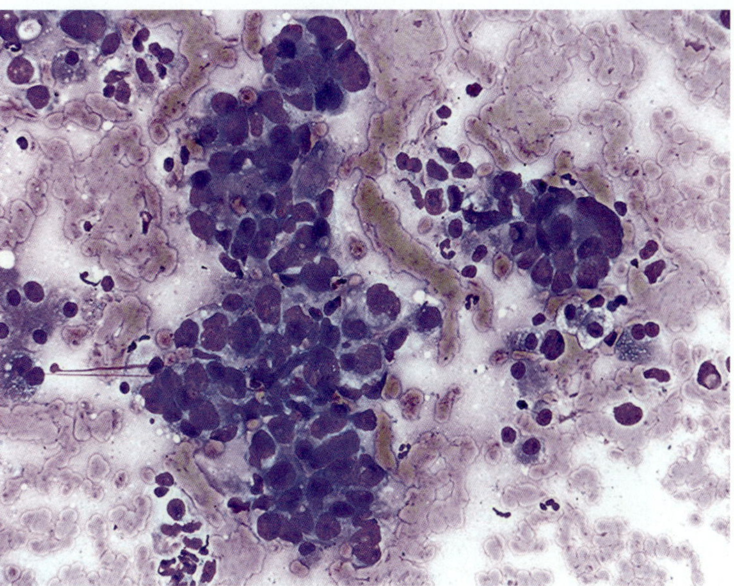

Figure 3.158 — Liver, Metastatic Pancreatic Adenocarcinoma. Fragments of malignant epithelium with three-dimensional gland-like architecture are present in a background of granular debris consistent with necrosis. Pancreatic adenocarcinoma frequently metastasizes to the liver. (Diff Quik stain, high power)

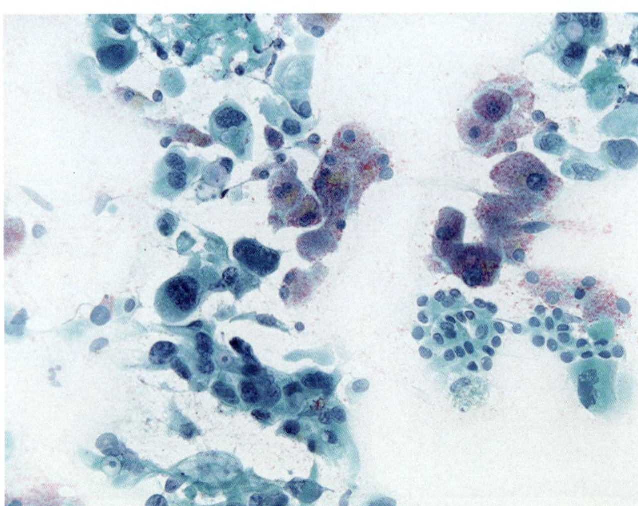

Figure 3.159 — Liver, Metastatic Pancreatic Adenocarcinoma. A fragment of poorly differentiated malignant epithelium is present with interspersed benign hepatic tissue. If material is present for immunostains, pancreatic adenocarcinoma will typically show positivity for cytokeratin 7, but does not have a specific immunoprofile. (Papanicolaou stain, high power)

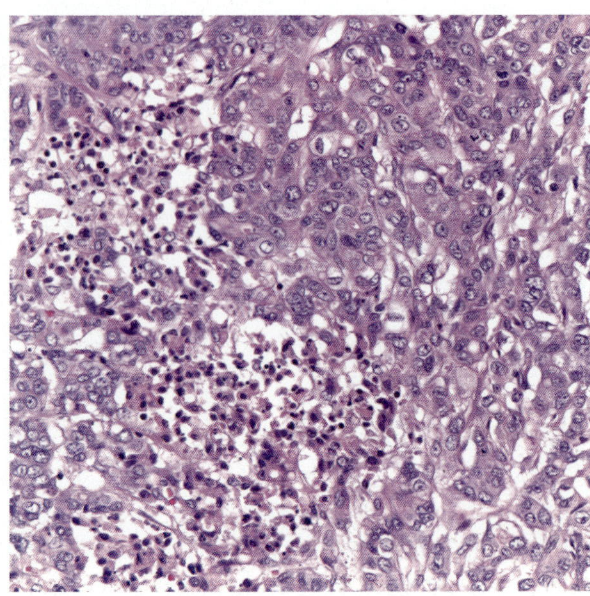

Figure 3.160 — Liver, Metastatic Pancreatic Adenocarcinoma (Histology). Poorly differentiated metastatic pancreatic adenocarcinoma is shown. The growth pattern is predominantly solid. There is significant cytological atypia with irregular nuclear outlines, prominent nucleoli, and necrosis and apoptosis. (Hematoxylin and eosin stain, medium power)

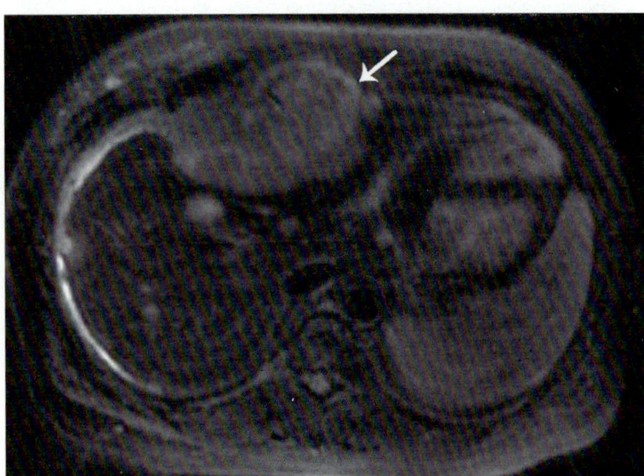

Figure 3.161 — Liver, Metastatic Gastrointestinal Stromal Tumor. This 55-year-old man with a history of a gastrointestinal stromal tumor resected from the greater curvature of the stomach presented with decreased appetite and increased abdominal distension. Axial T2-weighted MR image demonstrates multiple, heterogeneous T2 hyperintense masses in the liver with the largest located in the left lobe (arrow).

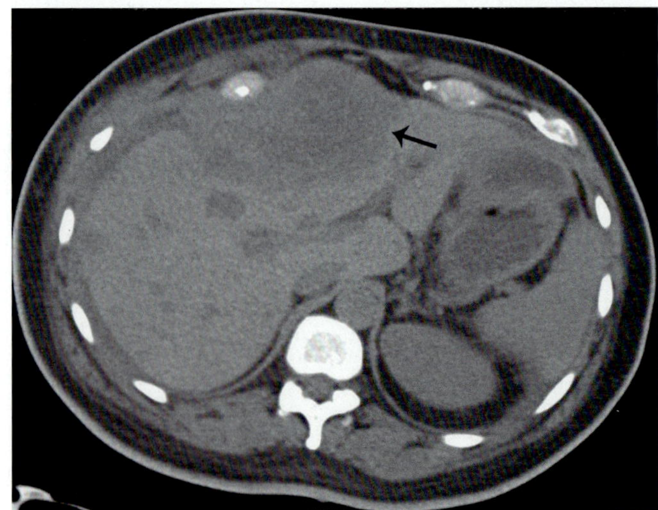

Figure 3.162 — Liver, Metastatic Gastrointestinal Stromal Tumor. Axial unenhanced CT image confirms a large hypodense liver mass in the left lobe containing a lower-density area of necrosis (arrow). Metastases from gastrointestinal stromal tumors are usually heterogeneous and mimic the original tumor.

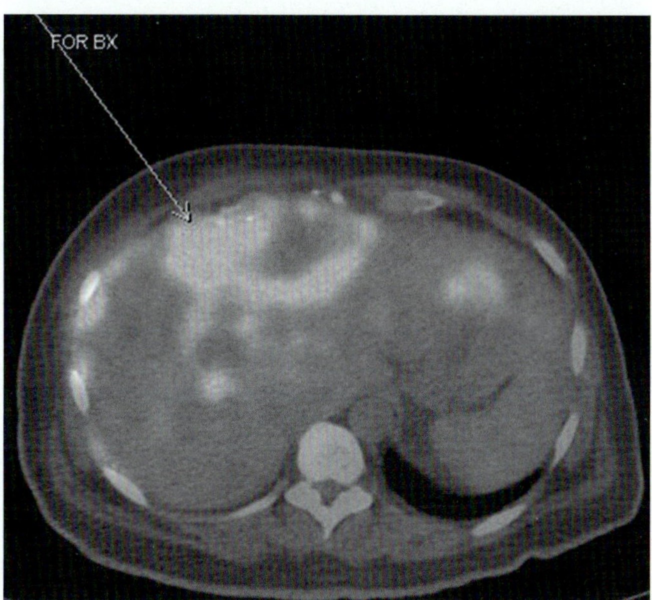

Figure 3.163 — Liver, Metastatic Gastrointestinal Stromal Tumor. Axial fused PET/CT scan confirms FDG uptake in the left hepatic lobe mass with focal area of decreased FDG activity consistent with necrosis (arrow).

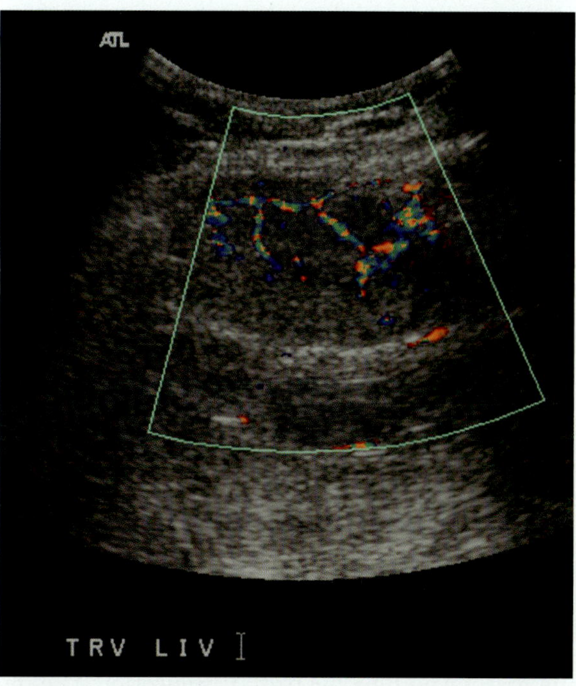

Figure 3.164 — Liver, Metastatic Gastrointestinal Stromal Tumor. Sonographic image confirms the presence of a left lobe liver mass with internal vascularity.

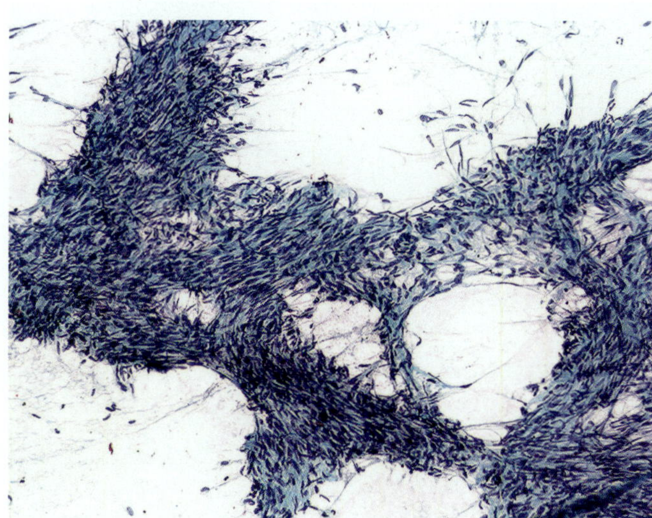

Figure 3.165 — Liver, Metastatic Gastrointestinal Stromal Tumor. On low power, the dense cellularity of this tissue is evident. The nuclei are spindled, consistent with a mesenchymal neoplasm. (Papanicolaou stain, low power)

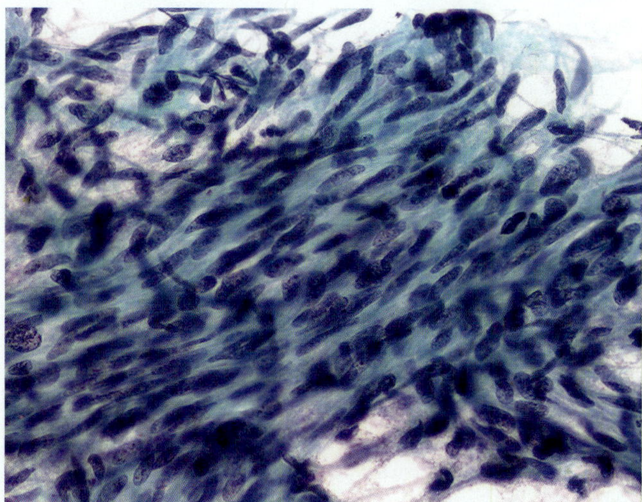

Figure 3.166 — Liver, Metastatic Gastrointestinal Stromal Tumor. The spindled tumor cells are densely packed and uniform in size. Metastatic spindle cell lesions are more common than primary mesenchymal liver lesions. (Papanicolaou stain, high power)

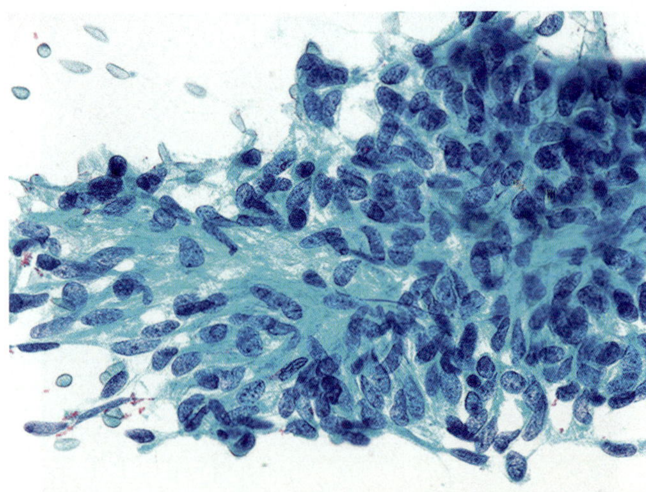

Figure 3.167 — Liver, Metastatic Gastrointestinal Stromal Tumor. These tumor cells demonstrate predominantly spindle cell features, with a few cells showing a more rounded, epithelioid configuration. Epithelioid gastrointestinal stromal tumors can be mistaken for primary or metastatic epithelial lesions. Immunostains are helpful in distinguishing the two. (Papanicolaou stain, medium power)

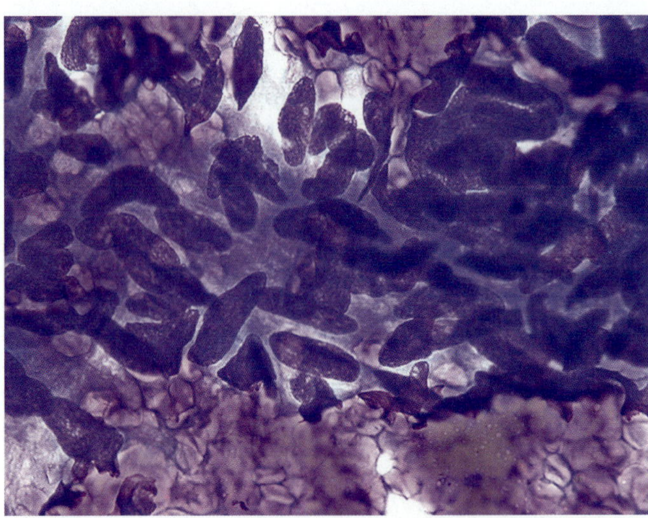

Figure 3.168 — Liver, Metastatic Gastrointestinal Stromal Tumor. Spindled nuclei showing rounded to tapered ends are present. The nuclei are crowded, but no marked atypia is noted. Gastrointestinal stromal tumors are immunoreactive for c-kit (CD117) and CD34. Ki-67, a proliferative marker, is often employed to determine tumor grade. (Diff Quik stain, medium power)

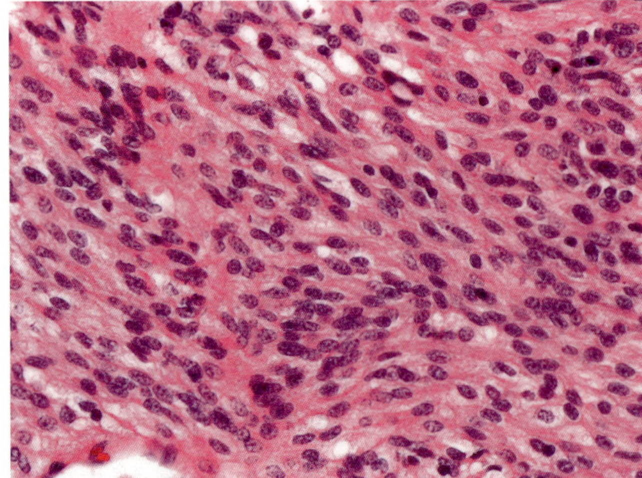

Figure 3.169 — Liver, Metastatic Gastrointestinal Stromal Tumor. The lesion consists of fascicles of bland spindle cells with eosinophilic cytoplasm. The nuclei range from ovoid to more elongated with blunt ends. A c-kit immunostain showed diffuse and strong labeling in the tumor cells (not shown). (Hematoxylin and eosin stain, high power)

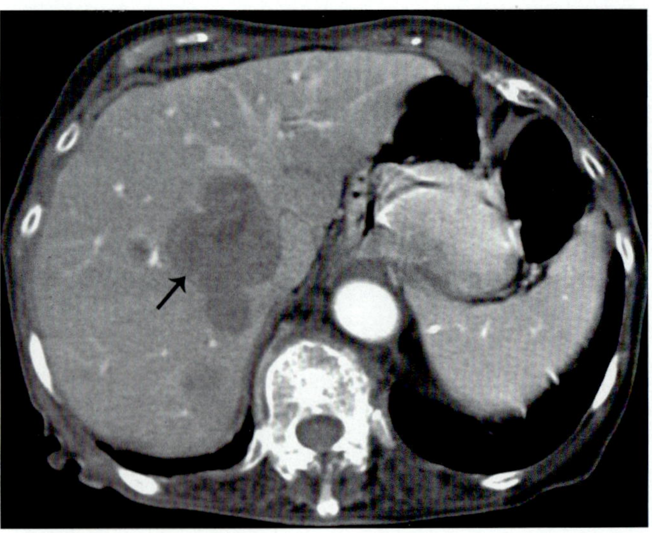

Figure 3.170 — Liver, Metastatic Melanoma. This 83-year-old female complained of weight loss and left-sided abdominal pain. Axial contrast-enhanced CT shows a lobulated, heterogeneous mass in the right lobe of the liver (arrow).

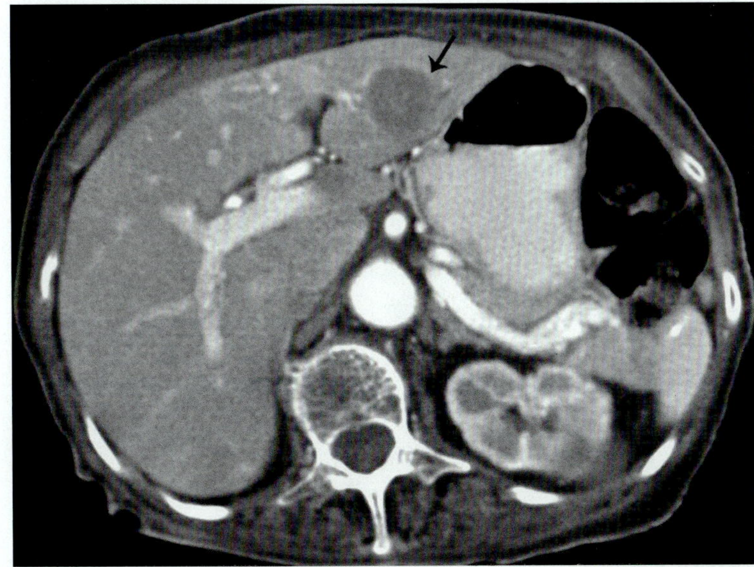

Figure 3.171 — Liver, Metastatic Melanoma. There are additional masses in the liver including the left lobe (arrow). Most hepatic metastases are hypovascular, as in this case.

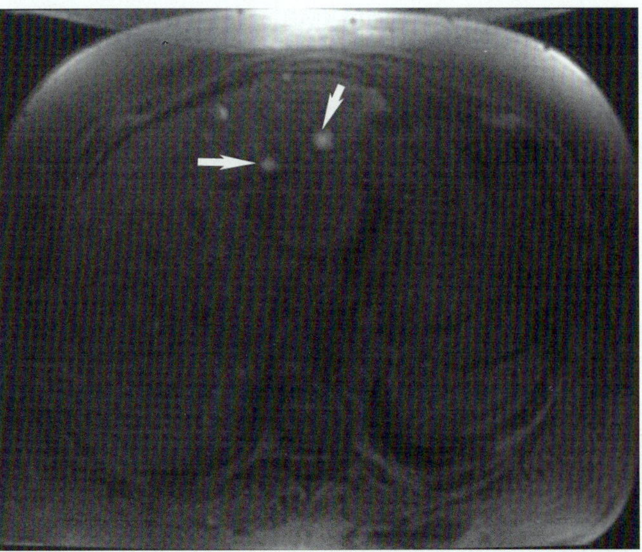

Figure 3.172 — Liver, Metastatic Melanoma. This 52-year-old man had a history of a renal transplant, with renal cell carcinoma present in his remaining native kidney 2 years ago, and a "skin lesion." He now presents with fever and right flank pain. A renal ultrasound incidentally noted multiple liver masses. Axial T1 fat-saturated precontrast MR image shows multiple T1 hyperintense small liver lesions (arrows).

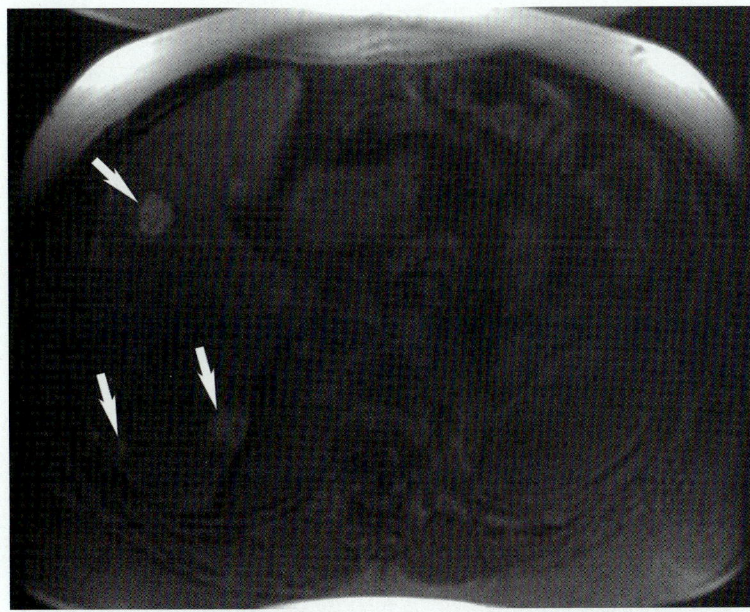

Figure 3.173 — Liver, Metastatic Melanoma. Additional T1 hyperintense liver lesions are seen more inferiorly in the right lobe of the liver (arrows). Metastases from malignant melanoma frequently are T1 hyperintense.

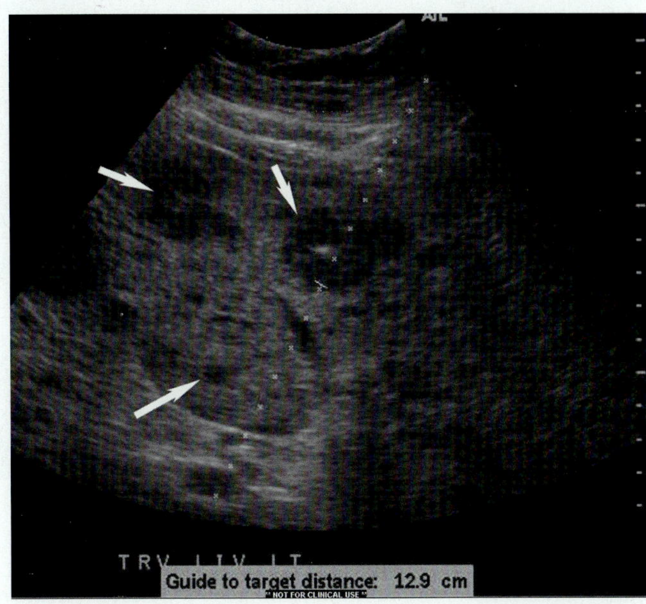

Figure 3.174 — Liver, Metastatic Melanoma. Sonographic image confirms multiple hypoechoic liver masses (arrows).

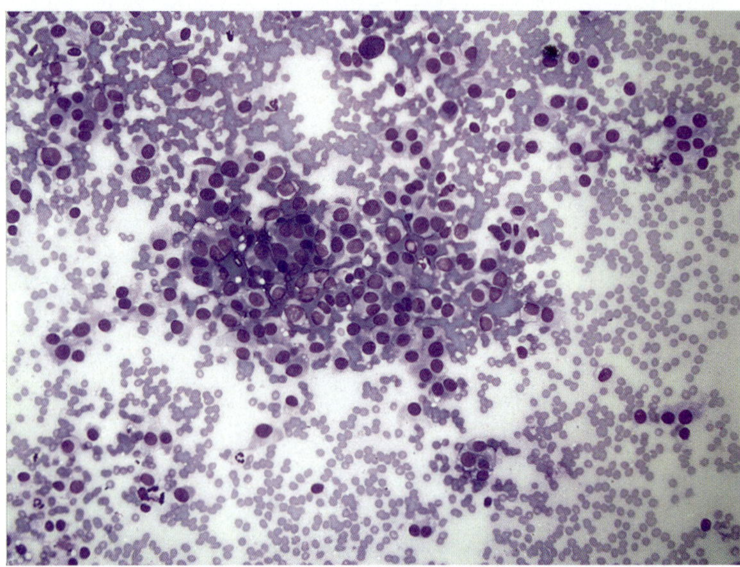

Figure 3.175 — Liver, Metastatic Melanoma. A dispersed, single-cell population is present. At low to medium magnification, these cells may be mistaken for hepatocytes. (Diff Quik stain, medium power)

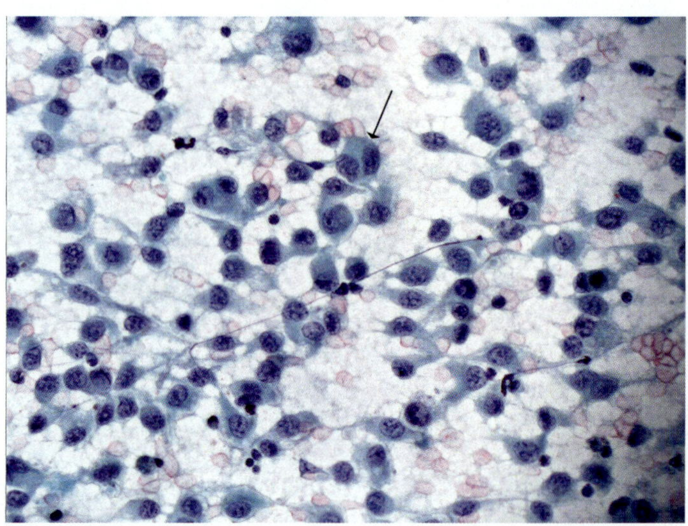

Figure 3.176 — Liver, Metastatic Melanoma. On higher power, atypical features are seen, including occasional binucleation (arrow). The nuclei are eccentrically placed (plasmacytoid appearance), characteristic of melanoma. (Papanicolaou stain, high power)

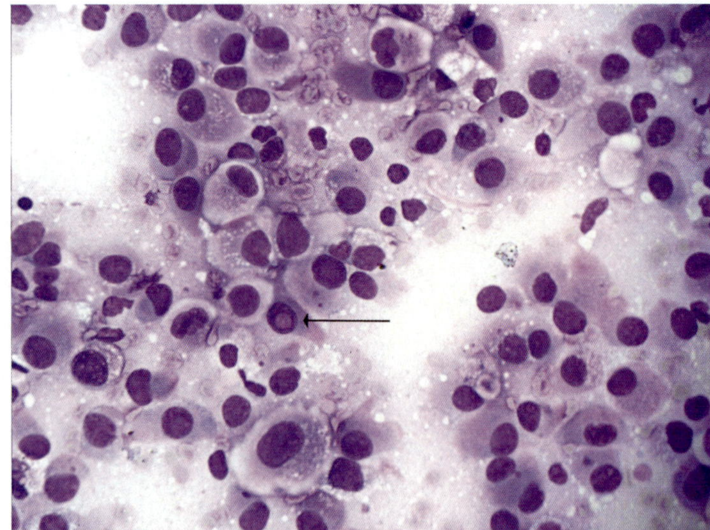

Figure 3.177 — Liver, Metastatic Melanoma. An intranuclear inclusion is present (arrow), which is consistent with melanoma, but may also be seen in hepatocellular carcinoma and other metastatic carcinomas. The dominant single-cell population shown here makes an epithelial malignancy unlikely. (Diff Quik stain, high power)

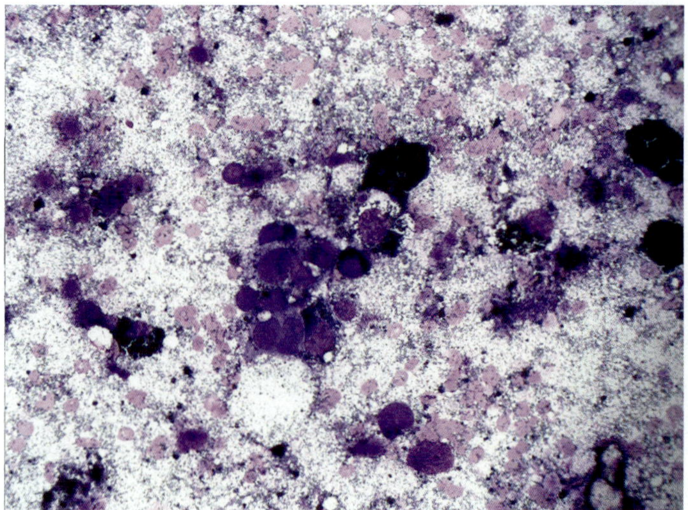

Figure 3.178 — Liver, Metastatic Melanoma. Abundant dark black, finely granular pigment is seen here within tumor cells, in macrophages, and dispersed in the background suggest a diagnosis of melanoma. Melanin pigment should be distinguished from bile and other pigments, which may also appear dark on Diff Quik staining. (Diff Quik stain, high power)

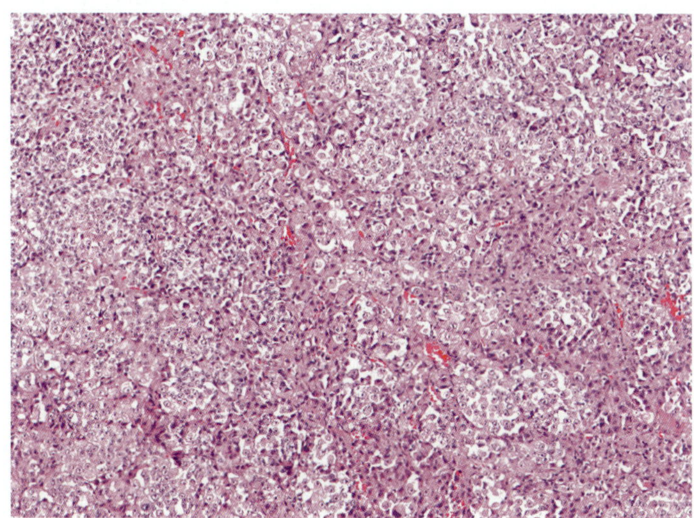

Figure 3.179 — Liver, Metastatic Melanoma. Nests of poorly differentiated neoplastic cells are present with abundant granular pink cytoplasm and prominent macronucleoli. The neoplastic cells are seen infiltrating the hepatic parenchyma. Poorly differentiated hepatocellular carcinoma is considered in the differential diagnosis. (Hematoxylin and eosin stain, medium power)

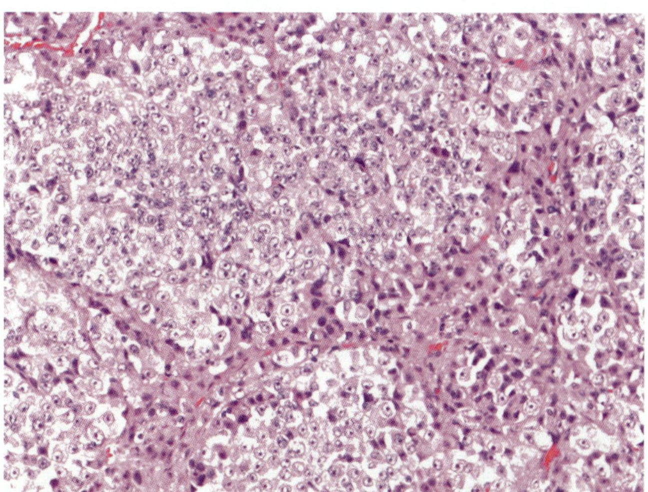

Figure 3.180 — Liver, Metastatic Melanoma. Sheets of neoplastic cells show prominent atypia with anisonucleosis and prominent nucleoli. The neoplastic cells are arranged in large solid sheets and cords. There is no evidence of any glandular or squamous differentiation. Immunostains for S-100 protein and Melan-A were positive in the tumor. (Hematoxylin and eosin stain, high power)

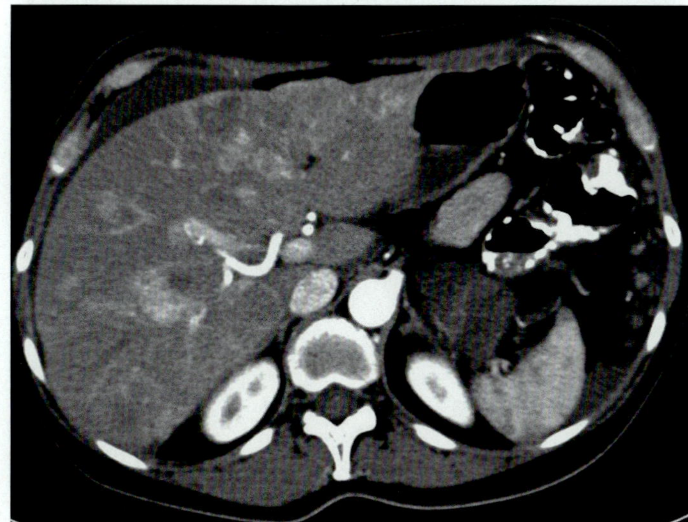

Figure 3.181 — Liver, Metastatic Neuroendocrine Tumor. A 49-year-old woman complained of diarrhea and abdominal pain. Axial contrast-enhanced CT image in the arterial phase shows multiple hypervascular liver masses.

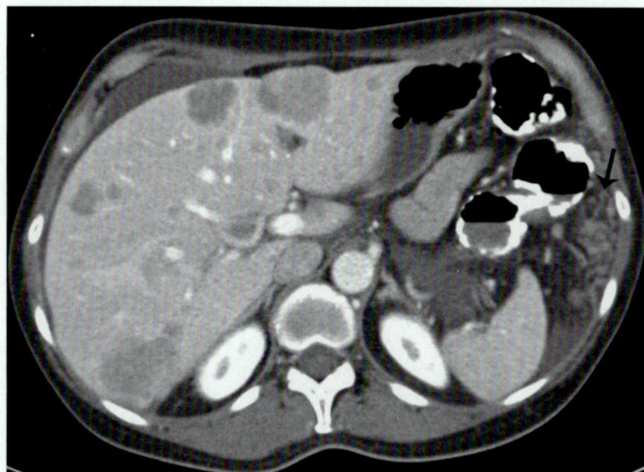

Figure 3.182 — Liver, Metastatic Neuroendocrine Tumor. The masses wash out in the venous phase. Hypervascular metastases can be seen with neuroendocrine tumors, sarcoma, carcinoids, renal cell carcinomas, and thyroid carcinomas. Note this patient also has ascites and multiple small soft tissue nodules in the left upper quadrant compatible with carcinomatosis (arrow).

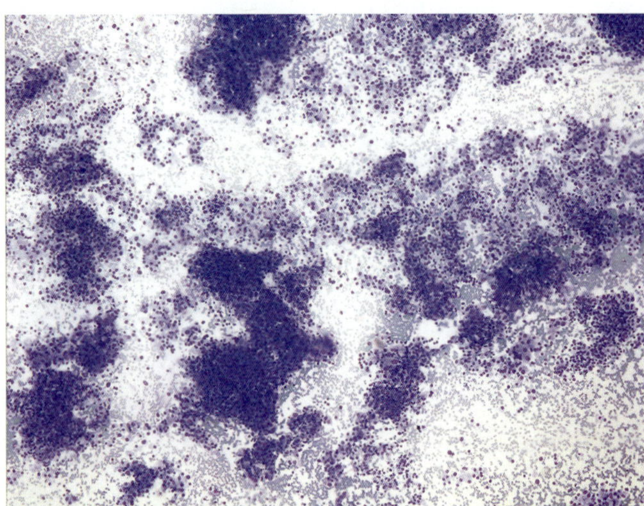

Figure 3.183 — Liver, Metastatic Neuroendocrine Tumor. A combination of cohesive fragments and single cells is present in this very cellular aspirate smear. At low power, the cells appear uniform and appear to have ample cytoplasm. (Diff Quik stain, low power)

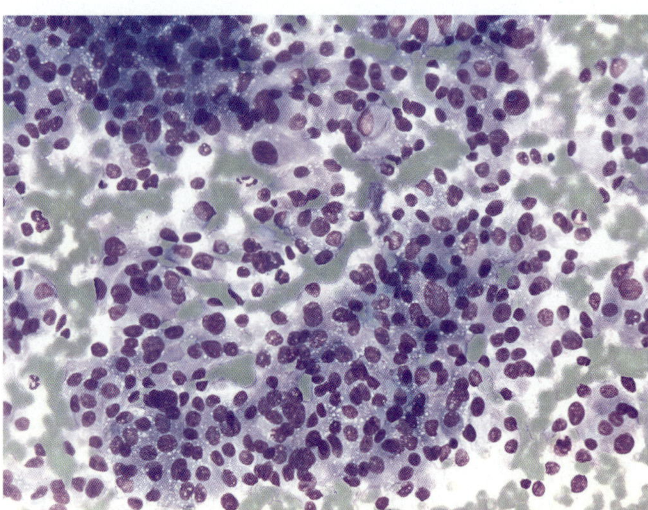

Figure 3.184 — Liver, Metastatic Neuroendocrine Tumor. A relatively uniform population of neoplastic cells is present with round to focally oval nuclei and ill-defined cell borders. Primary neuroendocrine tumors of the liver do occur, but are extremely rare. A metastasis from the pancreas or gastrointestinal tract is much more common. (Diff Quik stain, high power)

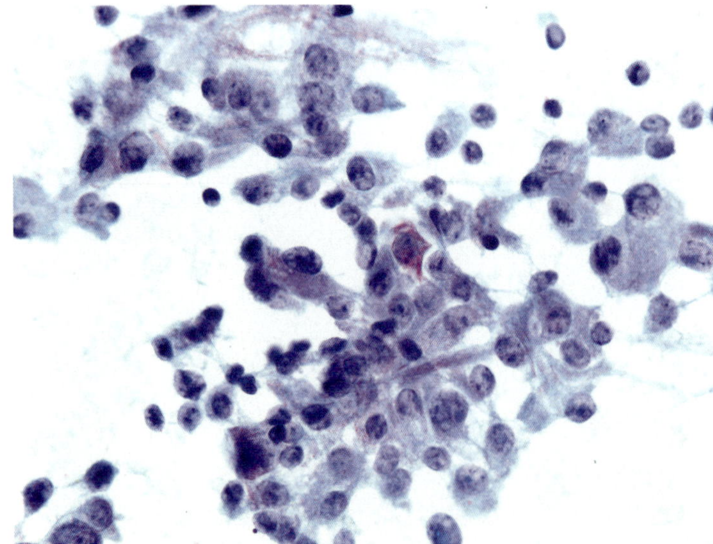

Figure 3.185 — Liver, Metastatic Neuroendocrine Tumor. These cells are monotonous and show abundant cytoplasm showing focal granularity. The nuclei are round and have stippled chromatin characteristic of neuroendocrine differentiation. (Papanicolaou stain, high power)

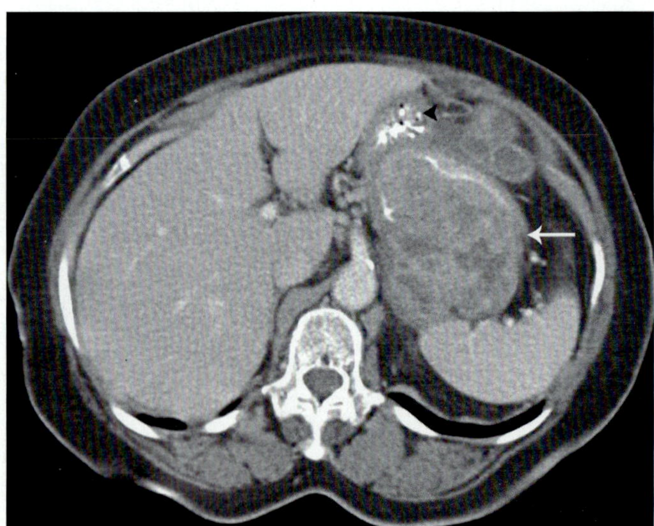

Figure 3.186 — Soft Tissue, Perigastric, Gastrointestinal Stromal Tumor. An 84-year-old woman presented with fatigue and abdominal pain. Axial contrast-enhanced CT image demonstrates an enhancing mass between the stomach and the spleen (arrow). The mass arises exophytically from the stomach (arrowhead).

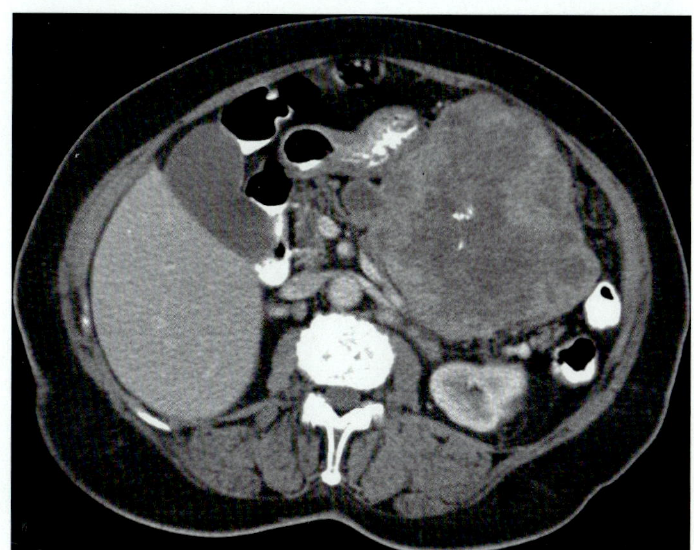

Figure 3.187 — Soft Tissue, Perigastric, Gastrointestinal Stromal Tumor. Axial contrast-enhanced CT shows the mass contains central calcifications. Gastrointestinal stromal tumors are commonly exophytic and can be heterogeneous when large.

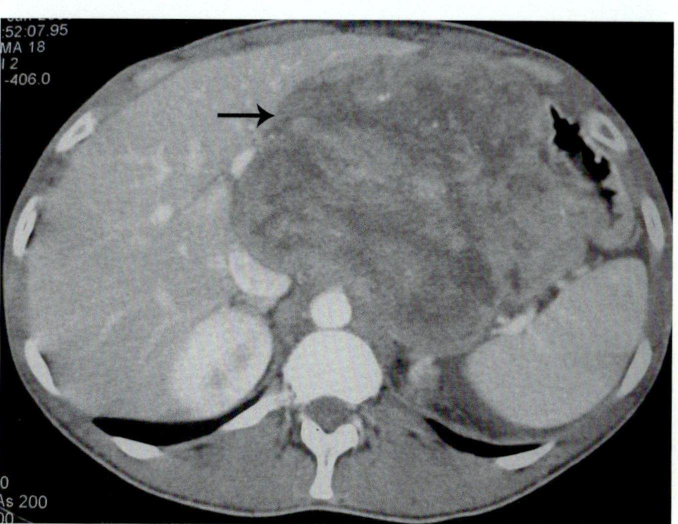

Figure 3.188 — Soft Tissue, Mesenteric, Gastrointestinal Stromal Tumor. This 42-year-old HIV-positive man presented with a 4-month history of upper abdominal pain, nausea, and vomiting. Axial contrast-enhanced CT shows a large, markedly heterogeneous soft tissue mass in the upper abdomen (arrow).

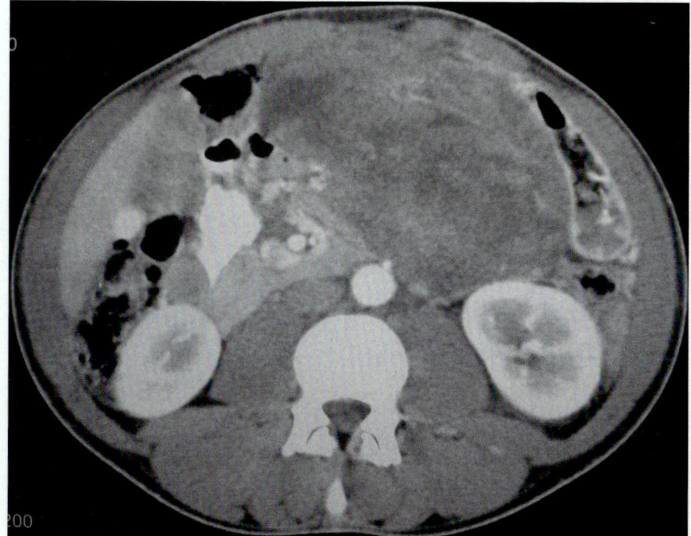

Figure 3.189 — Soft Tissue, Mesenteric, Gastrointestinal Stromal Tumor. Axial contrast-enhanced CT demonstrates that the epicenter of the mass appears in the mesentery. Gastrointestinal stromal tumors can be predominantly exophytic or occur primarily in the mesentery.

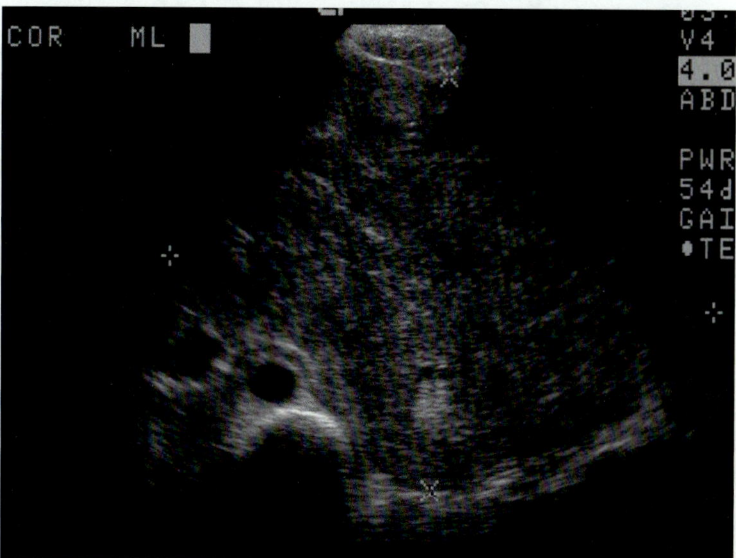

Figure 3.190 — Soft Tissue, Mesenteric, Gastrointestinal Stromal Tumor. Sonographic image at the time of ultrasound-guided biopsy shows the heterogeneous abdominal mass.

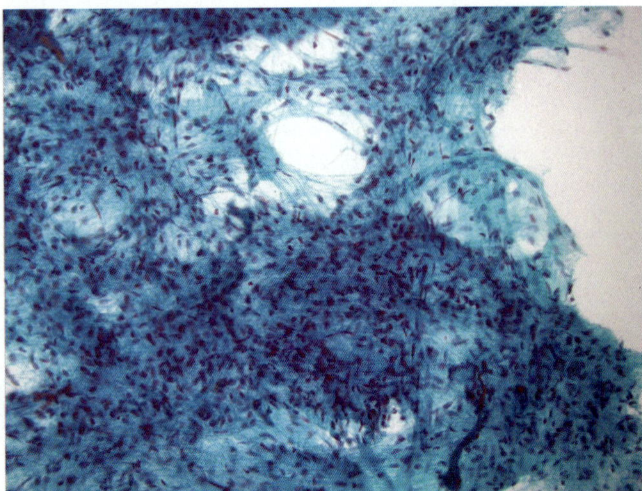

Figure 3.191 — Soft Tissue, Perigastric, Gastrointestinal Stromal Tumor. A large fragment of fibrous stroma is present containing many densely packed spindled nuclei. The differential for a perigastric stromal nodule includes gastrointestinal stromal tumor, schwannoma, and leiomyoma. (Papanicolaou stain, medium power)

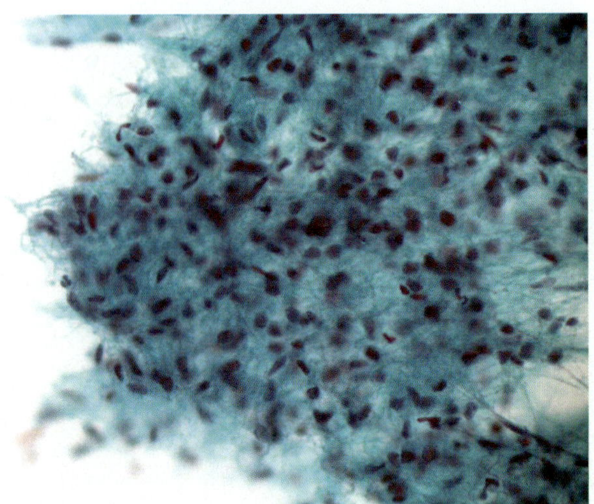

Figure 3.192 — Soft Tissue, Perigastric, Gastrointestinal Stromal Tumor. The spindle cells are densely packed, but have very small, bland nuclei. Most gastrointestinal stromal tumors are benign, but malignant tumors do occur. Malignant potential is related to tumor location, size, necrosis, and mitotic index. (Papanicolaou stain, high power)

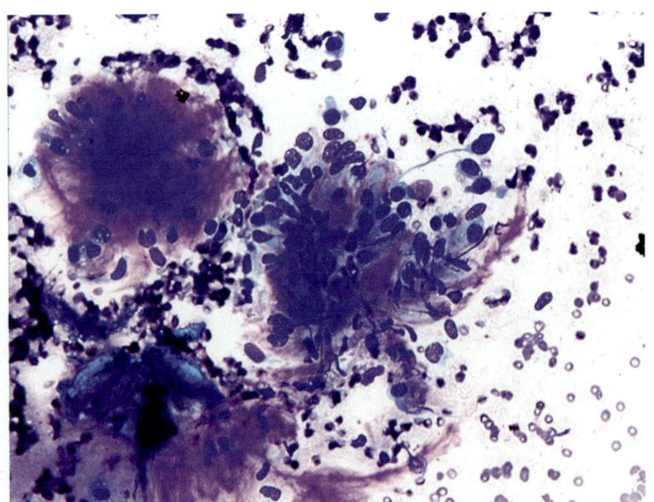

Figure 3.193 — Soft Tissue, Perigastric, Gastrointestinal Stromal Tumor. Myxoid stroma is seen admixed with epithelioid- to spindle-shaped cells, characteristic of gastrointestinal stromal tumor. The tumor cells may be quite epithelioid, morphologically suggesting an epithelial or neuroendocrine neoplasm. (Diff Quik stain, high power)

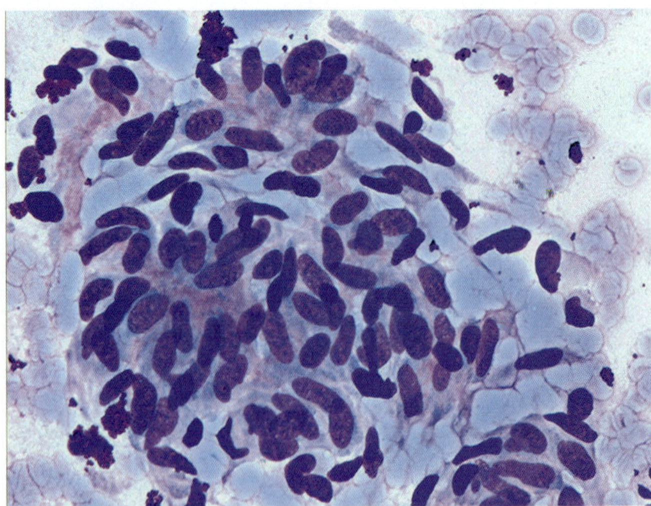

Figure 3.194 — Soft Tissue, Perigastric, Gastrointestinal Stromal Tumor. The tumor cells show a spindle cell morphology here. Gastrointestinal stromal tumors are often aspirated via endoscopic ultrasound; thus, care must be taken not to interpret normal bowel wall as a spindle cell neoplasm. (Diff Quik stain, high power)

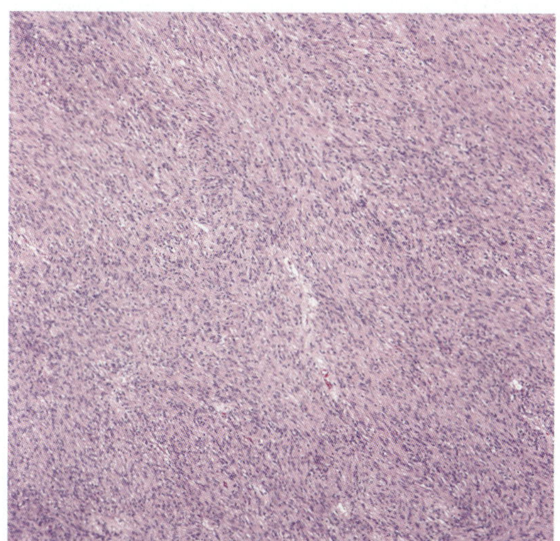

Figure 3.195 — Soft Tissue, Perigastric, Gastrointestinal Stromal Tumor (Histology). Sheets of neoplastic spindle cells are shown. Histologically, gastrointestinal stromal tumors most commonly have a spindle cell morphology, but may be epithelioid or have a pleomorphic/mixed morphology. The tumor cell morphology does not convey any prognostic significance. (Hematoxylin and eosin stain, low power)

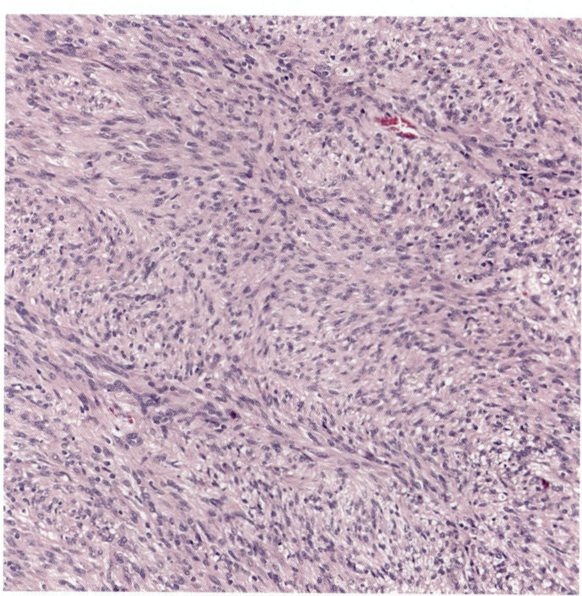

Figure 3.196 — Soft Tissue, Perigastric, Gastrointestinal Stromal Tumor (Histology). The neoplastic spindle cells are arranged in a fascicular pattern. Features that are predictive of aggressive behavior in gastrointestinal stromal tumors are mitotic rates greater than 5 per 10 high-power fields, size, and location. Immunohistochemical stains are positive c-kit (CD117), and CD34. (Hematoxylin and eosin stain, medium power)

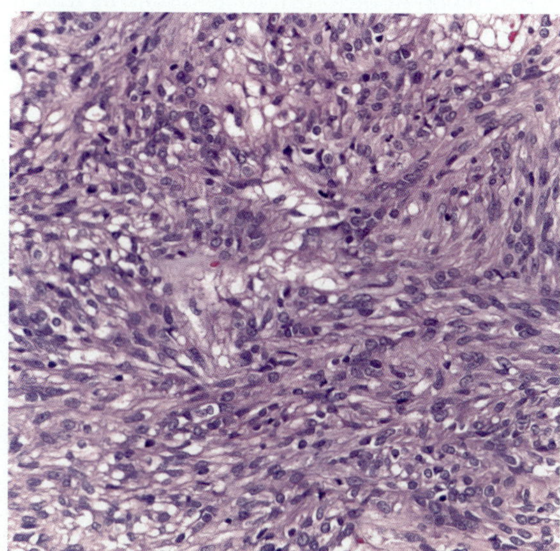

Figure 3.197 — Soft Tissue, Perigastric, Gastrointestinal Stromal Tumor (Histology). The tumor shows predominantly spindle-shaped cells with foci of epithelioid cells. The epithelioid tumor cells are round with clear cytoplasm and have a clearly demarcated cell membrane. The spindled cells have a fascicular growth pattern. (Hematoxylin and eosin stain, high power)

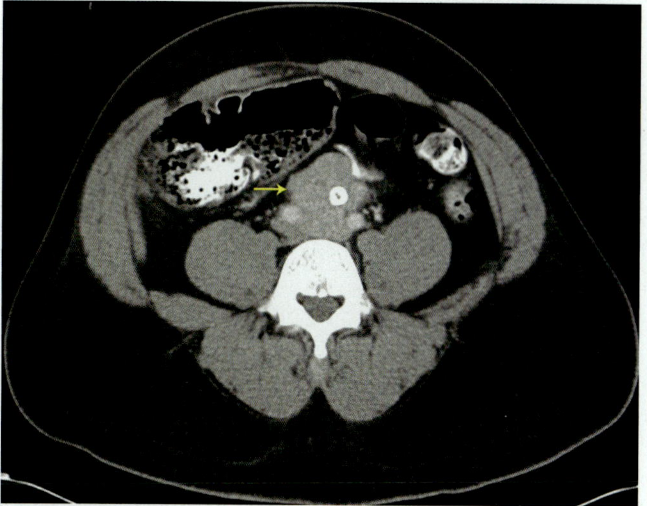

Figure 3.198 — Soft Tissue, Retroperitoneal, Paraganglioma. This 34-year-old man presented with left shoulder pain. Axial contrast-enhanced CT demonstrates a mass in the retroperitoneum (arrow).

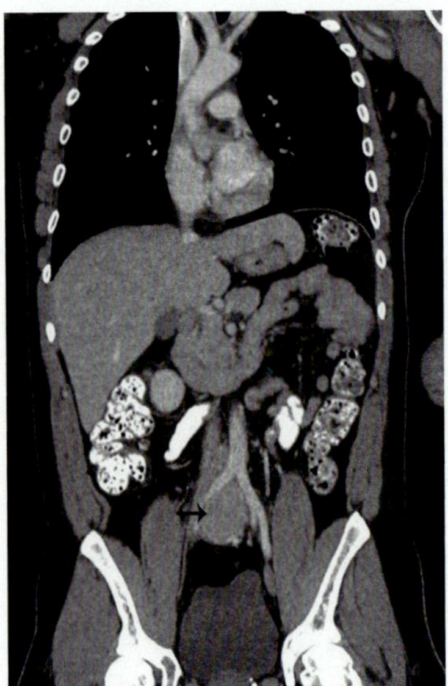

Figure 3.199 — Soft Tissue, Retroperitoneal, Paraganglioma. Coronal contrast-enhanced CT shows the mass (arrow) encases the common iliac vessels at the aortic bifurcation. Ten percent of pheochromocytomas are extra-adrenal, termed paragangliomas, with most occurring in the aorta near the origin of the inferior mesenteric artery.

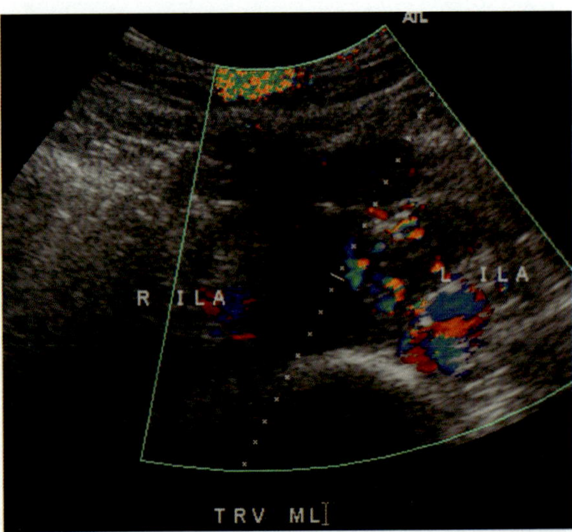

Figure 3.200 — Soft Tissue, Retroperitoneal, Paraganglioma. Sonographic image at the time of ultrasound-guided biopsy shows the hypoechoic mass encasing the common iliac vessels. Extra-adrenal paragangliomas are associated with Carney syndrome, NF1, and von Hippel–Lindau disease.

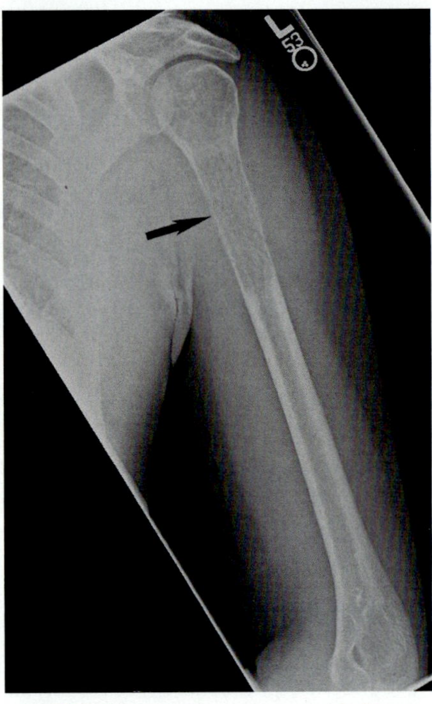

Figure 3.201 — Soft Tissue, Retroperitoneal, Paraganglioma. X-ray of the left shoulder in the same patient demonstrates a permeative lytic lesion in the proximal left humerus with thinning of the cortex, which was found to represent metastatic pheochromocytoma (arrow). Although rare, paragangliomas can metastasize.

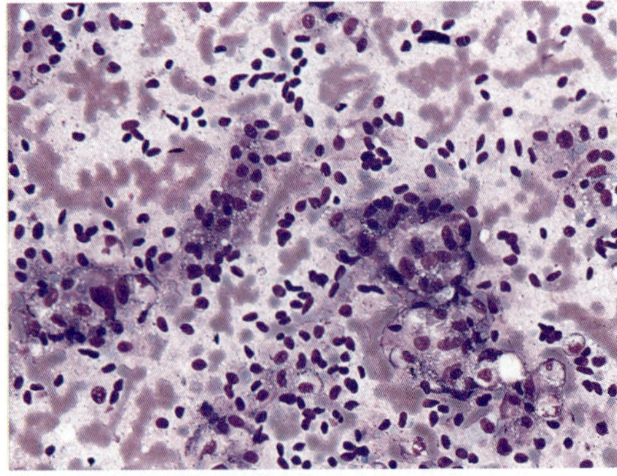

Figure 3.202 — Soft Tissue, Abdomen, Paraganglioma. Neoplastic cells with ample granular cytoplasm and ill-defined cell borders are shown. Note the numerous bare oval- to spindle-shaped nuclei in the background. (Diff Quik stain, high power)

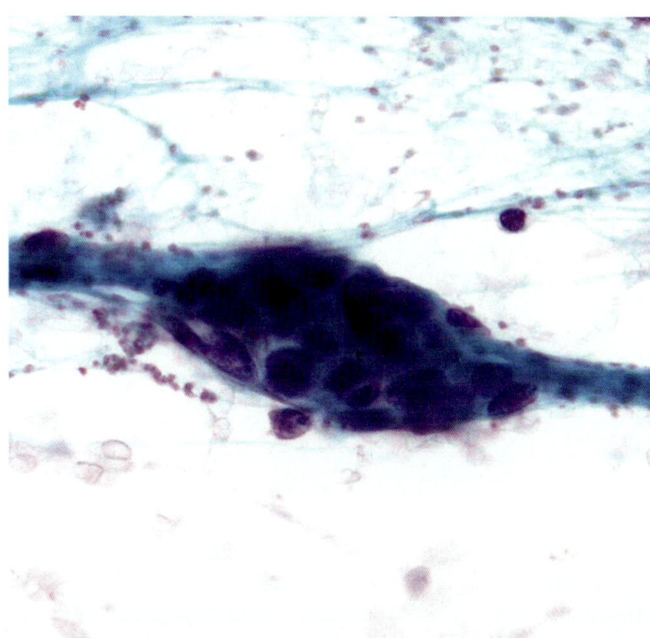

Figure 3.203 — Soft Tissue, Abdomen, Paraganglioma. A single nest of tumor cells is seen showing slight nuclear enlargement. Marked nuclear atypia may be present, but does not indicate malignancy. (Papanicolaou stain, high power)

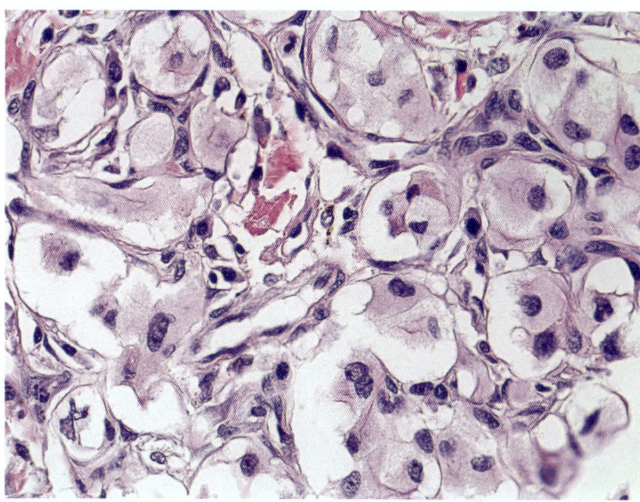

Figure 3.204 — Soft Tissue, Abdomen, Paraganglioma (Core Biopsy). A small core biopsy was obtained in this case and shows the characteristic nested architecture of paraganglioma. Tumor cells with abundant clear to finely granular cytoplasm and round to oval nuclei are separated by spindle-shaped sustentacular cells. (Hematoxylin and eosin stain, high power)

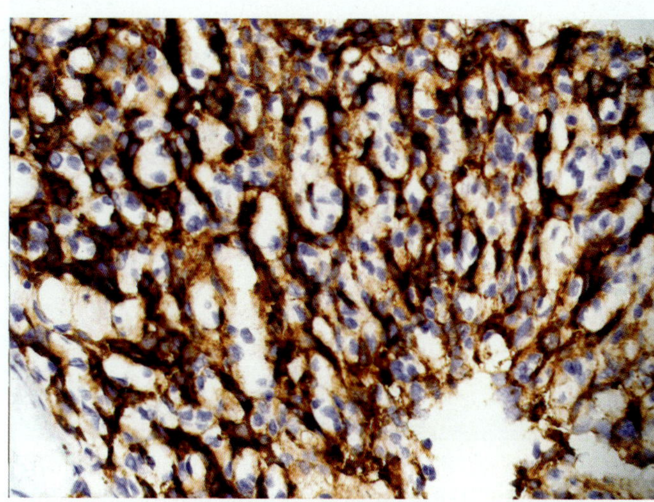

Figure 3.205 — Soft Tissue, Abdomen, Paraganglioma (Core Biopsy). The nested architecture, called Zellballen, is nicely highlighted with synaptophysin immunostaining. Chromogranin was also positive. (Synaptophysin immunostain, high power)

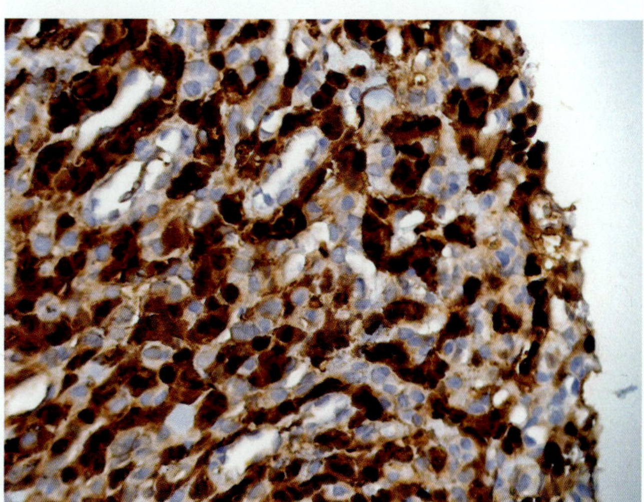

Figure 3.206 — Soft Tissue, Abdomen, Paraganglioma (Core Biopsy). S-100 protein immunostain highlights the sustentacular cells between the nests of tumor cells. Immunostains were also performed to rule out clear cell renal cell carcinoma and were negative. (S-100 protein immunostain, high power)

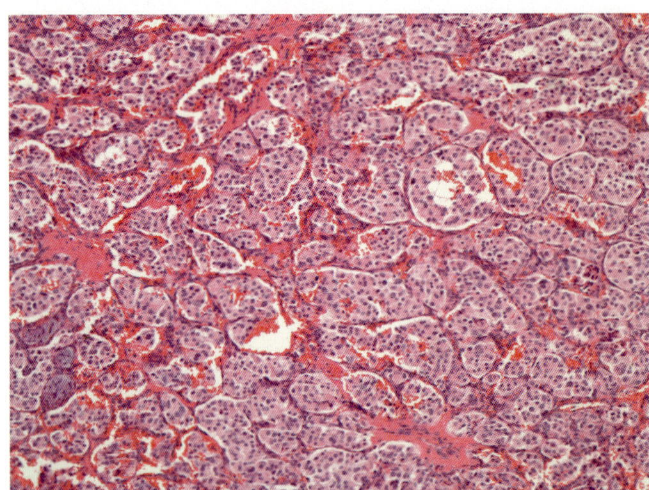

Figure 3.207 — Soft Tissue, Retroperitoneal, Paraganglioma (Histology). A nested or alveolar growth pattern is apparent. The tumor has a highly vascular stroma. Characteristically, the tumor cells are positive for synaptophysin and chromogranin, and negative for cytokeratin. S-100 protein labels the sustentacular cells. (Hematoxylin and eosin stain, low power)

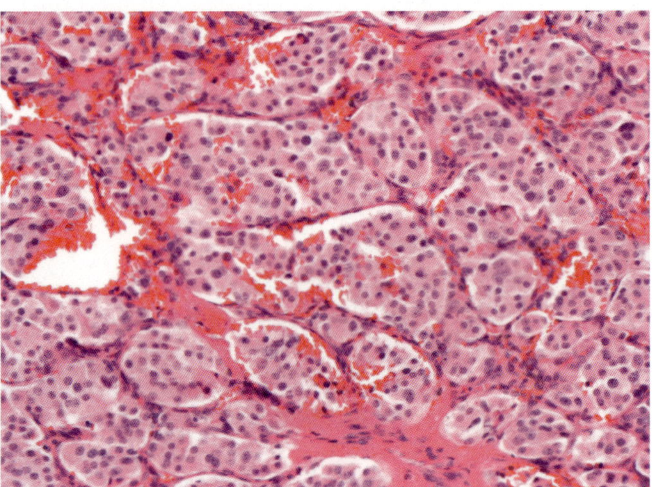

Figure 3.208 — Soft Tissue, Retroperitoneal, Paraganglioma (Histology). The neoplastic cells in a paraganglioma tend to cluster in nests (Zellballen). The tumor cells are large and polygonal and have abundant amphophilic cytoplasm with a uniform, "salt and pepper" type chromatin pattern. (Hematoxylin and eosin stain, high power)

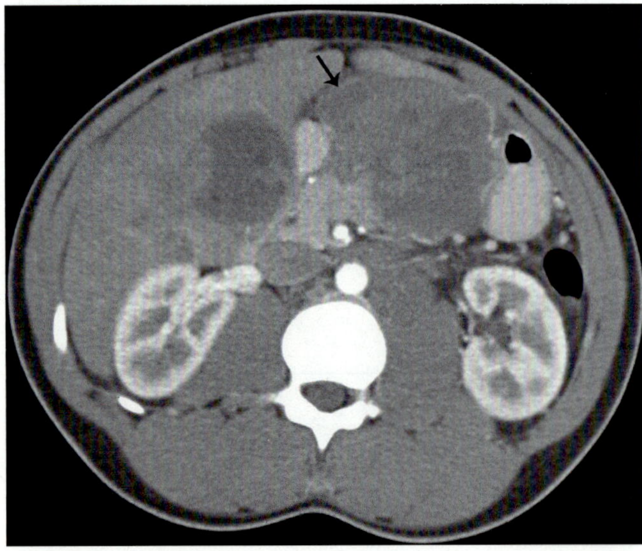

Figure 3.209 — Soft Tissue, Abdomen, Desmoplastic Small Round Cell Tumor. Axial contrast-enhanced CT shows a large, heterogeneous mass in the upper abdomen (arrow). Desmoplastic small round cell tumor is seen most often in young men, but is also seen in children.

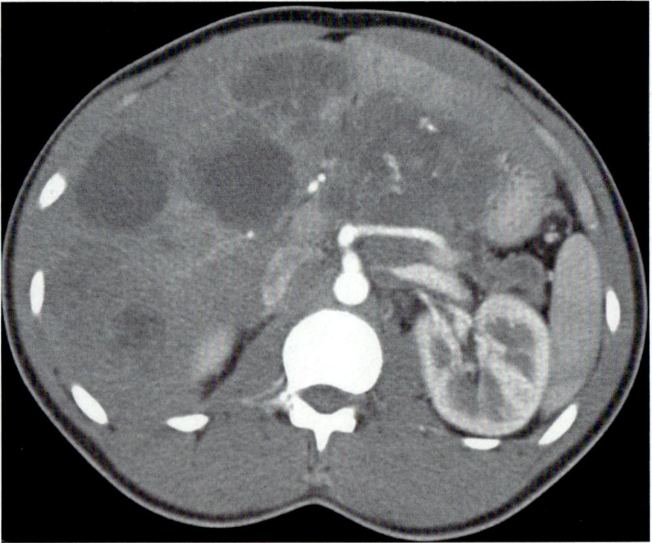

Figure 3.210 — Soft Tissue, Abdomen, Desmoplastic Small Round Cell Tumor. There are also multiple heterogeneous masses in the liver representing metastatic disease. Desmoplastic small round cell tumor typically presents as a large abdominal or pelvic mass, often with multiple peritoneal tumor implants at the time of presentation.

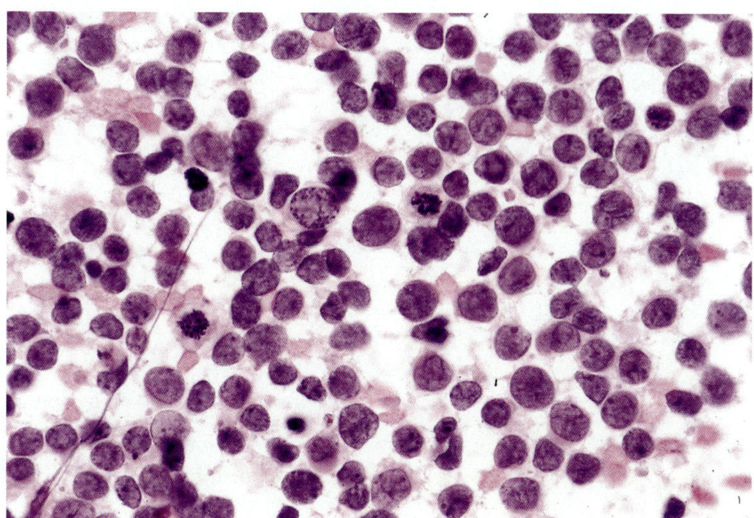

Figure 3.211 — Soft Tissue, Abdomen, Desmoplastic Small Round Cell Tumor. Numerous dispersed, single malignant cells are shown with at least two mitotic figures present. The differential diagnosis would include lymphoma and small cell carcinoma. (Diff Quik stain, high power)

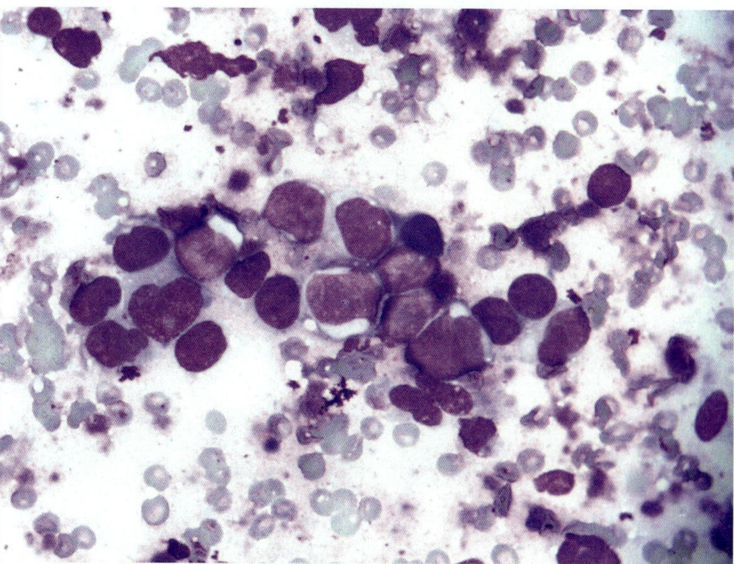

Figure 3.212 — Soft Tissue, Abdomen, Desmoplastic Small Round Cell Tumor. A cluster of tumor cells is shown with high nuclear-to-cytoplasmic ratios and irregular nuclear contours. Chromatin is evenly dispersed and nucleoli are not prominent. Tumor cells are actually quite large, despite the tumor name. (Diff Quik stain, high power)

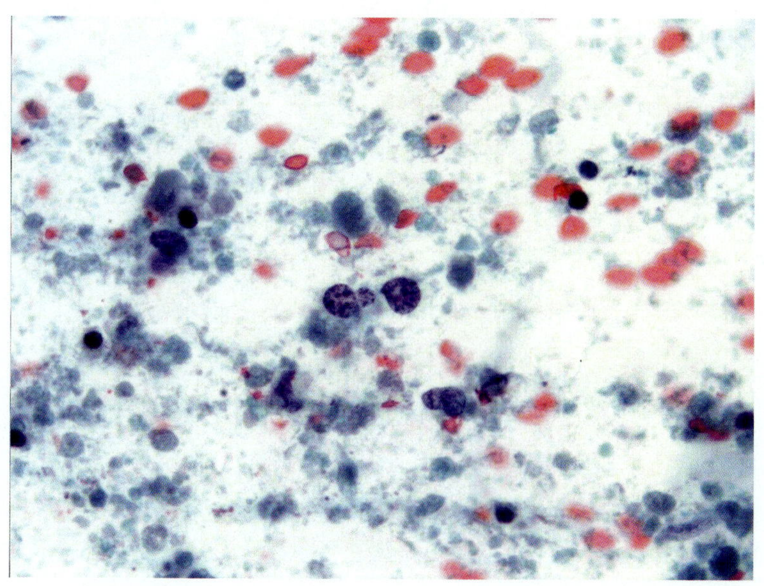

Figure 3.213 — Soft Tissue, Abdomen, Desmoplastic Small Round Cell Tumor. The Papanicolaou stained slide shows predominantly necrosis admixed with few single tumor cells. Desmoplastic small round cell tumor is associated with a characteristic translocation involving the EWS gene, t(11;22)(p13;q12). (Papanicolaou stain, high power)

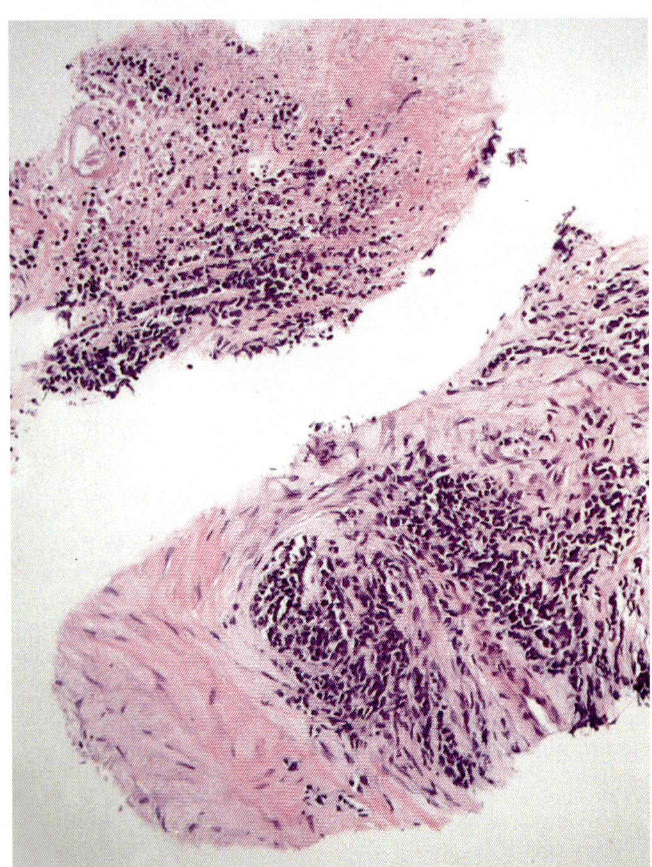

Figure 3.214 — Soft Tissue, Abdomen, Desmoplastic Small Round Cell Tumor (Core Biopsy). Two small core biopsies are shown. The top core shows necrosis, as was seen in the Papanicolaou stain. The bottom core shows the characteristic admixture of dense fibrous tissue with islands of poorly differentiated tumor cells. (Hematoxylin and eosin stain, medium power)

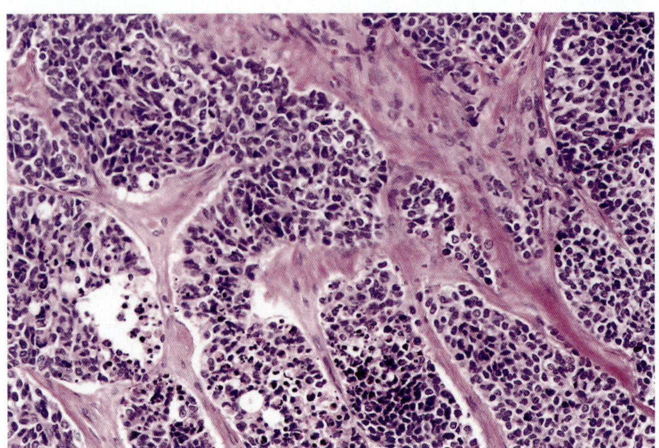

Figure 3.215 — Soft Tissue, Abdomen, Desmoplastic Small Round Cell Tumor (Core Biopsy). On high power, the desmoplastic stroma is evident surrounding nests of round to oval cells with scant cytoplasm. The cells are immunoreactive for desmin (in a characteristic punctate perinuclear pattern), as well as WT1. CD99 can be positive, although typically in a cytoplasmic pattern. (Hematoxylin and eosin stain, high power)

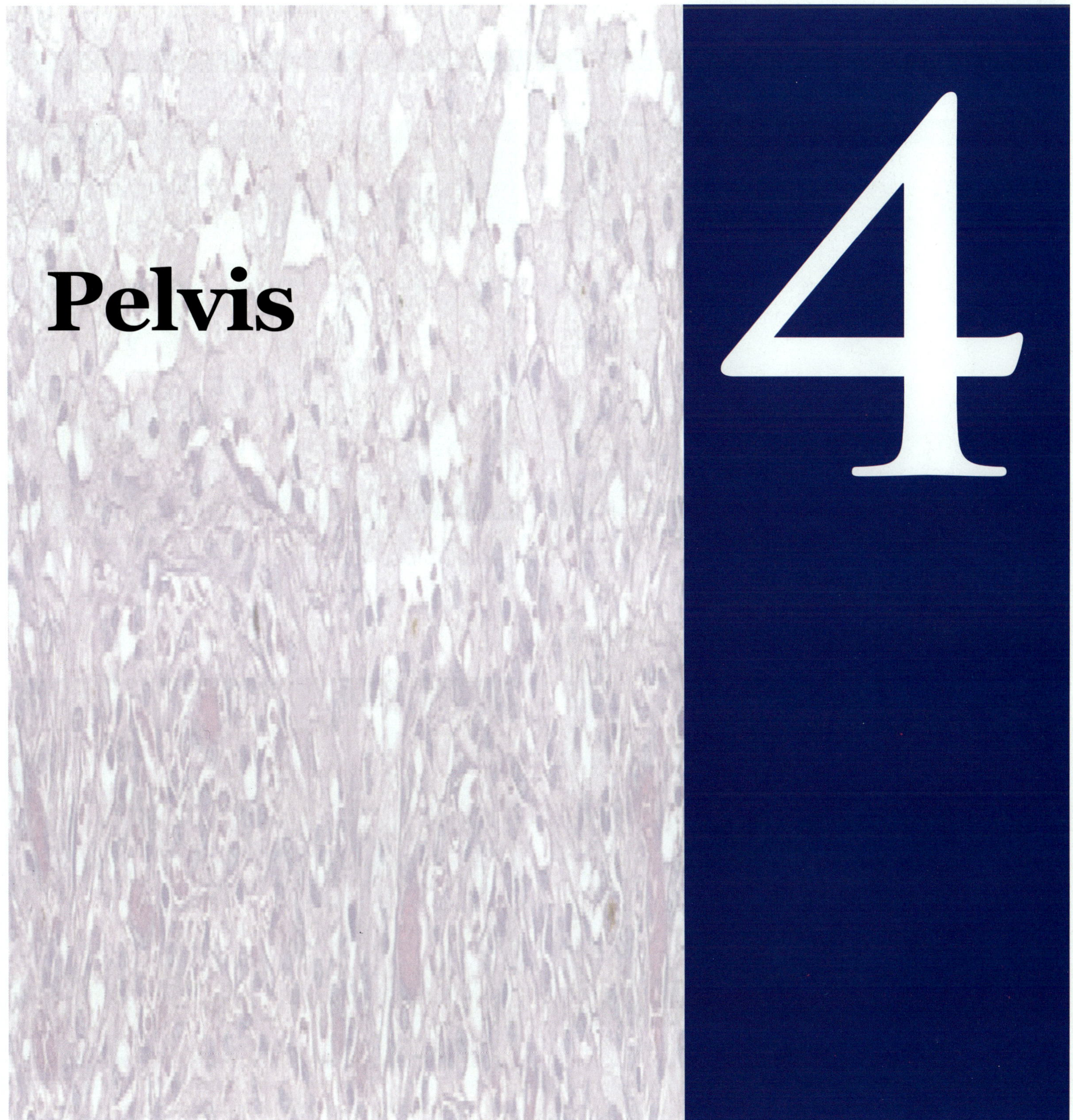

Pelvis

4

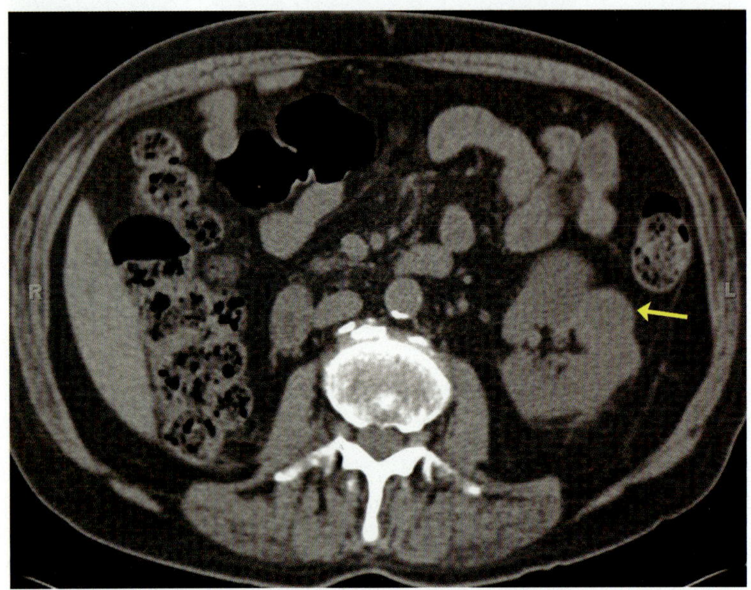

Figure 4.1 — Kidney, Oncocytoma. Axial noncontrast CT shows a small mass in the mid left kidney (arrow).

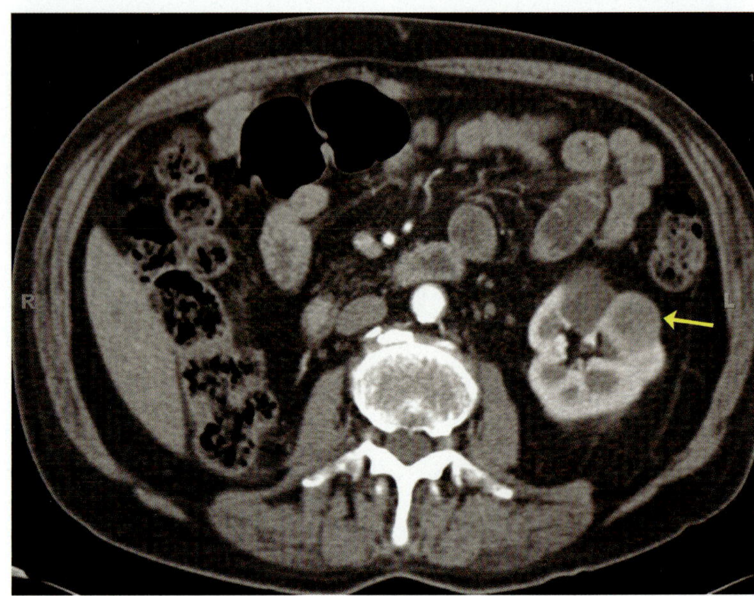

Figure 4.2 — Kidney, Oncocytoma. Axial contrast-enhanced CT in the arterial phase shows the mass mildly enhances (arrow).

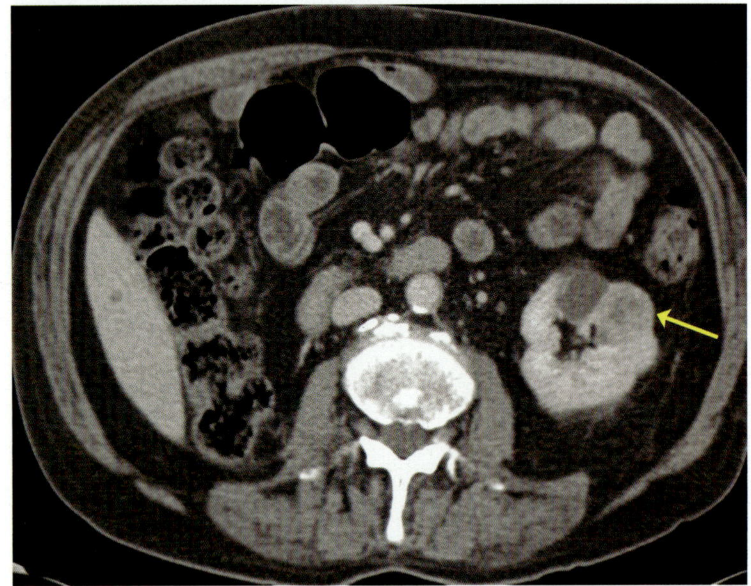

Figure 4.3 — Kidney, Oncocytoma. Axial contrast-enhanced CT in the venous phase also shows mild enhancement in the mass (arrow) with minimal central low density, which could represent a central scar. Oncocytomas characteristically have a stellate central scar.

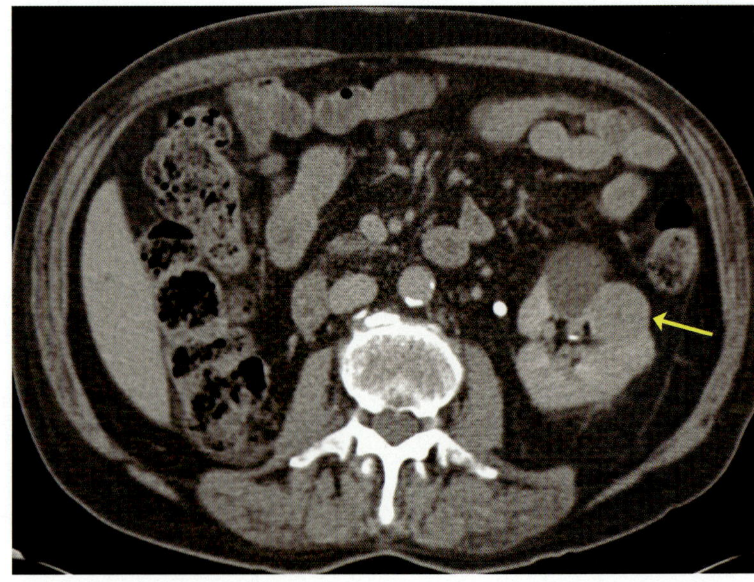

Figure 4.4 — Kidney, Oncocytoma. Axial contrast-enhanced CT in the delayed phase shows mild de-enhancement of the mass (arrow).

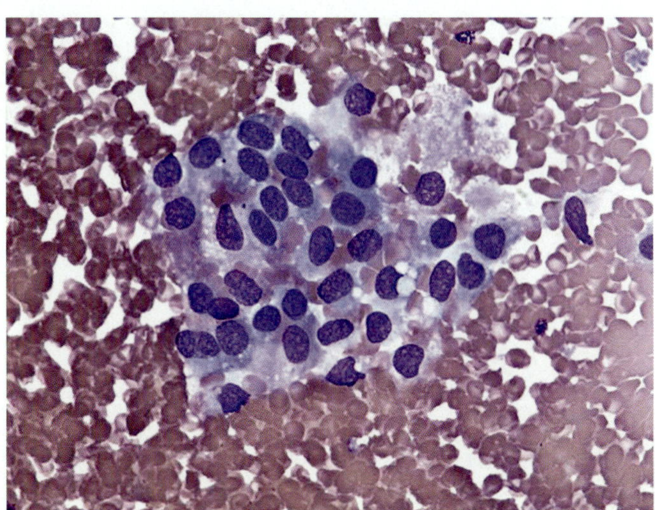

Figure 4.5 — Kidney, Oncocytoma. This group of epithelial cells shows uniform round to oval nuclei with abundant granular cytoplasm consistent with oncocytes. Focal oncocytes may occur in renal cell carcinoma; thus, a definitive diagnosis of oncocytoma should not be made on FNA or core biopsy. Oncocytosis should also be entertained in the differential diagnosis. (Diff Quik stain, medium power)

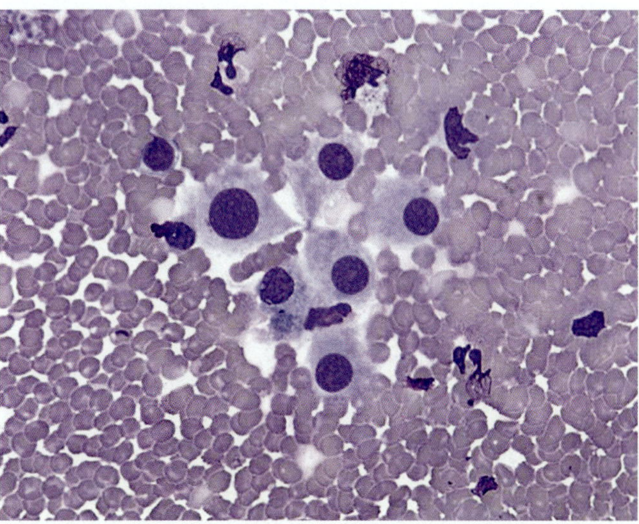

Figure 4.6 — Kidney, Oncocytoma. This group of loosely cohesive cells show centrally placed, round nuclei and abundant granular cytoplasm. The cytoplasmic granularity in oncocytoma represents abundant mitochondria. (Diff Quik stain, high power)

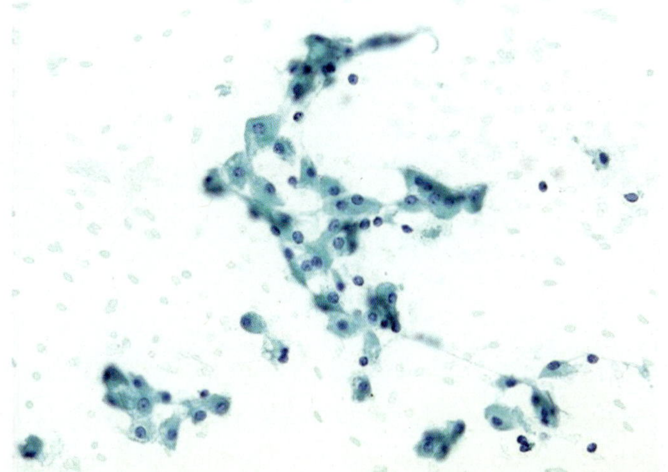

Figure 4.7 — Kidney, Oncocytoma. This fragment of neoplastic cells shows a uniform population of oncocytes. Oncocytoma cannot be reliably differentiated from a chromophobe renal cell carcinoma on cytologic material; thus, this morphology warrants a diagnosis of "oncocytic neoplasm" on FNA. (Papanicolaou stain, high power)

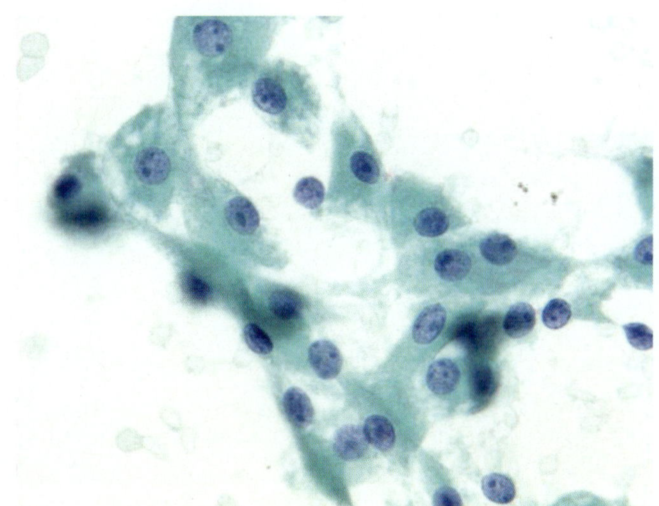

Figure 4.8 — Kidney, Oncocytoma. These cells have abundant granular cytoplasm and round nuclei with occasional prominent nucleoli. Renal oncocytoma is associated with the rare Birt–Hogg–Dubé syndrome. (Papanicolaou stain, high power)

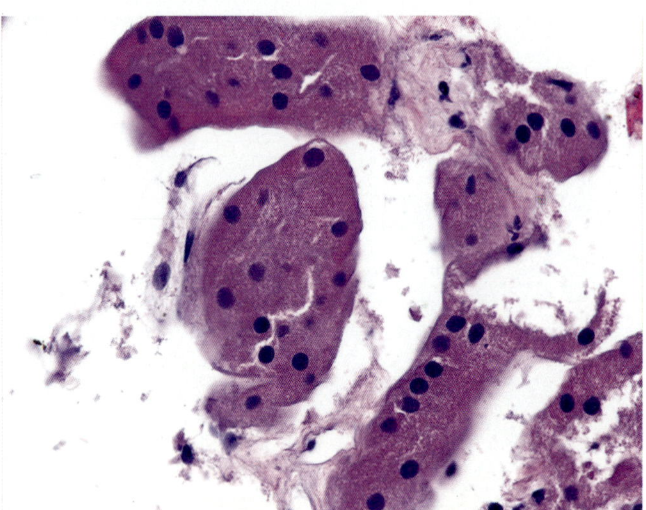

Figure 4.9 — Kidney, Oncocytoma (Core Biopsy). A core biopsy of the lesion shows bland round nuclei, surrounded by abundant finely granular cytoplasm. Chromophobe renal cell carcinoma remains in the differential diagnosis. Surgical excision, often a partial nephrectomy if possible, is indicated for both diagnoses. (Hematoxylin and eosin stain, high power)

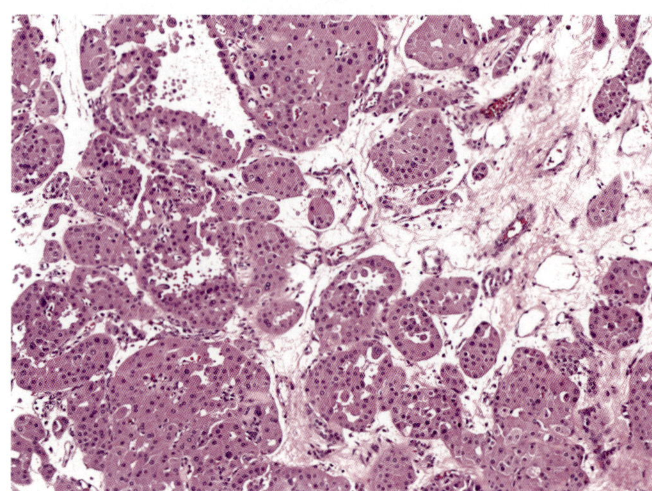

Figure 4.10 — Kidney, Oncocytoma (Histology). Tumor cells show abundant eosinophilic granular cytoplasm and small, round uniform nuclei. The neoplastic cells are arranged in nests and tubules. The background shows a loose fibromyxoid stroma that is characteristic of oncocytoma. (Hematoxylin and eosin stain, low power)

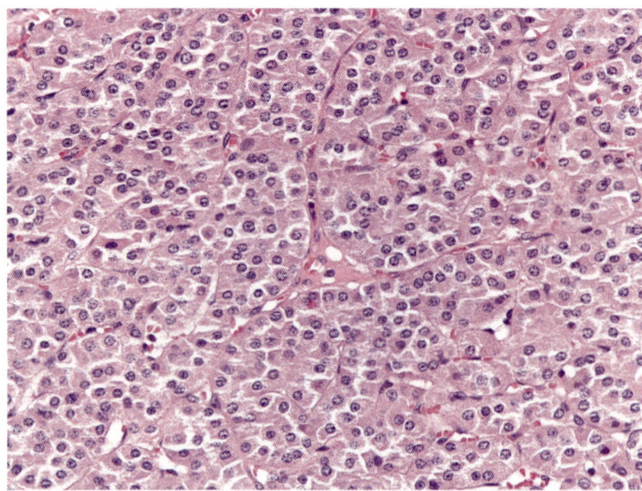

Figure 4.11 — Kidney, Oncocytoma (Histology). An oncocytoma with a prominent solid growth pattern is shown. The tumor shows uniform cells with low nuclear-to-cytoplasmic ratios and uniform, round nuclei. In some nuclei there are small inconspicuous nucleoli. (Hematoxylin and eosin stain, medium power)

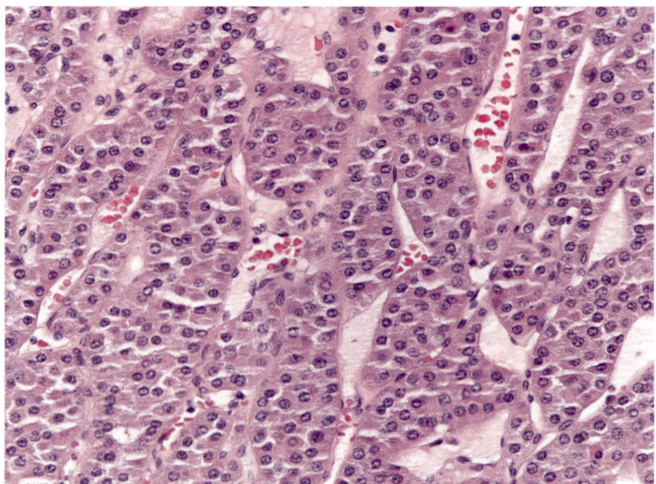

Figure 4.12 — Kidney, Oncocytoma (Histology). Oncocytoma may display several phenotypic patterns: nesting, alveolar, or tubular. In this case, the neoplastic cells are forming cords or tubule-like structures of uniform round/polygonal cells with abundant, intensely eosinophilic and granular cytoplasm. Nuclei are uniform, round, and central with evenly dispersed chromatin and smooth contours. (Hematoxylin and eosin stain, medium power)

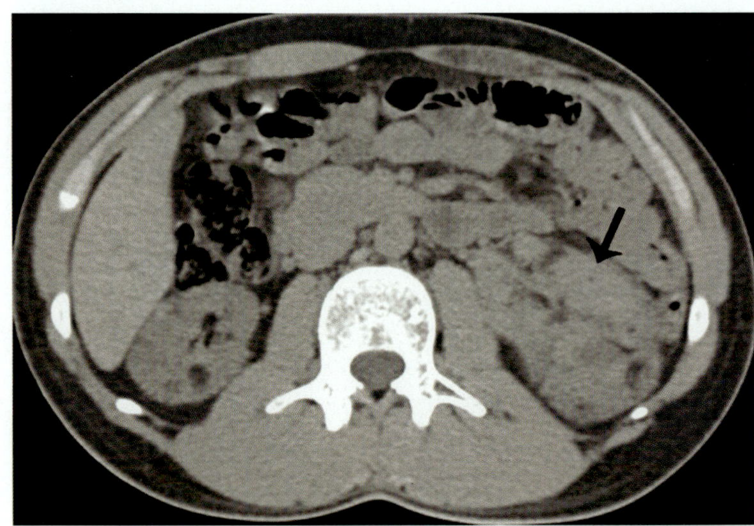

Figure 4.13 — Kidney, Angiomyolipoma. Axial CT without contrast shows a large soft tissue mass in the left kidney (arrow) and multiple small bilateral angiomyolipomas. This patient has a history of tuberous sclerosis which is associated with multiple, bilateral angiomyolipomas.

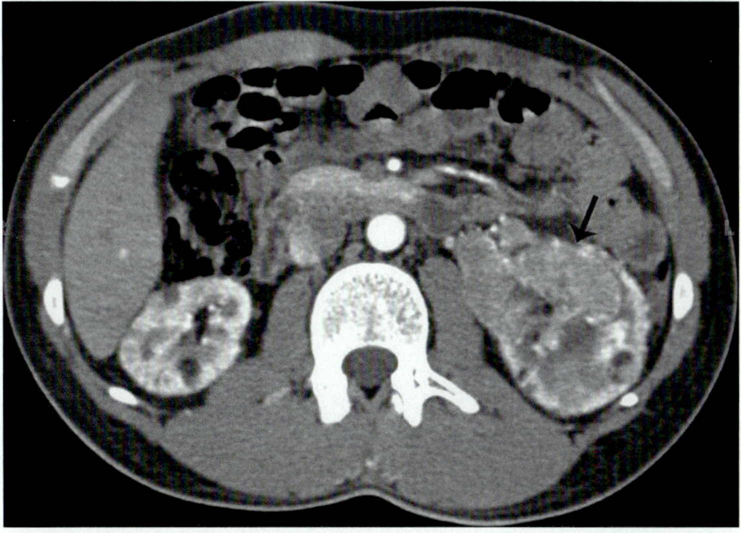

Figure 4.14 — Kidney, Angiomyolipoma. Contrast-enhanced CT shows the mass in the left kidney enhances in the arterial phase (arrow) and also contains small fatty components which are characteristic of angiomyolipoma. The mass involves the left renal sinus.

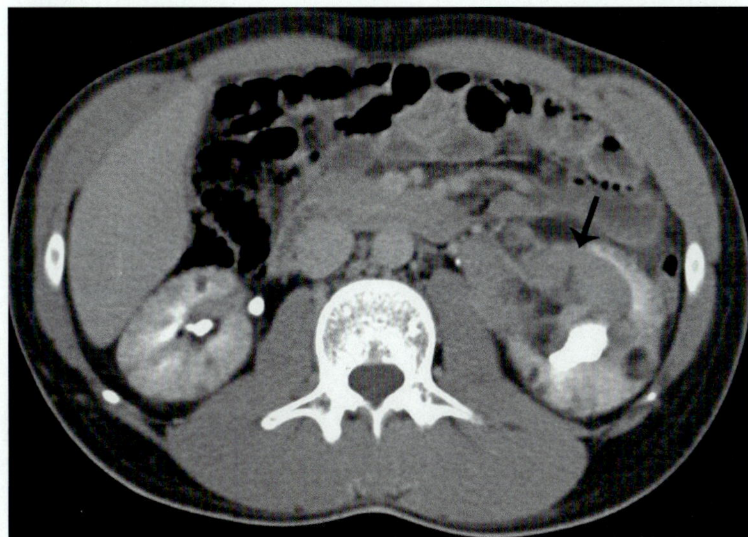

Figure 4.15 — Kidney, Angiomyolipoma. Axial contrast-enhanced CT in the delayed phase shows the enhancing soft tissue mass in the left kidney (arrow) containing fatty components. The mass involves the left renal sinus. There are also multiple additional smaller bilateral angiomyolipomas.

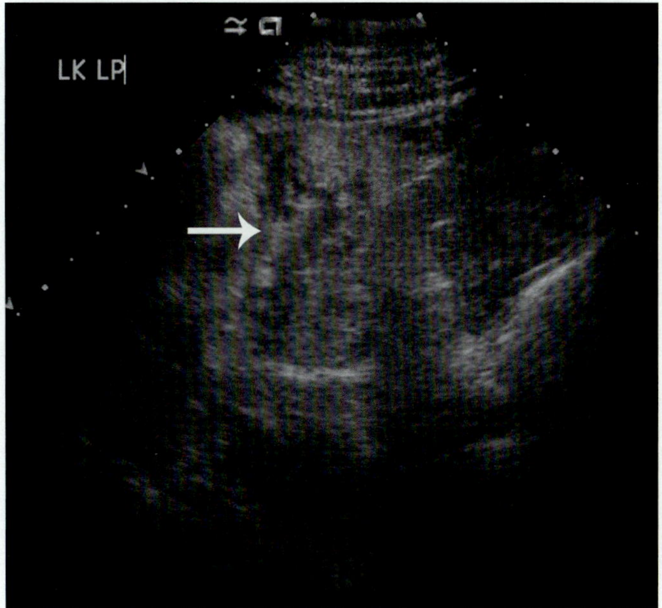

Figure 4.16 — Kidney, Angiomyolipoma. Sonographic image confirms echogenic mass in the left kidney (arrow). The imaging characteristics of angiomyolipoma are often so characteristic that tissue diagnosis is not required.

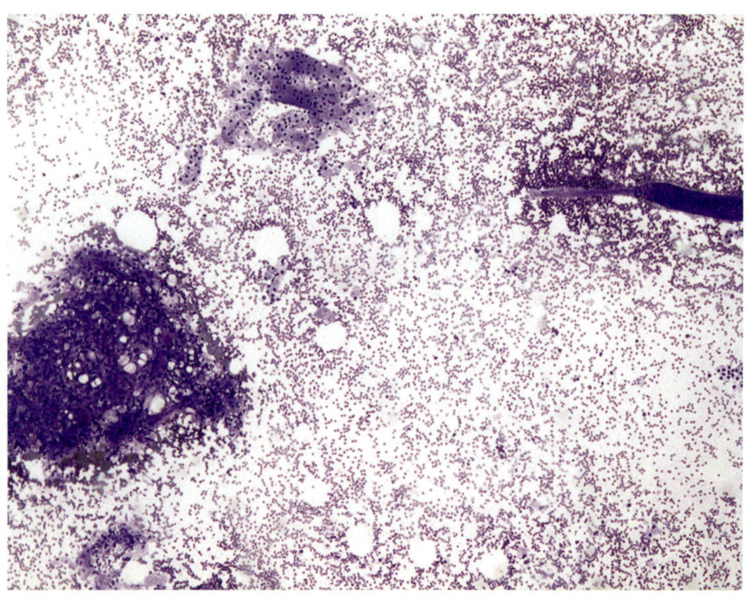

Figure 4.17 — Kidney, Angiomyolipoma. A polymorphic appearance is often appreciated in this tumor. At low power, several different cell types are appreciated. There is adipose tissue present in the left portion of the field, epithelioid cells in the top center, and a medium-sized vessel present at right. (Diff Quik stain, low power)

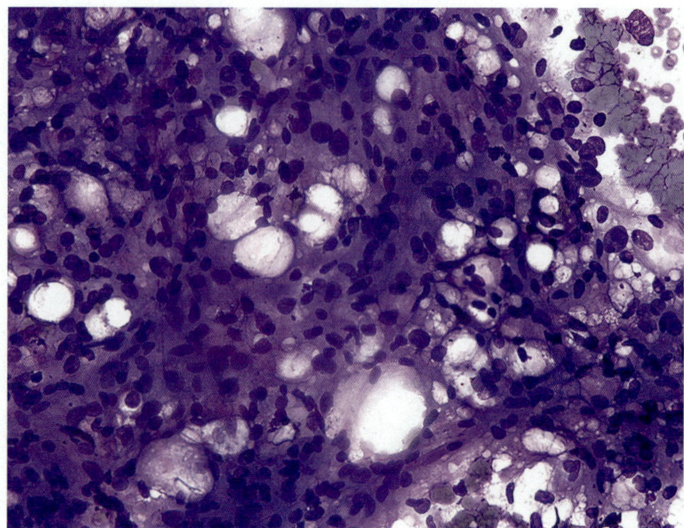

Figure 4.18 — Kidney, Angiomyolipoma. On higher magnification, small, bland spindle cells representing smooth muscle cells are admixed with adipose tissue. Angiomyolipoma is a member of the group of neoplasms known as perivascular epithelioid cell (PEC) tumors, or PEComas. (Diff Quik stain, high power)

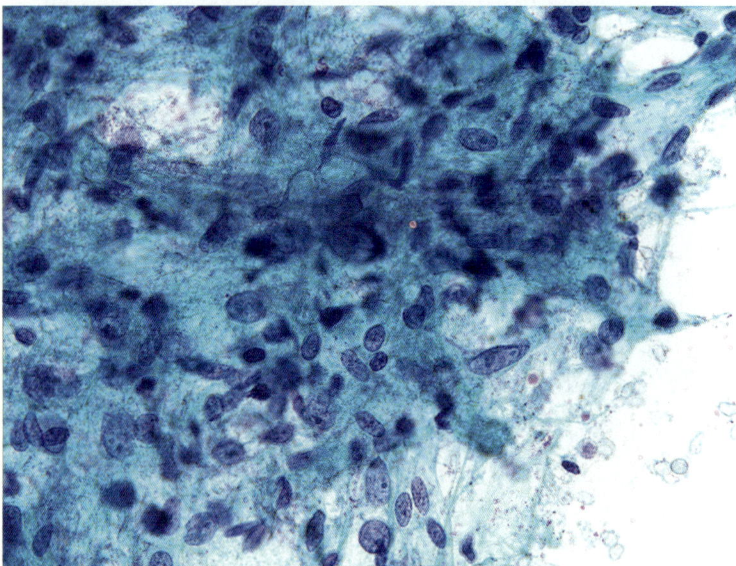

Figure 4.19 — Kidney, Angiomyolipoma. The spindle cells show minimal nuclear atypia. The differential diagnosis includes leiomyoma, particularly when the spindle cell component is prominent. (Papanicolaou stain, high power)

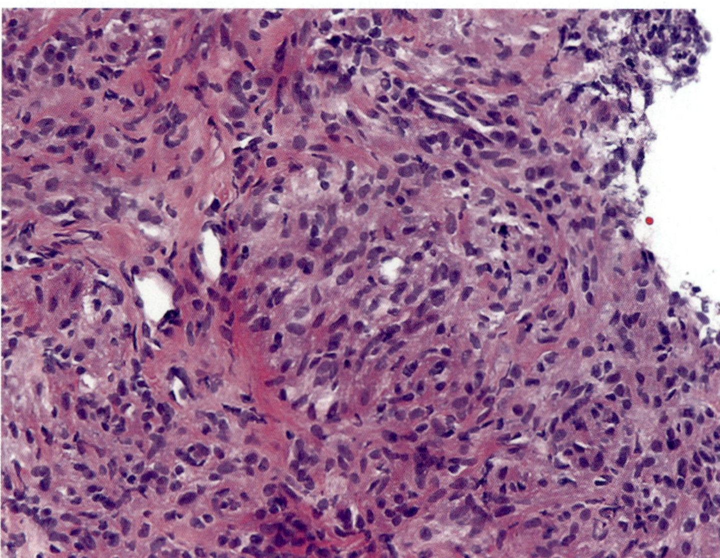

Figure 4.20 — Kidney, Angiomyolipoma (Core Biopsy). Bland spindle cells are admixed with small blood vessels. The adipocytic component may be scant, making a morphologic definitive diagnosis more difficult. (Hematoxylin and eosin stain, high power)

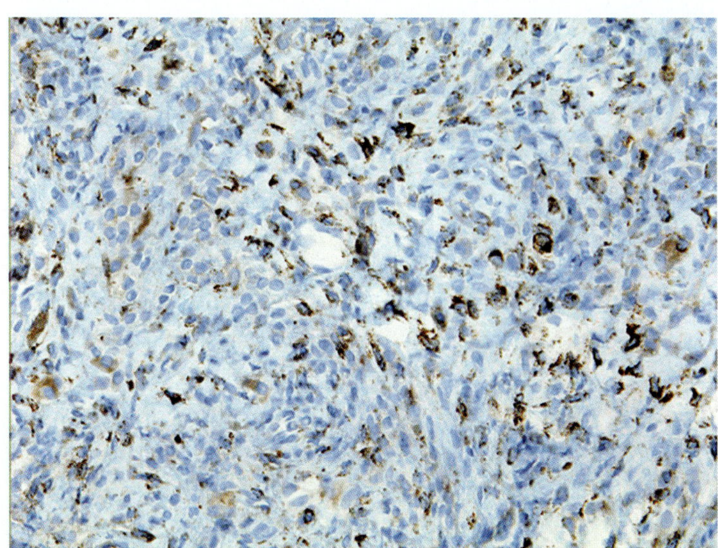

Figure 4.21 — Kidney, Angiomyolipoma (Core Biopsy). PEComas are characterized by positivity for HMB45, as is seen here. Renal cell carcinoma, which is often in the differential diagnosis, is negative for HMB45. (HMB45 immunostain, high power)

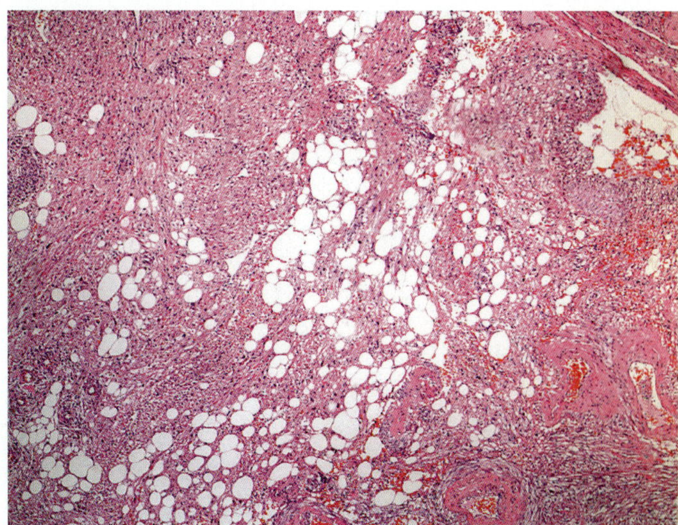

Figure 4.22 — Kidney, Angiomyolipoma. The tumor is composed of a mixture of blood vessels, fat, and smooth muscle. Grossly, this tumor, because of its yellow color, may be mistaken for a renal cell carcinoma. The blood vessels in angiomyolipomas often are tortuous and thick walled. Mitotic activity is not observed. There is no true capsule. (Hematoxylin and eosin stain, low power)

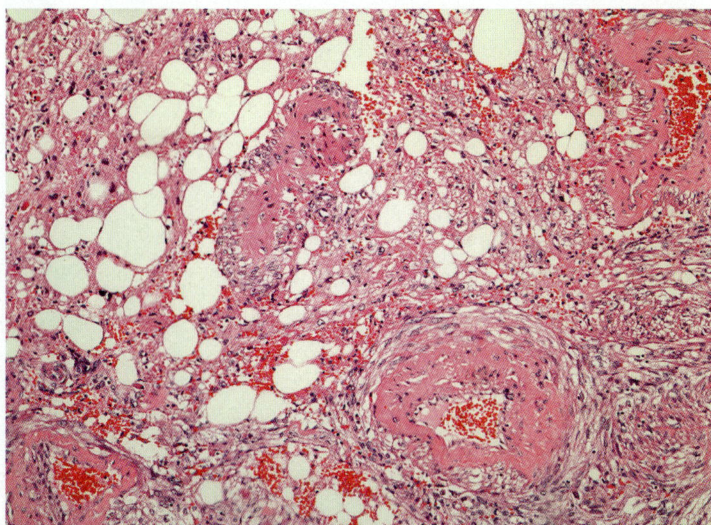

Figure 4.23 — Kidney, Angiomyolipoma. This tumor shows a mixture of benign-appearing mature fat, smooth muscle, and aggregates of thick-walled blood vessels. There is often degenerative-type atypia in the smooth muscle component with enlarged and sometimes multinucleated cells. (Hematoxylin and eosin stain, high power)

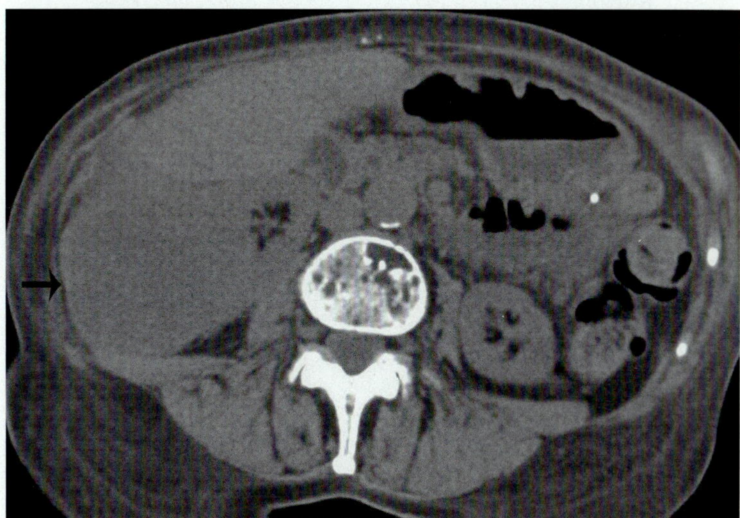

Figure 4.24 — Kidney, Inflammatory Myofibroblastic Tumor. This 66-year-old woman had a history of inflammatory myofibroblastic tumor in the right lung status post-resection 4 years prior and was found to have an abdominal mass on follow-up imaging. Axial noncontrast CT of the abdomen shows a large mass in the outer portion of the right kidney (arrow).

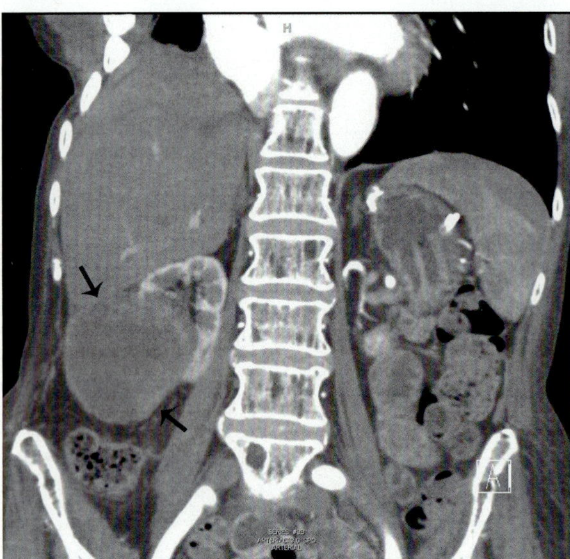

Figure 4.25 — Kidney, Inflammatory Myofibroblastic Tumor. Coronal contrast-enhanced CT in the arterial phase shows several areas of enhancement within the mass (arrows).

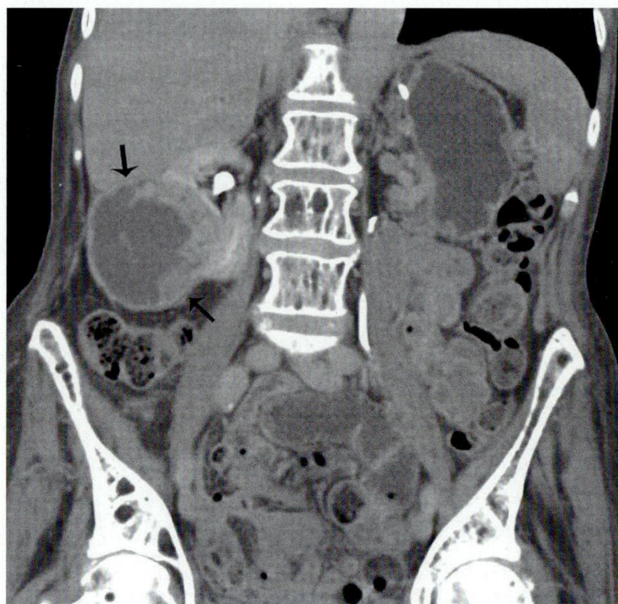

Figure 4.26 — Kidney, Inflammatory Myofibroblastic Tumor. Coronal contrast-enhanced CT in the delayed phase shows the large mass in the right kidney with prominent enhancing soft tissue component and a large area of necrosis (arrows).

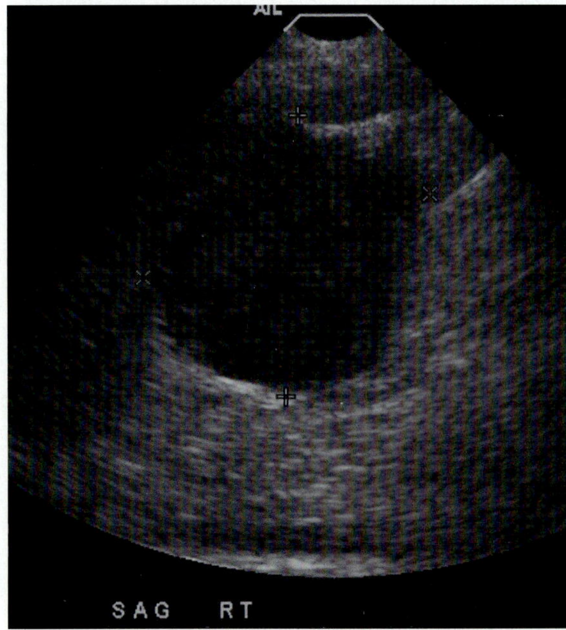

Figure 4.27 — Kidney, Inflammatory Myofibroblastic Tumor. Sonographic image at the time of ultrasound-guided biopsy shows the hypoechoic right renal mass. Although these tumors usually behave in a benign fashion, this mass represented a metastatic lesion from the patient's known lung primary.

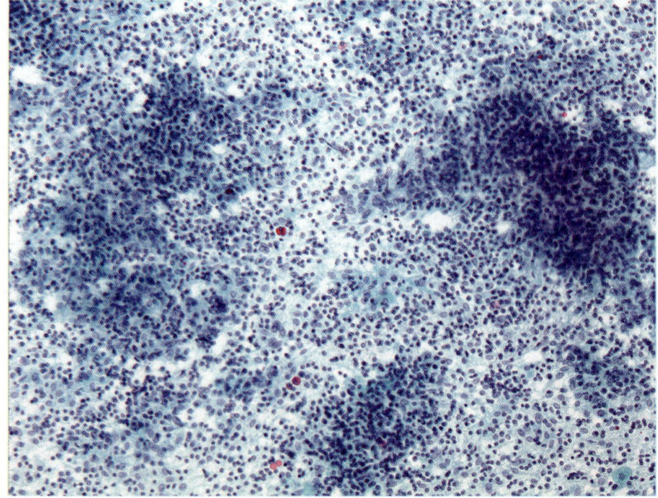

Figure 4.28 — Kidney, Inflammatory Myofibroblastic Tumor. A mixture of spindled myofibroblastic cells are seen surrounded by an inflammatory infiltrate composed predominantly of plasma cells and small lymphocytes. Although this lesion represented a metastasis, primary inflammatory myofibroblastic tumors of the kidney do occur. (Papanicolaou stain, medium power)

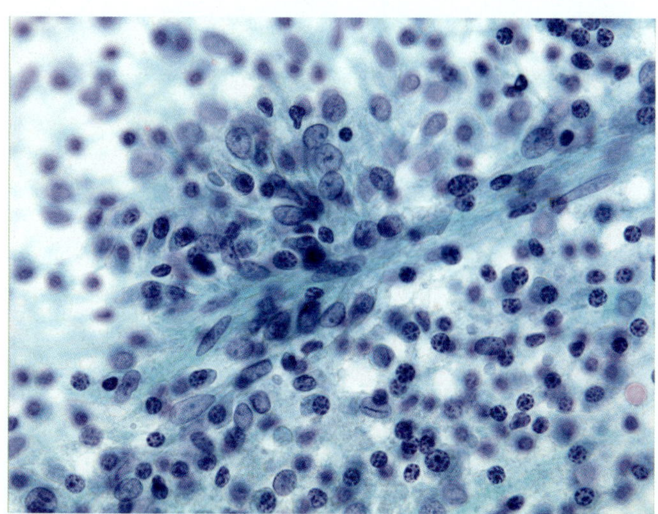

Figure 4.29 — Kidney, Inflammatory Myofibroblastic Tumor. Bland spindle cells with pale chromatin and smooth nuclear borders are practically obscured by abundant inflammatory cells. Inflammatory myofibroblastic tumors are also referred to as "inflammatory pseudotumors." (Papanicolaou stain, high power)

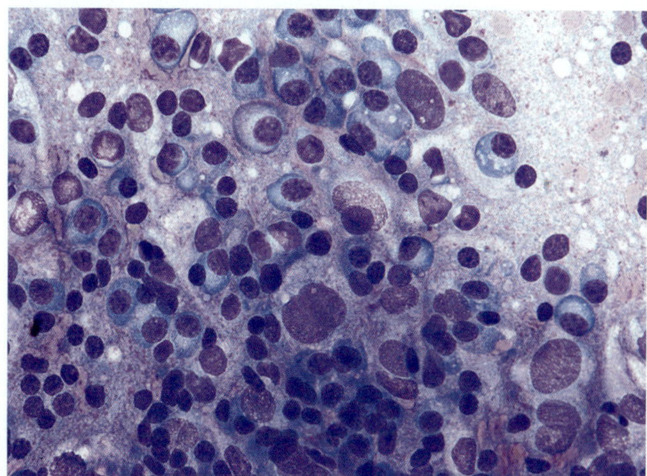

Figure 4.30 — Kidney, Inflammatory Myofibroblastic Tumor. Numerous plasma cells are identified by their basophilic cytoplasm and perinuclear clearing (hof). Few myofibroblastic cells are scattered among the inflammation. The differential diagnosis includes fibromatosis and granulation tissue. (Diff Quik stain, medium power)

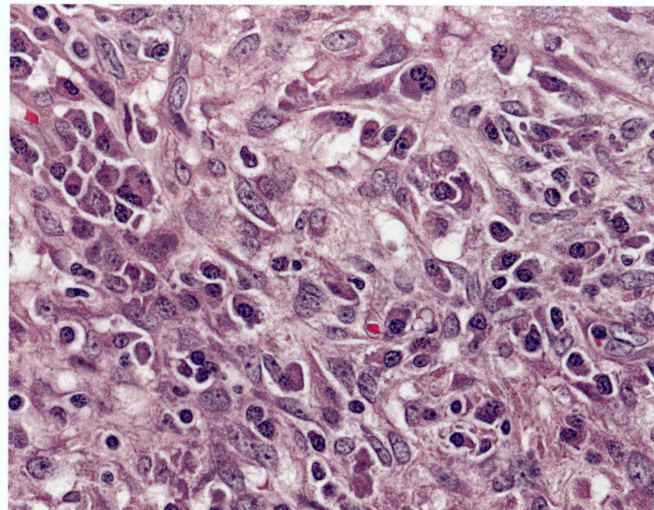

Figure 4.31 — Kidney, Inflammatory Myofibroblastic Tumor (Core Biopsy). On high power, spindle cells are seen in a background of numerous plasma cells and lymphocytes. Inflammatory myofibroblastic tumors are immunoreactive for smooth muscle actin and over half of the cases are positive for ALK, which portends a worse prognosis. (Hematoxylin and eosin stain, high power)

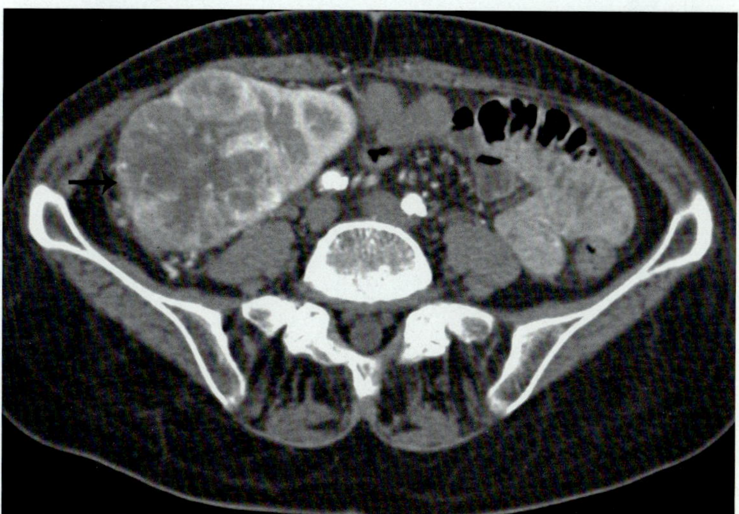

Figure 4.32 — Kidney, Renal Cell Carcinoma, Conventional (Clear Cell) Type. This 69-year-old woman had no pertinent past medical history. Axial contrast-enhanced CT image in the arterial phase shows a large, heterogeneous, hypervascular right renal mass (arrow). Clear cell carcinomas are the most common subtype of renal cell carcinoma and are commonly hypervascular.

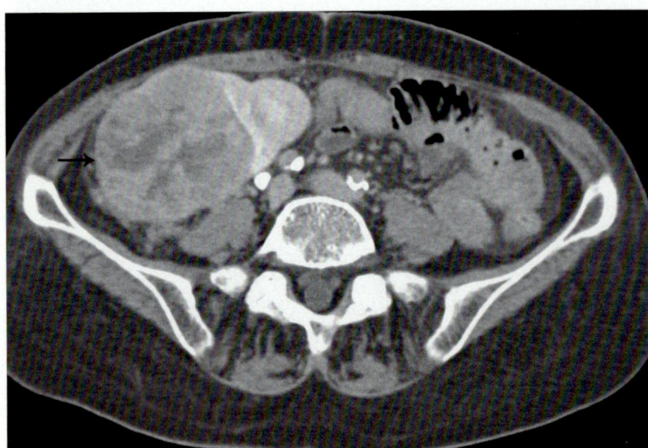

Figure 4.33 — Kidney, Renal Cell Carcinoma, Conventional (Clear Cell) Type. There is a prominent soft tissue component within the mass in the delayed phase (arrow). Clear cell carcinomas are commonly heterogeneous due to hemorrhage and necrosis.

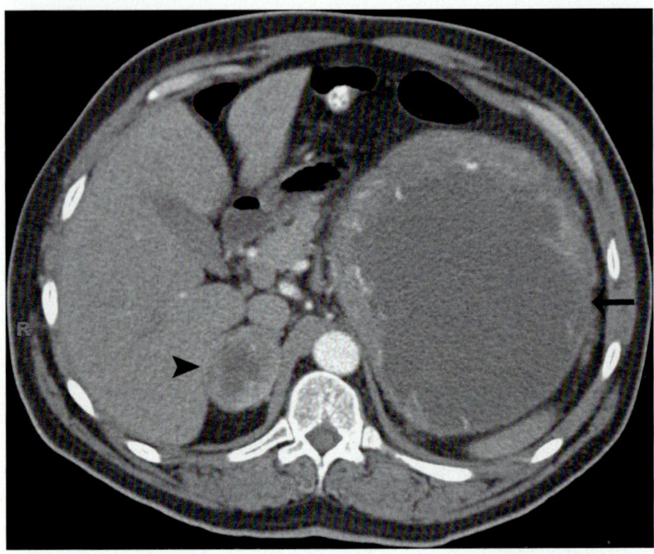

Figure 4.34 — Kidney, Renal Cell Carcinoma, Conventional (Clear Cell) Type. This 52-year-old man presented with shortness of breath and respiratory distress and a CT was performed. Axial contrast-enhanced CT image in the arterial phase shows a large, peripherally enhancing left renal mass (arrow) containing a large central area of necrosis. There is soft tissue component in the mass predominantly in the periphery. A right adrenal mass representing a metastasis is also present (arrowhead).

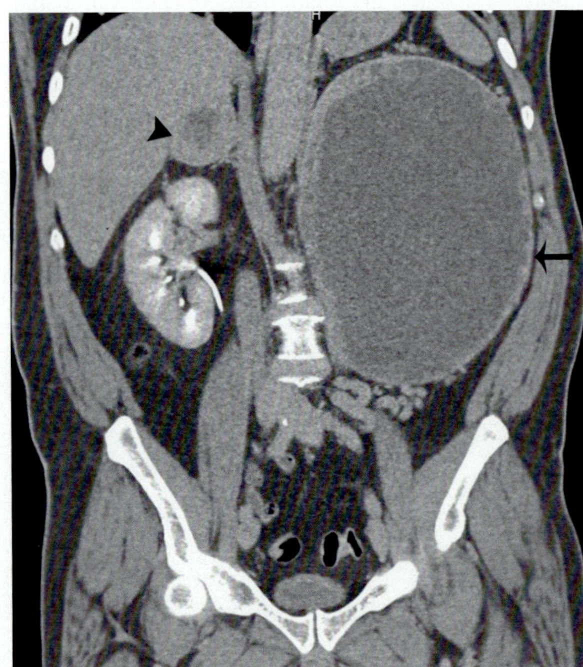

Figure 4.35 — Kidney, Renal Cell Carcinoma, Conventional (Clear Cell) Type. Coronal contrast-enhanced CT in the delayed phase confirms the large, necrotic enhancing left renal mass (arrow) as well as a small amount of soft tissue component in the mass predominantly in the periphery. A right adrenal heterogeneous mass is also present and is suspicious for a metastasis (arrowhead).

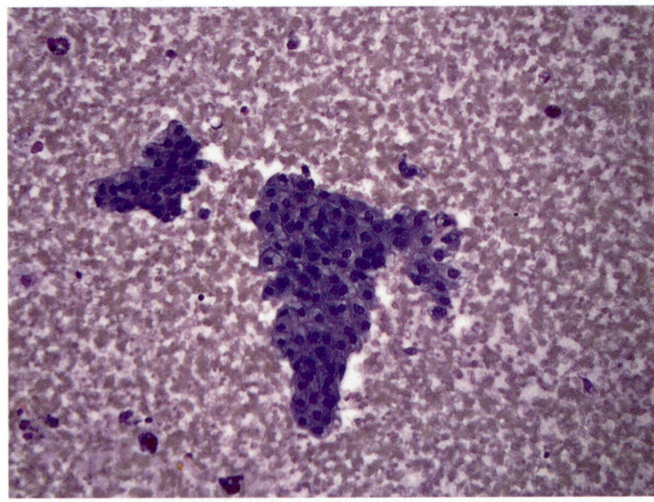

Figure 4.36 — Kidney, Renal Cell Carcinoma, Conventional (Clear Cell) Type. Two fragments of epithelial cells are present. The nuclei are round, N/C ratios are low, and there is abundant vacuolated cytoplasm. (Diff Quik stain, medium power)

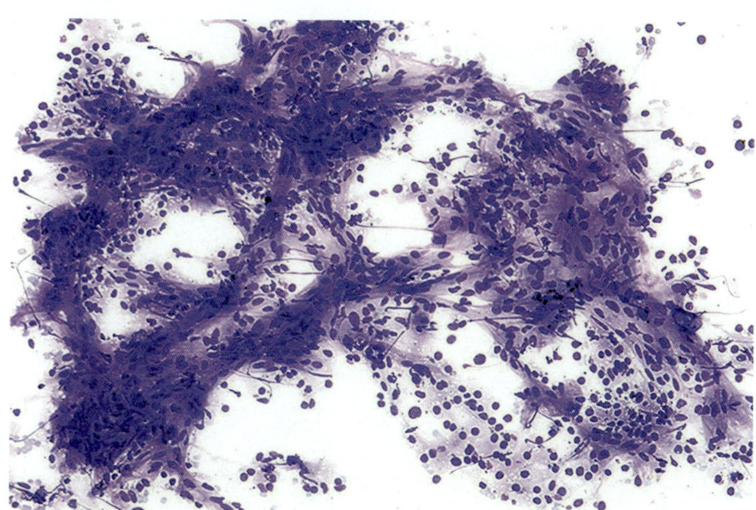

Figure 4.37 — Kidney, Renal Cell Carcinoma, Conventional (Clear Cell) Type. A complex matrix containing numerous small capillaries is shown. Scattered single tumor cells are evident, particularly in the lower portion of the field. A large population of stripped-off "naked" nuclei is almost always present in the smear background, which may have a finely vacuolated "foamy" appearance. (Diff Quik stain, medium power)

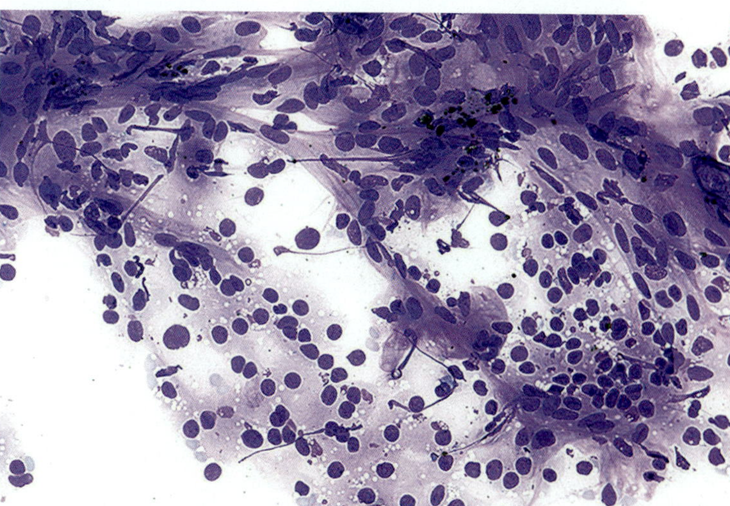

Figure 4.38 — Kidney, Renal Cell Carcinoma, Conventional (Clear Cell) Type. Small spindled endothelial cells line the capillary network. Tumor cells show abundant finely vacuolated cytoplasm and small round nuclei, suggesting a low Fuhrman grade. Fuhrman grading is not typically performed on cytologic specimens. (Diff Quik stain, high power)

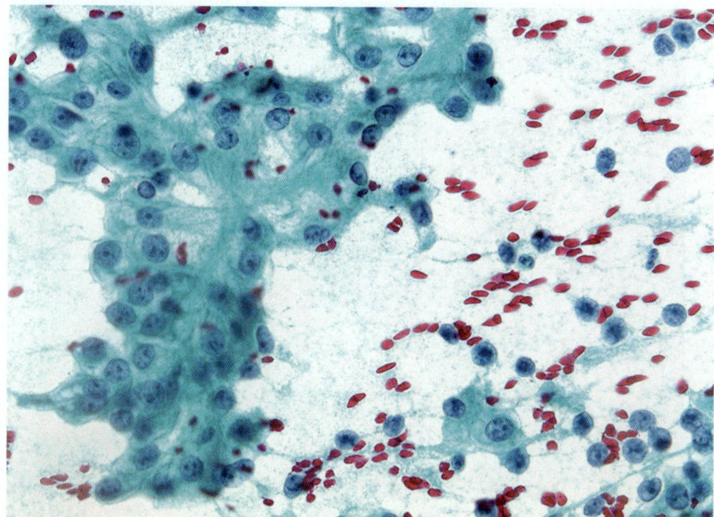

Figure 4.39 — Kidney, Renal Cell Carcinoma, Conventional (Clear Cell) Type. Cytoplasmic vacuolization, representing either fat or glycogen, is apparent. Sampling of benign adrenal cortical cells should be considered in the differential. However, in this case, the nuclei are enlarged and display prominent nucleoli. Background has a distinct granular appearance. (Papanicolaou stain, high power)

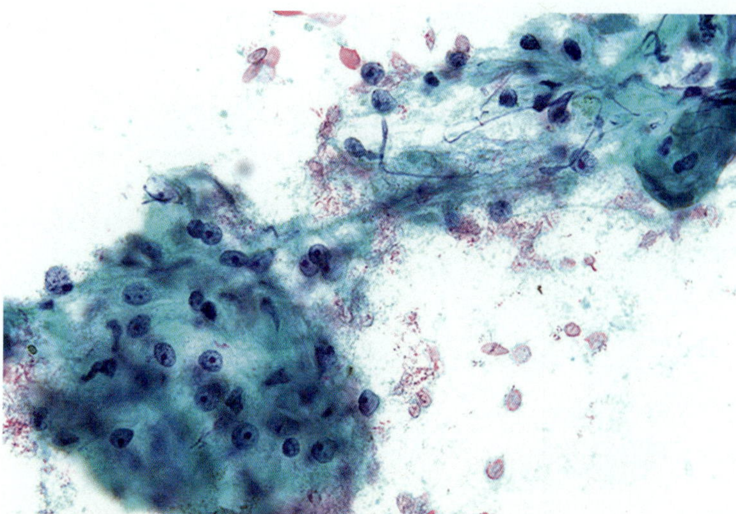

Figure 4.40 — Kidney, Renal Cell Carcinoma, Conventional (Clear Cell) Type. A cohesive fragment of cells with abundant cytoplasm and ill-defined cell borders is present. Histiocytes are also considered in the differential, but the round nuclei and prominent nucleoli seen here are not features of histiocytes. (Papanicolaou stain, high power)

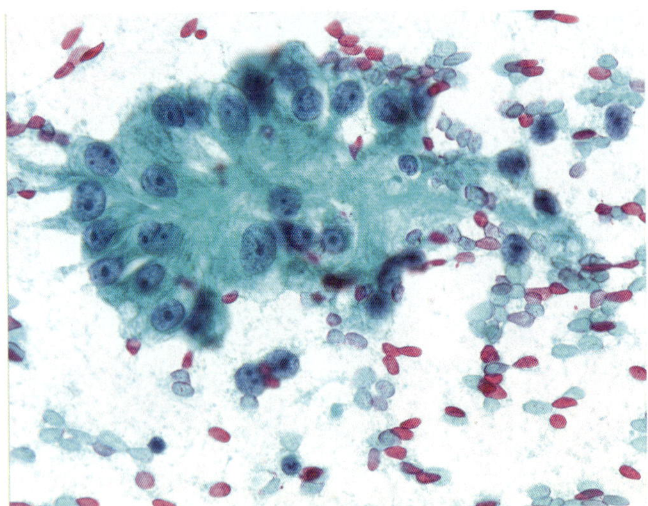

Figure 4.41 — Kidney, Renal Cell Carcinoma, Conventional (Clear Cell) Type. The neoplastic cells have delicate cytoplasm and round to oval, bland nuclei with prominent nucleoli. Bare nuclei may be present in the background due to the delicate nature of the cytoplasm, which is easily stripped (not shown). (Papanicolaou stain, high power)

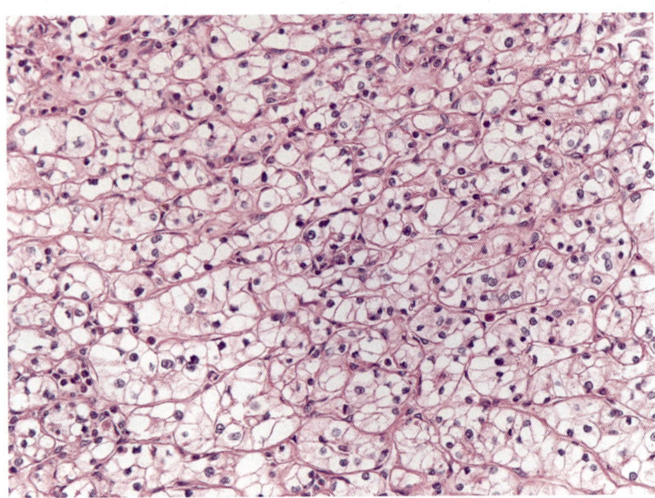

Figure 4.42 — Kidney, Renal Cell Carcinoma, Conventional (Clear Cell) Type (Histology). Clear cell renal cell carcinoma is the most common renal malignancy in adults. Malignant epithelial cells show clear cytoplasm and nested growth pattern. The neoplasm has characteristic delicate and extensive arborizing vasculature. Grossly, the tumor is typically well circumscribed with prominent cystic or hemorrhagic areas. (Hematoxylin and eosin stain, medium power)

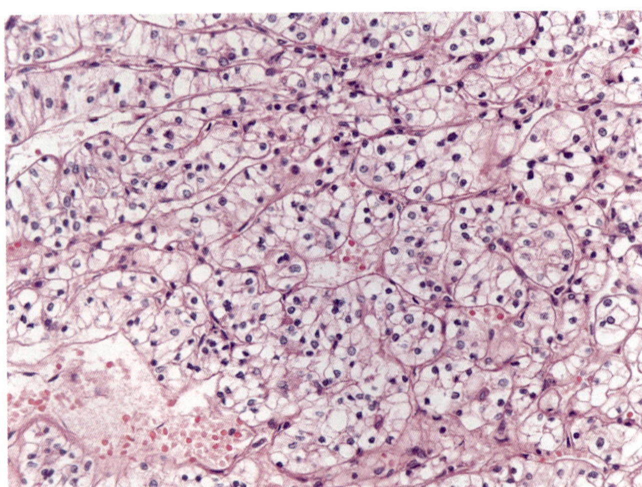

Figure 4.43 — Kidney, Renal Cell Carcinoma, Conventional (Clear Cell) Type (Histology). Tumor cells are arranged in nests and separated from each other by an extensive network of delicate sinusoidal capillaries. Some patients with renal cell carcinoma may have a paraneoplastic syndrome leading to the production of hormones such as erythropoietin causing polycythemia. (Hematoxylin and eosin stain, medium power)

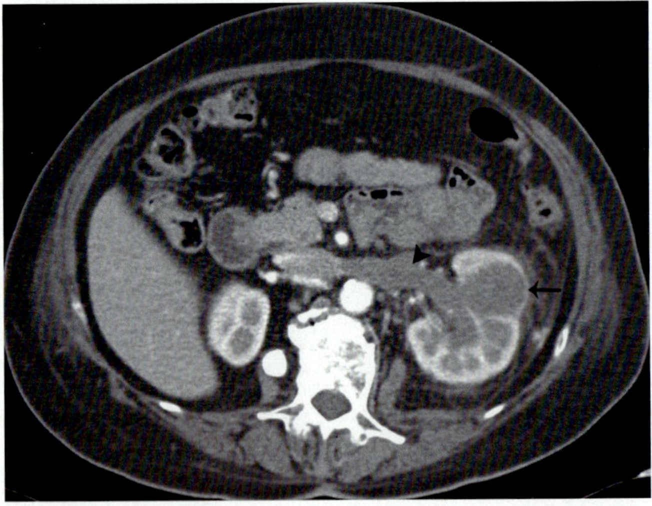

Figure 4.44 — Kidney, Renal Cell Carcinoma, Papillary Type. This 71-year-old female presented with acute onset left-sided pain. Axial contrast-enhanced CT in the arterial phase shows a hypovascular left renal mass (arrow) extending into the left renal vein (arrowhead). Papillary renal cell carcinomas are commonly hypovascular and are the second most common type of primary renal cell carcinoma after clear cell type.

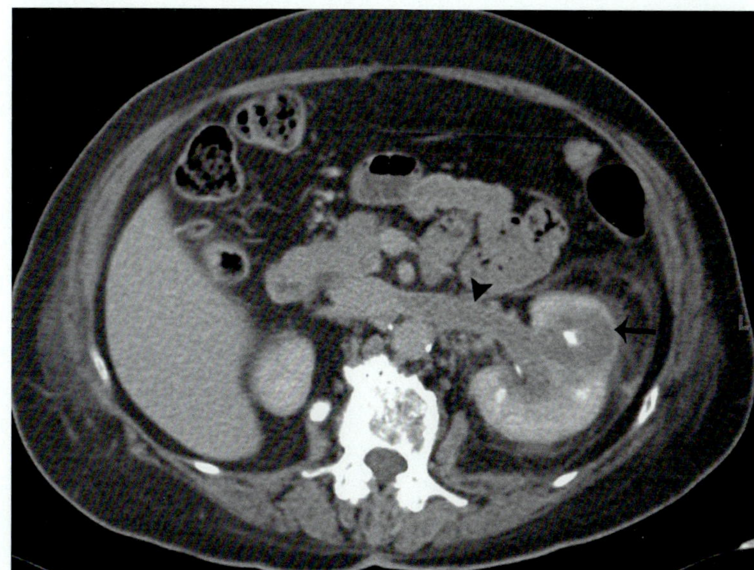

Figure 4.45 — Kidney, Renal Cell Carcinoma, Papillary Type. The mass is hypovascular in the delayed phase (arrow) and extends into the left renal vein (arrowhead).

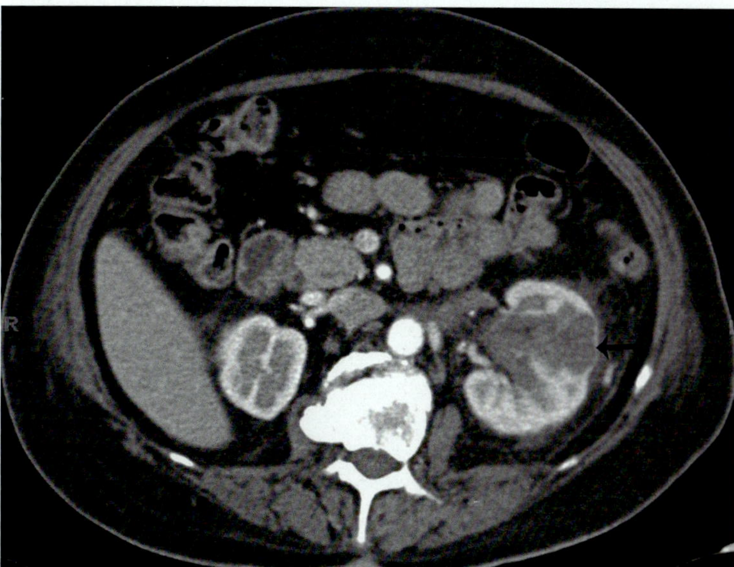

Figure 4.46 — Kidney, Renal Cell Carcinoma, Papillary Type. Axial contrast-enhanced CT in the arterial phase more inferiorly shows further extent of the mass in the renal parenchyma (arrow).

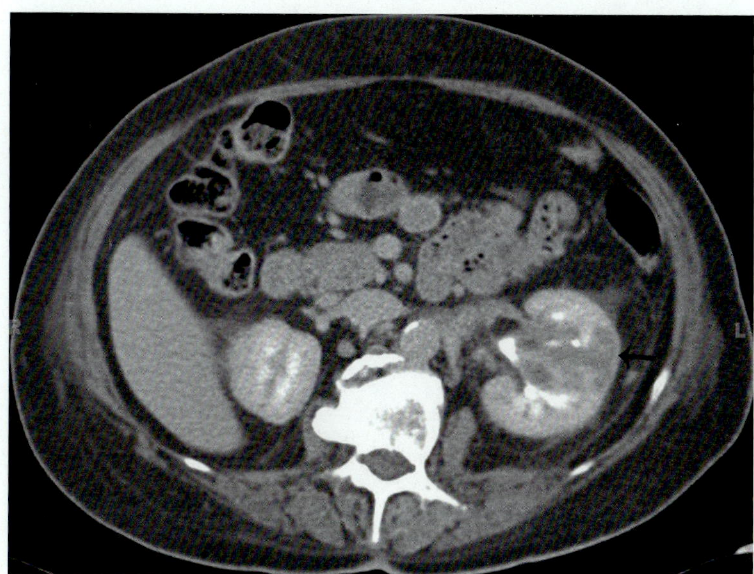

Figure 4.47 — Kidney, Renal Cell Carcinoma, Papillary Type. Axial contrast-enhanced CT in the delayed phase at the same level shows minimal enhancement of the mass (arrow).

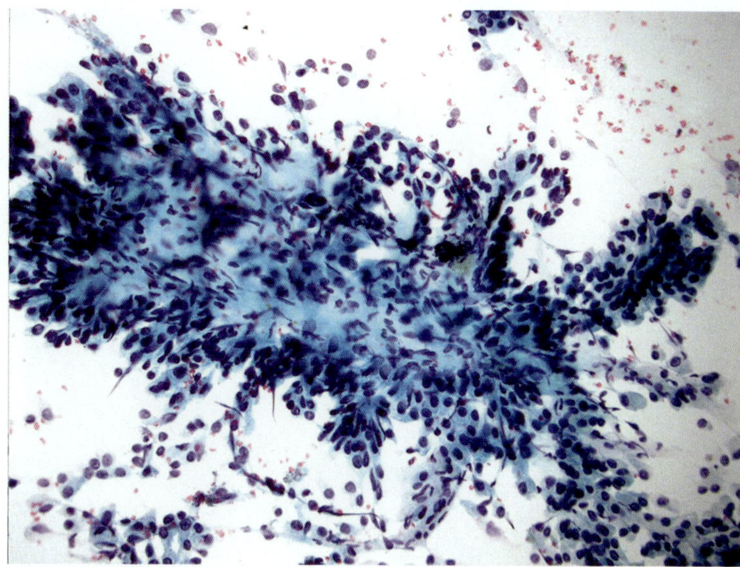

Figure 4.48 — Kidney, Renal Cell Carcinoma, Papillary Type. A cellular fragment with a papillary configuration is shown. There is a central fibrovascular core surrounded by a uniform population of neoplastic cells with round to oval nuclei and ample cytoplasm. (Papanicolaou stain, medium power)

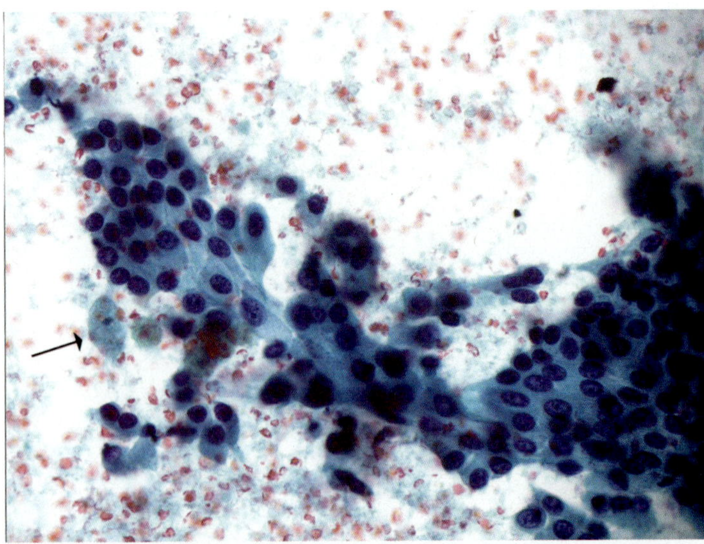

Figure 4.49 — Kidney, Renal Cell Carcinoma, Papillary Type. These tumor cells show abundant granular to opaque cytoplasm and round to oval nuclei. Note that nucleoli are not as prominent as in clear cell renal cell carcinoma. Scattered macrophages are present (arrow). (Papanicolaou stain, high power)

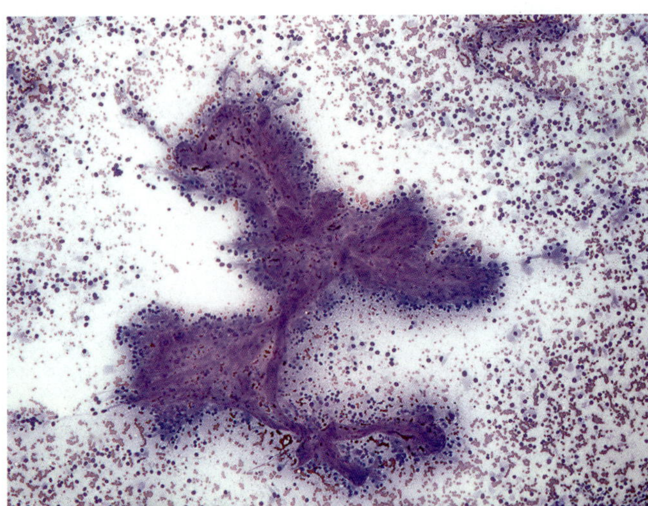

Figure 4.50 — Kidney, Renal Cell Carcinoma, Papillary Type. The papillary architecture of this fragment of malignant cells is evident with a well-defined fibrovascular core. The presence of a papillary architecture alone is insufficient for a diagnosis of papillary type renal cell carcinoma. (Diff Quik stain, medium power)

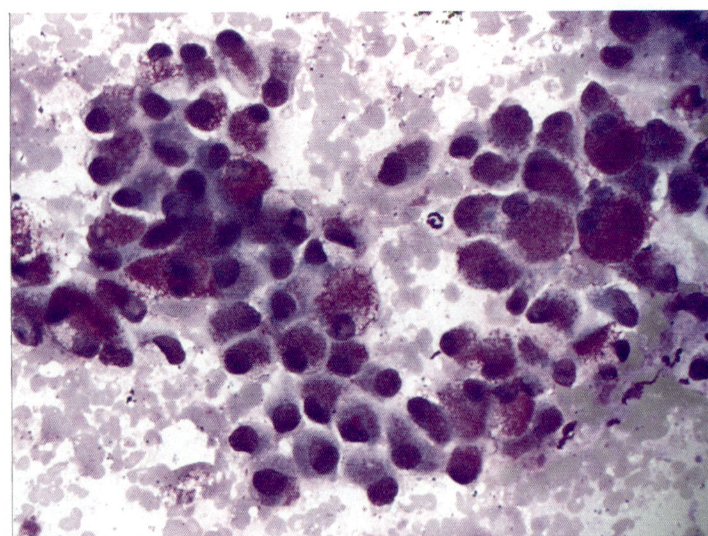

Figure 4.51 — Kidney, Renal Cell Carcinoma, Papillary Type. The tumor cells demonstrate a characteristic cytoplasmic granularity on Diff Quick stain. This likely reflects the type 2 or eosinophilic type of papillary renal cell carcinoma. (Diff Quik stain, high power)

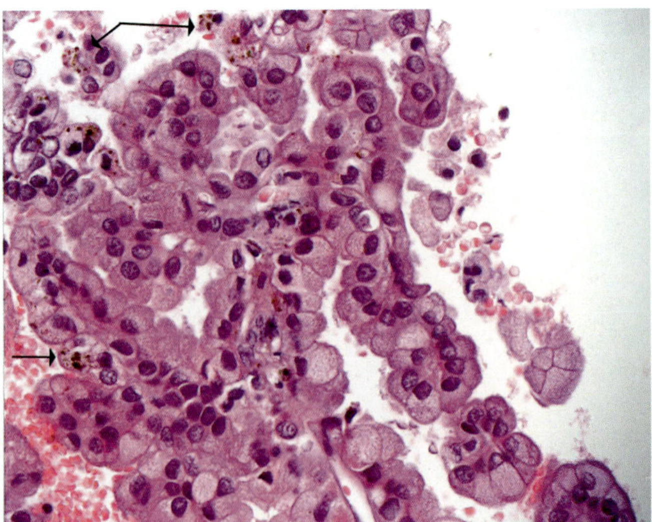

Figure 4.52 — Kidney, Renal Cell Carcinoma, Papillary Type (Cell Block). A cell block section highlights the papillary architecture. Cytoplasmic hemosiderin (arrows) and numerous foam cells are typical of papillary type renal cell carcinoma. Note the granularity of the tumor cell cytoplasm. (Hematoxylin and eosin stain, high power)

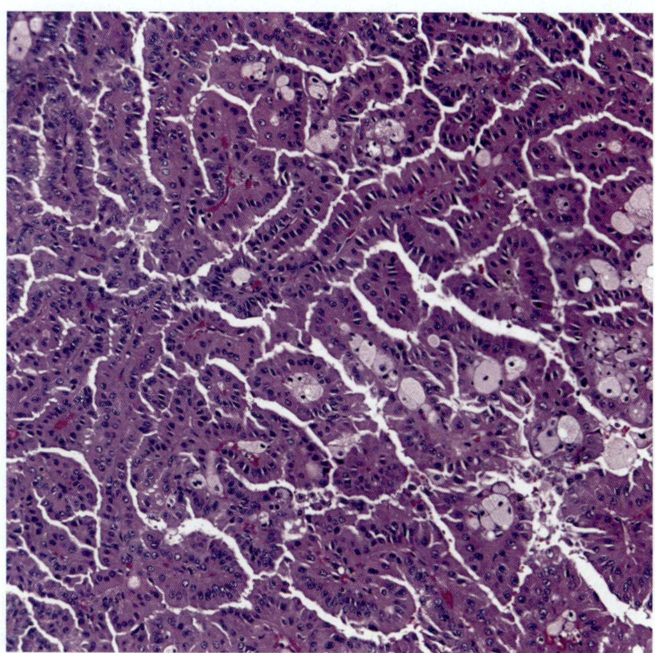

Figure 4.53 — Kidney, Renal Cell Carcinoma, Papillary Type (Histology). Papillary renal cell carcinoma is associated with gains of chromosome 7 or 17. The tumor has a distinct papillary architecture with cells showing mild to moderate pleomorphism and occasional nucleoli. (Hematoxylin and eosin stain, low power)

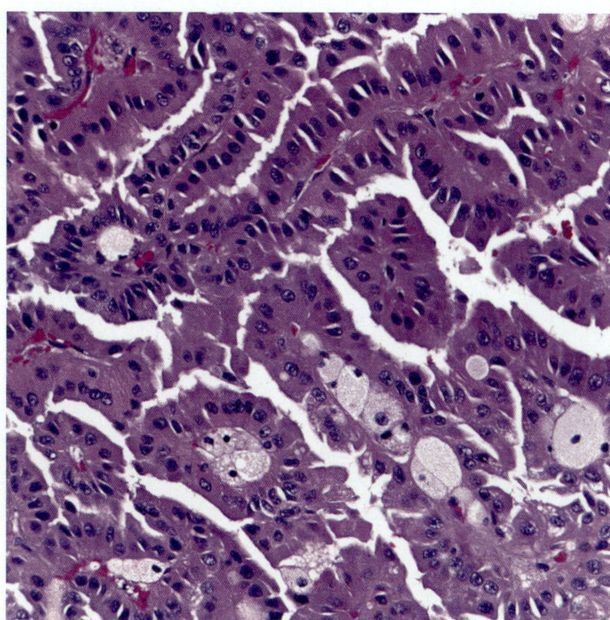

Figure 4.54 — Kidney, Renal Cell Carcinoma, Papillary Type (Histology). The papillary subtype of renal cell carcinoma is the most common subtype to present with bilateral tumors. The neoplasm is composed of papillae covered by large eosinophilic cells with round to oval nuclei and prominent nucleoli. Occasional foam cell are present in the fibrovascular cores. (Hematoxylin and eosin stain, medium power)

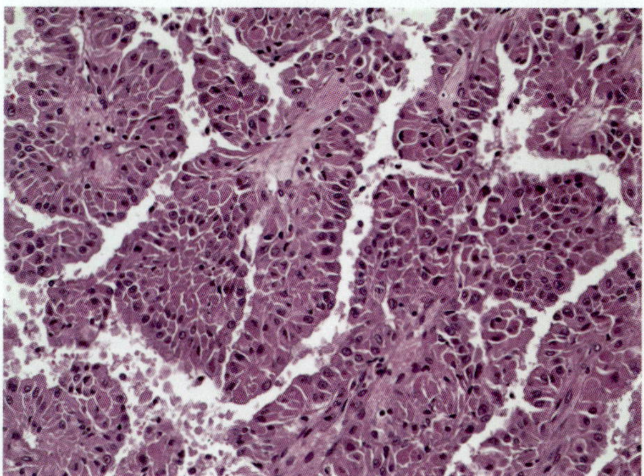

Figure 4.55 — Kidney, Renal Cell Carcinoma, Papillary Type (Histology). Papillary renal cell carcinoma, type 2 shows tall columnar cells with eosinophilic cytoplasm. Note the pseudostratified nuclei and prominent nucleoli. Fibrovascular papillary cores are present. (Hematoxylin and eosin stain, medium power)

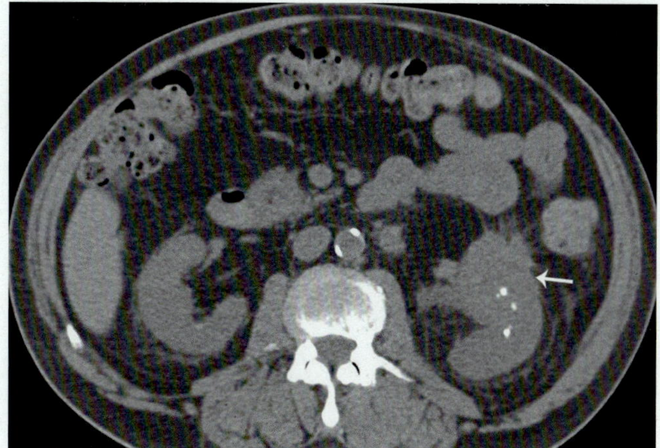

Figure 4.56 — Kidney, Urothelial Carcinoma. This 71-year-old man with a history of nephrolithiasis treated with extracorporeal shock wave lithotripsy presented with hematuria. Axial noncontrast CT shows an irregular mass in the left kidney (arrow). There are also several coarse calcifications in the left kidney.

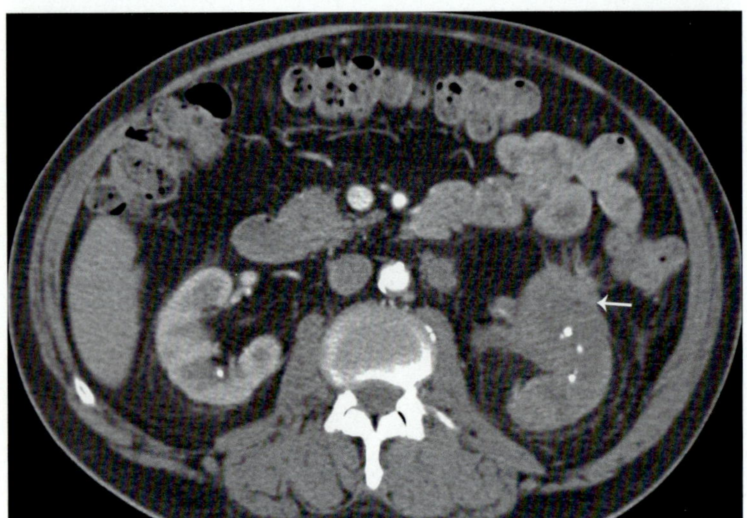

Figure 4.57 — Kidney, Urothelial Carcinoma. Axial contrast-enhanced CT in the arterial phase confirms an ill-defined, infiltrative mass in the left kidney (arrow) with mild enhancement.

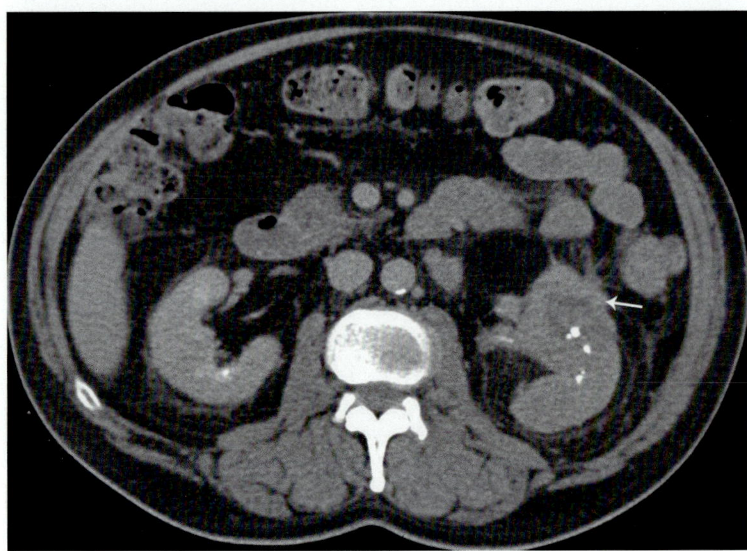

Figure 4.58 — Kidney, Urothelial Carcinoma. Axial contrast-enhanced CT in the delayed phase shows the ill-defined, infiltrative mass with mild enhancement (arrow) in the left kidney. There is perinephric extension of tumor anteriorly.

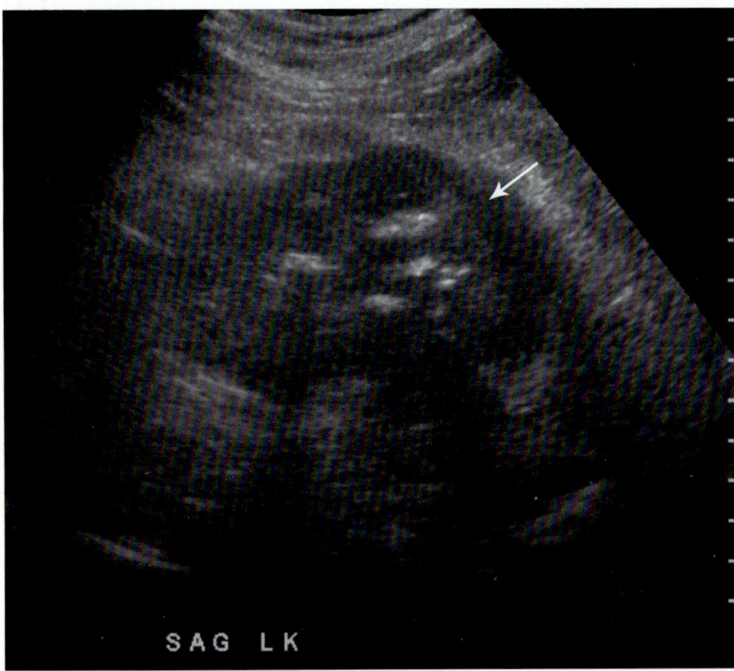

Figure 4.59 — Kidney, Urothelial Carcinoma. Sonographic image at the time of ultrasound-guided biopsy shows the infiltrative mass (arrow) in the left kidney. Urothelial carcinomas are commonly ill defined and infiltrative.

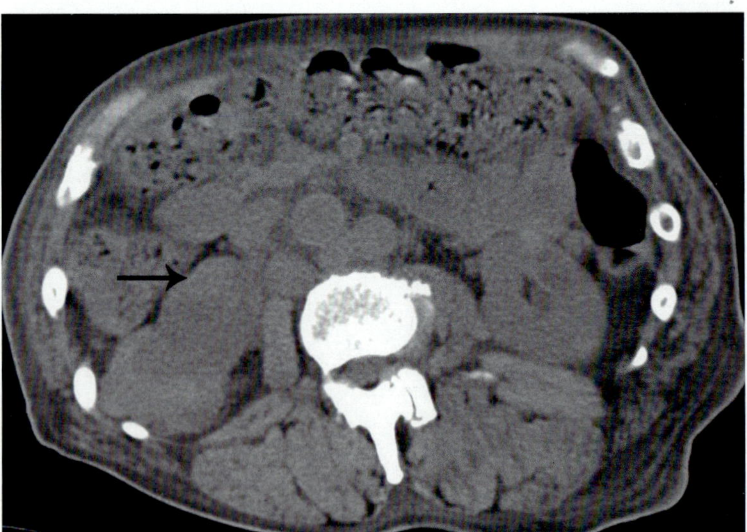

Figure 4.60 — Kidney, Urothelial Carcinoma. This patient presented with abdominal pain. Axial noncontrast CT shows moderate right hydronephrosis due to a soft tissue mass in the right renal pelvis and proximal right ureter (arrow).

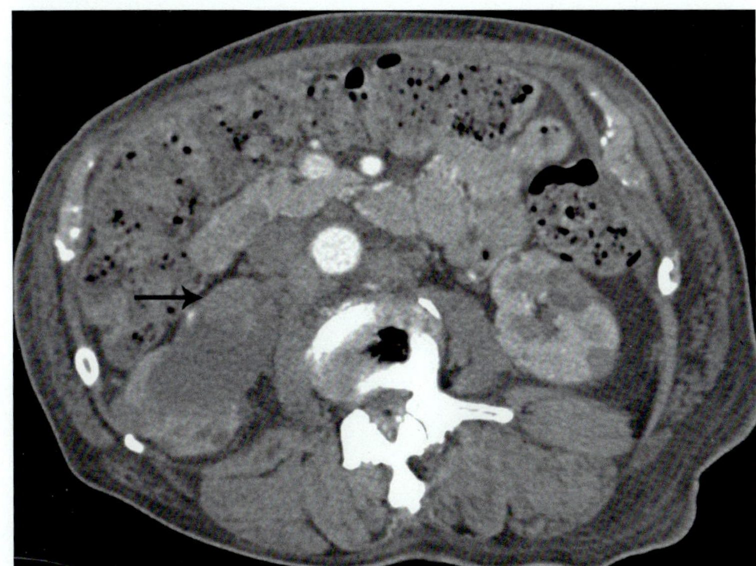

Figure 4.61 — Kidney, Urothelial Carcinoma. Axial contrast-enhanced CT in the arterial phase is shown. There is enhancement of the soft tissue mass in the right renal pelvis and proximal right ureter in the arterial phase (arrow).

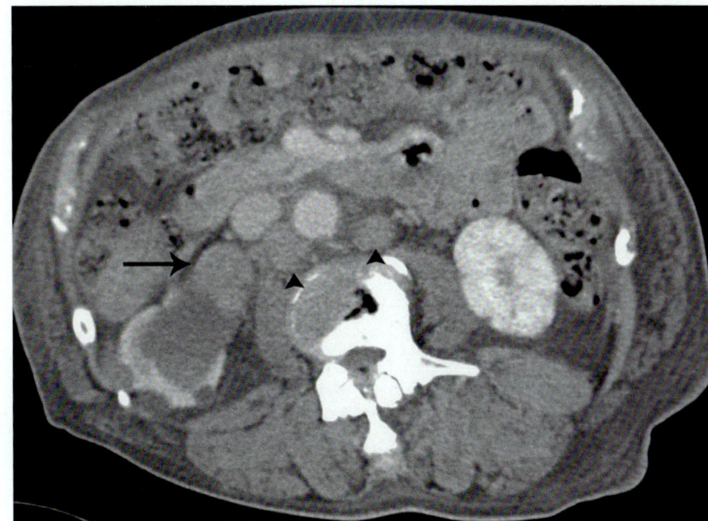

Figure 4.62 — Kidney, Urothelial Carcinoma. Axial contrast-enhanced CT in the venous phase also shows moderate right hydronephrosis due to the obstructing soft tissue mass in the right renal pelvis and proximal right ureter (arrow). There is also retroperitoneal adenopathy (arrowheads) representing metastatic disease.

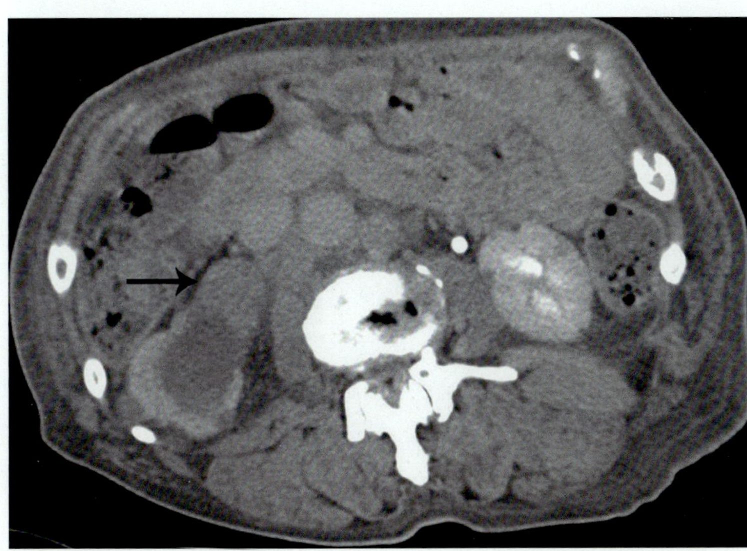

Figure 4.63 — Kidney, Urothelial Carcinoma. Axial contrast-enhanced CT in the delayed phase shows persistent enhancement of obstructing soft tissue mass in the right renal pelvis and proximal right ureter (arrow). An enhancing soft tissue mass in the renal collecting system is suggestive of malignancy.

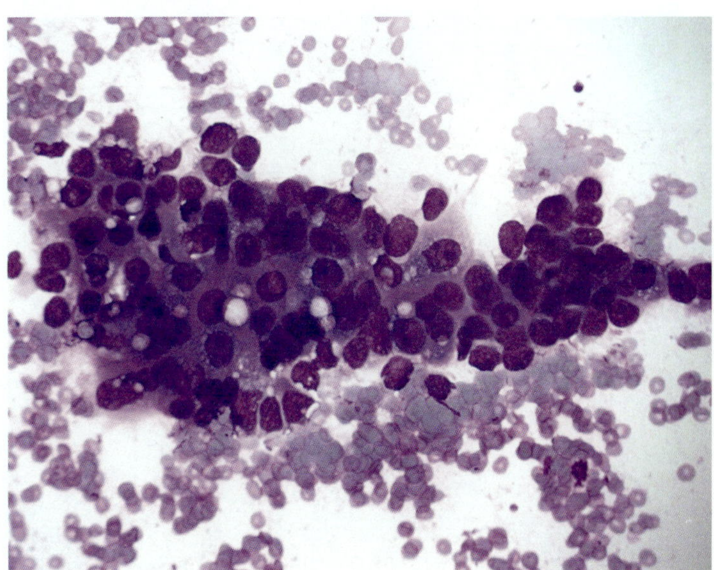

Figure 4.64 — Kidney, Urothelial Carcinoma. A cohesive fragment of epithelial cells shows high nuclear-to-cytoplasmic ratio and hyperchromatic oval-shaped nuclei. Urothelial carcinomas account for 5–10% of renal malignancies. (Diff Quik stain, high power)

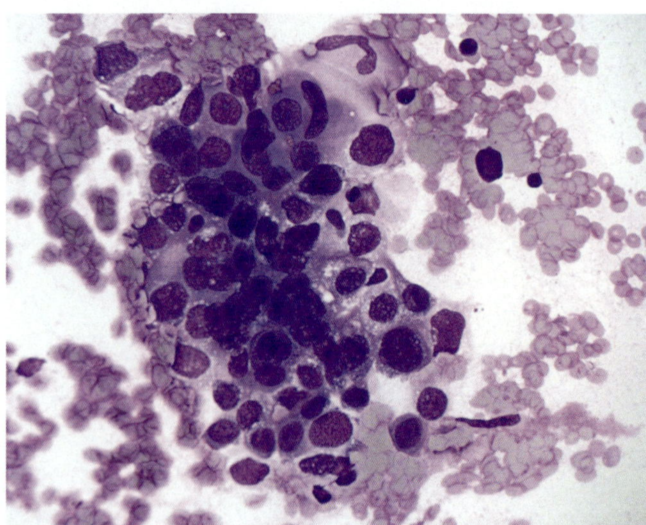

Figure 4.65 — Kidney, Urothelial Carcinoma. These nuclei show variation in size and hyperchromasia. High-grade urothelial carcinoma is often difficult to distinguish morphologically from high-grade renal cell carcinoma or metastatic neoplasms. (Diff Quik stain, high power)

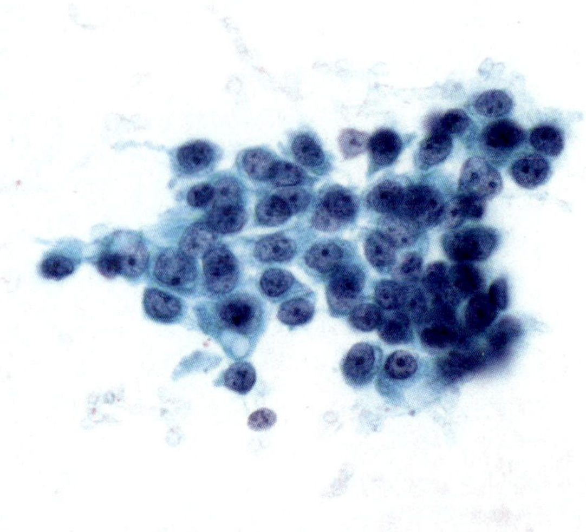

Figure 4.66 — Kidney, Urothelial Carcinoma. This group of malignant epithelial cells shows coarse chromatin and small- to medium-sized nucleoli. Urothelial carcinoma is frequently multifocal; thus, a diagnosis of urothelial carcinoma of the renal pelvis often prompts evaluation of the bladder and ureters for additional lesions. (Papanicolaou stain, high power)

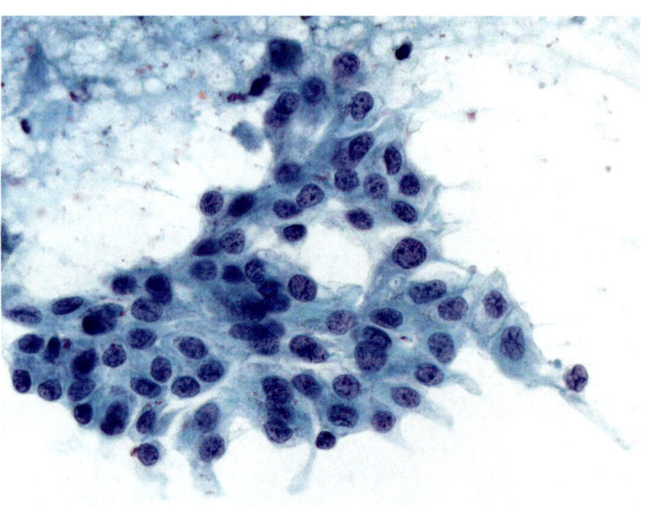

Figure 4.67 — Kidney, Urothelial Carcinoma. Malignant urothelial cells may have oval-shaped nuclei with intranuclear grooves, although this is not specific. Urothelial carcinoma frequently shows squamous cell differentiation (not shown). Pure squamous cell carcinoma of the kidney is extremely rare. (Papanicolaou stain, high power)

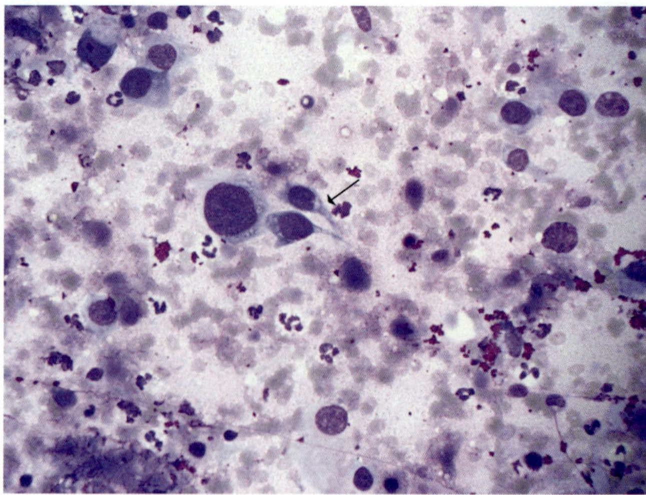

Figure 4.68 — Kidney, Urothelial Carcinoma. Scattered single malignant cells are shown. Some show cytoplasmic "tails," or polarized wisps of cytoplasm (arrow), characteristic of urothelial cells. (Diff Quik stain, high power)

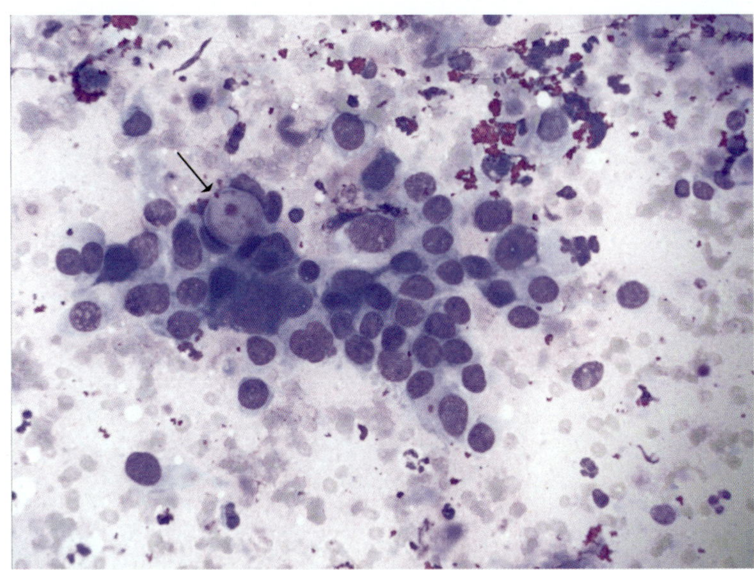

Figure 4.69 — Kidney, Urothelial Carcinoma. A cytoplasmic mucin droplet is present (arrow), causing formation of a signet-ring cell. Urothelial carcinoma may have focal glandular differentiation, which is more common than primary signet ring cell carcinoma or metastatic signet ring cell carcinoma. (Diff Quik stain, high power)

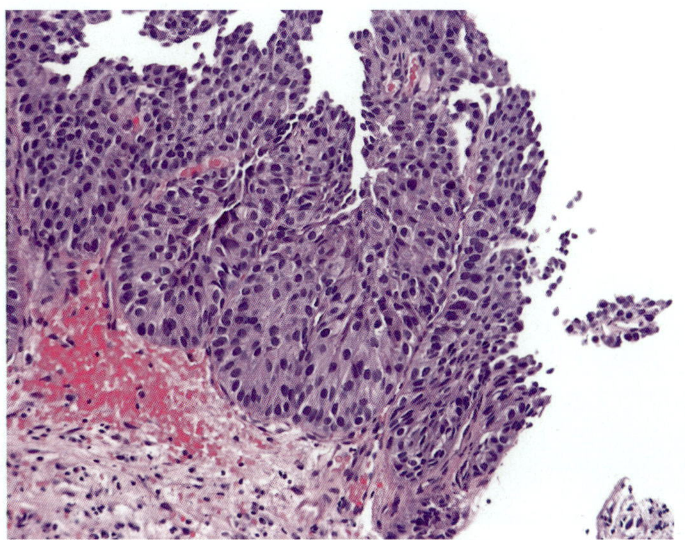

Figure 4.70 — Kidney, Urothelial Carcinoma (Histology). High-grade papillary urothelial carcinoma arising in the renal pelvis is shown. The neoplasm has well-formed papillary structures. The cells lining the papillae show moderate cytologic atypia with hyperchromasia and are overlapping. (Hematoxylin and eosin stain, medium power)

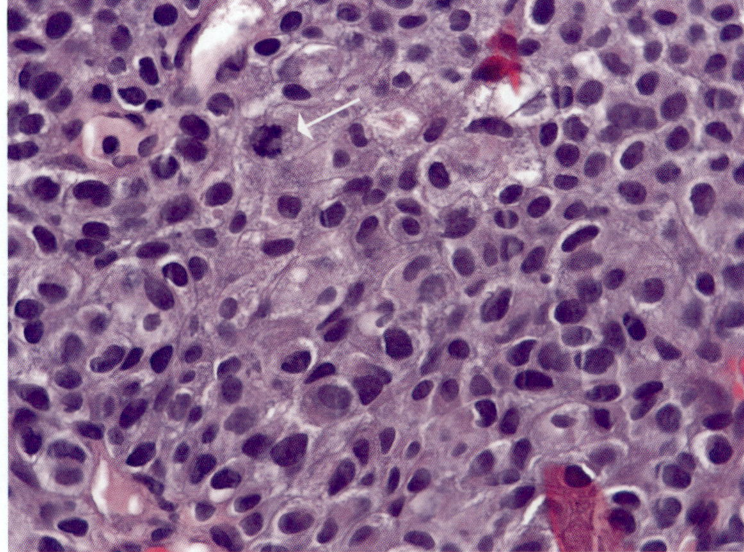

Figure 4.71 — Kidney, Urothelial Carcinoma (Histology). This high-grade urothelial carcinoma shows moderate to marked nuclear atypia, although the nuclear-to-cytoplasmic ratios are still relatively low. A mitotic figure is present (arrow). (Hematoxylin and eosin stain, high power)

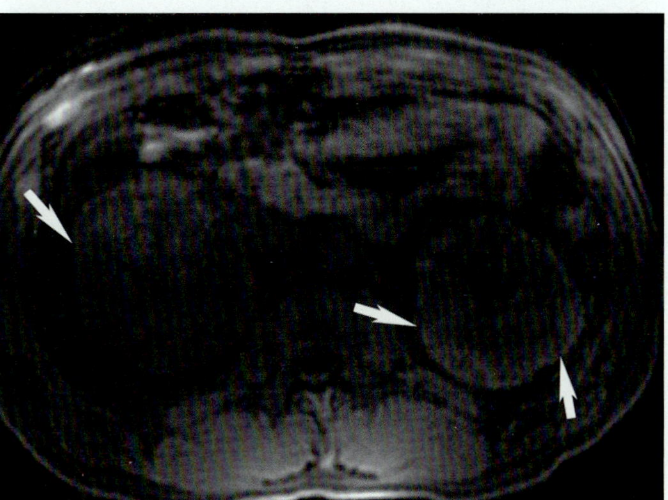

Figure 4.72 — Kidney, Burkitt-Like Lymphoma. This 40-year-old man with newly diagnosed HIV presented with a several month history of flank pain and acute renal failure. Axial T1 fat-saturated precontrast MR image shows enlarged kidneys bilaterally containing large hypointense areas (arrows).

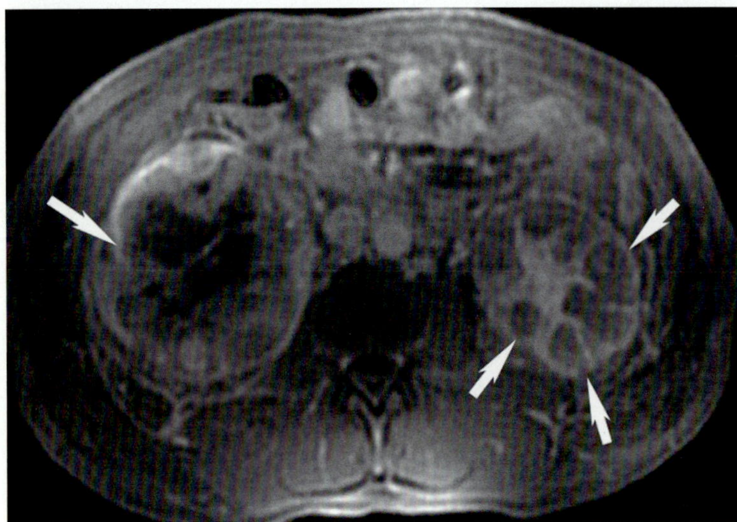

Figure 4.73 — Kidney, Burkitt-Like Lymphoma. Axial T1 fat-saturated post-contrast MR image shows that the heterogeneous enlarged kidneys are replaced by multiple hypointense masses (arrows).

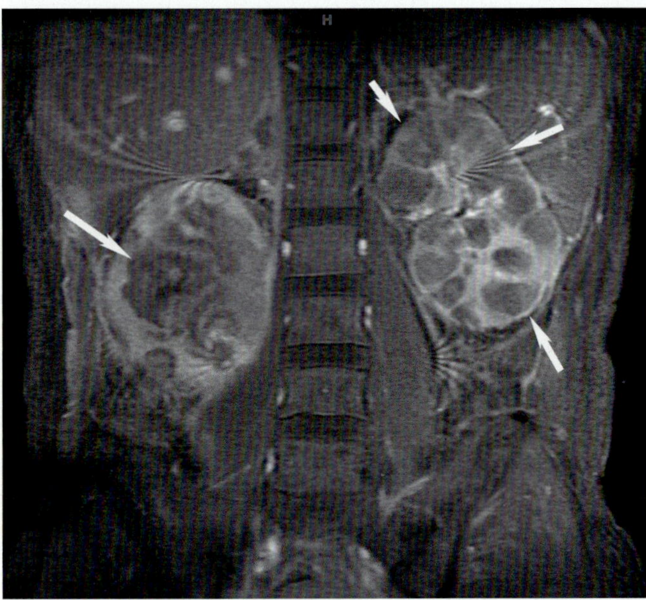

Figure 4.74 — Kidney, Burkitt-Like Lymphoma. Coronal T1 fat-saturated post-contrast MR image also depicts heterogeneous enlarged kidneys replaced by multiple hypointense masses (arrows). Involvement of the kidney by lymphoma is usually hypodense and can be multifocal or cause enlargement of the kidney.

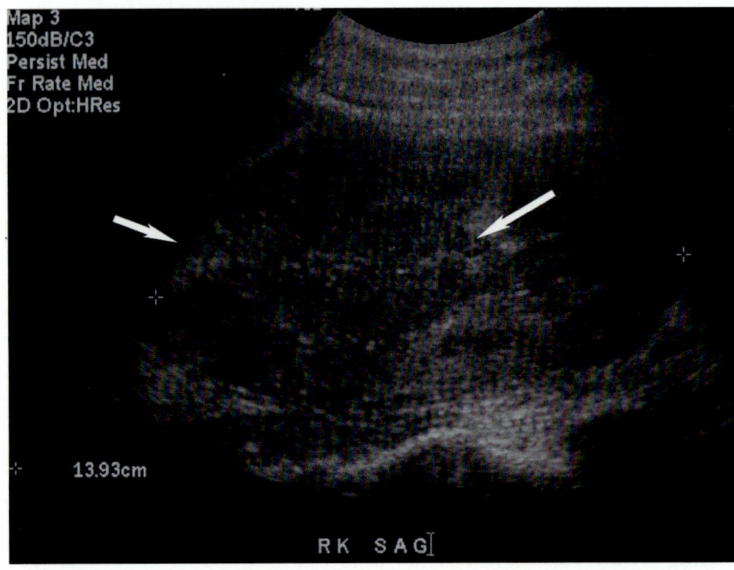

Figure 4.75 — Kidney, Burkitt-Like Lymphoma. Sonographic image of the right kidney at the time of ultrasound-guided biopsy shows a heterogeneously enlarged kidney which was targeted for biopsy (arrows).

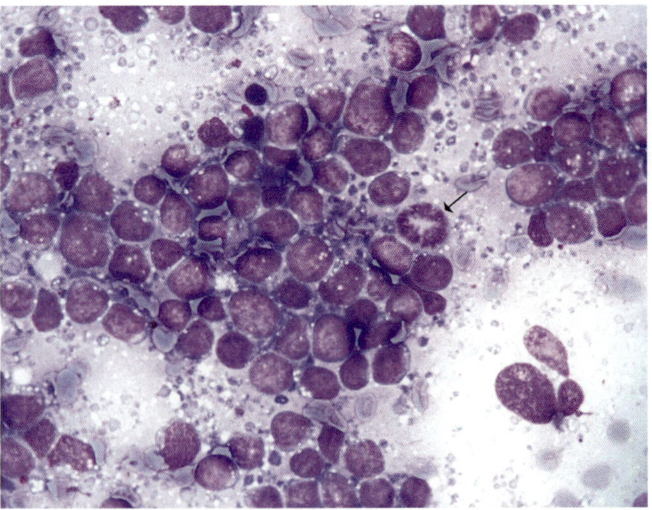

Figure 4.76 — Kidney, Burkitt-Like Lymphoma. A population of densely packed single cells is shown. The neoplastic cells have large nuclei and scant basophilic cytoplasm with scattered vacuoles. A mitotic figure is present (arrow). (Diff Quik stain, high power)

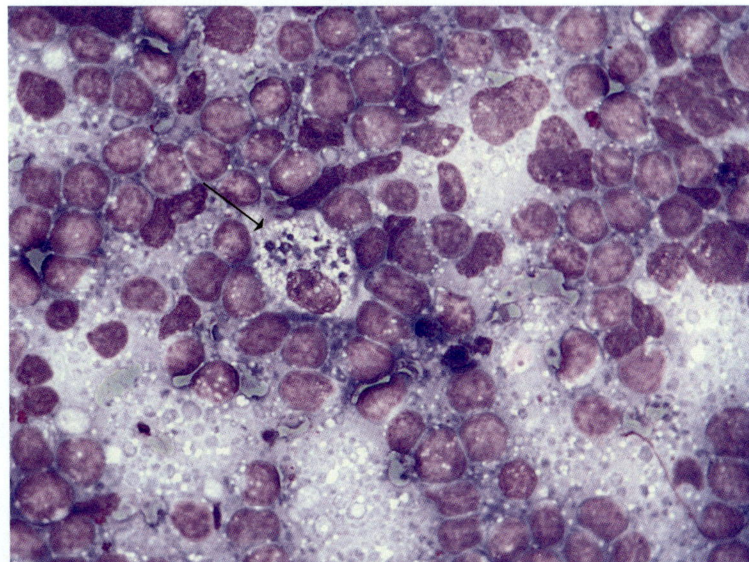

Figure 4.77 — Kidney, Burkitt-Like Lymphoma. A tingible body macrophage is present in the center of the field and shows cytoplasm stuffed with cellular debris (arrow). Burkitt-like lymphoma has a high cell turnover and tingible body macrophages are common. (Diff Quik stain, high power)

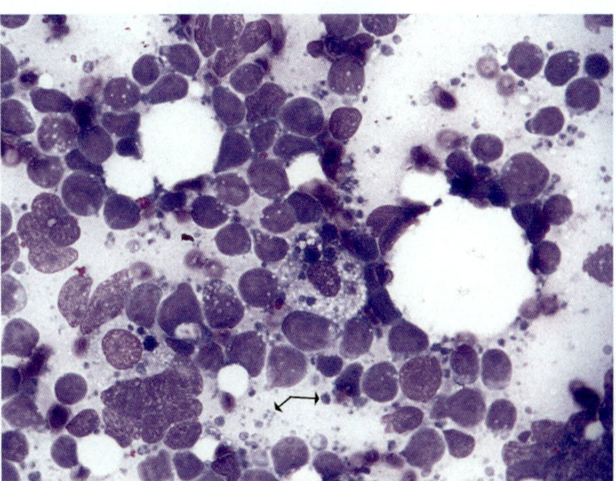

Figure 4.78 — Kidney, Burkitt-Like Lymphoma. Another tingible body macrophage is present in the center of the field surrounded by malignant lymphoid cells which have a very high nuclear-to-cytoplasmic ratio and a thin rim of basophilic cytoplasm. Scattered, small, round blue fragments present in the background (arrows), termed lymphoglandular bodies, are associated with hematolymphoid cells, although they are not specific. (Diff Quik stain, high power)

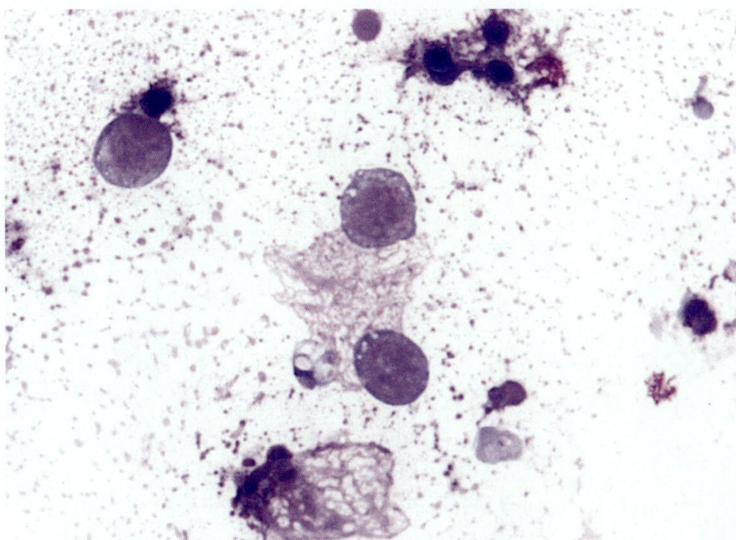

Figure 4.79 — Kidney, Burkitt-Like Lymphoma. These neoplastic cells have large nuclei and a thin rim of basophilic cytoplasm with small vacuoles. Cytoplasmic vacuoles are characteristic of Burkitt lymphoma, but can be seen in any hematopoietic neoplasm with a high turnover rate. (Diff Quik stain, high power)

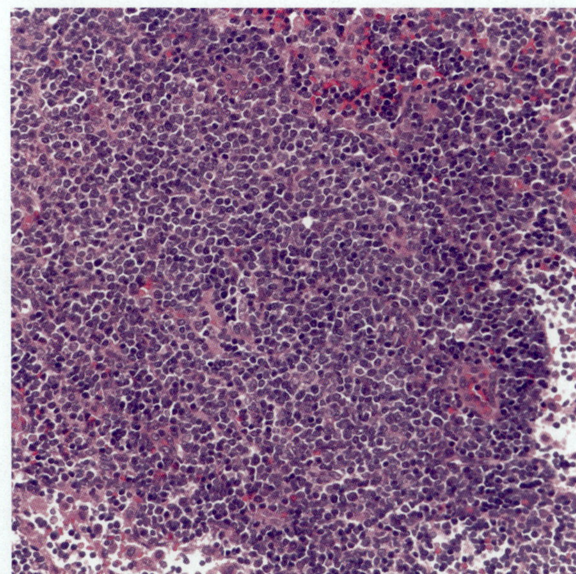

Figure 4.80 — Kidney, Burkitt-Like Lymphoma (Histology). A monotonous proliferation of lymphocytes shows scant basophilic cytoplasm and a high mitotic rate. The neoplastic cells of Burkitt lymphoma usually have membranous IgM with light chain restriction and are positive for CD19, CD20, CD22, CD10, and BCL6. (Hematoxylin and eosin stain, low power)

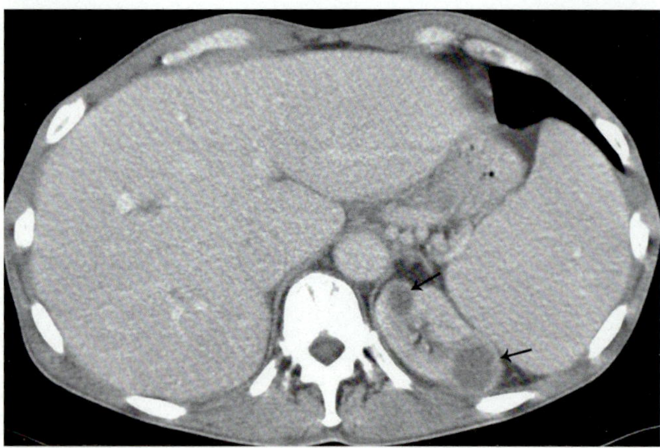

Figure 4.81 — Kidney, Aspergillus Fungal Infection. This 62-year-old male had a history of chronic lymphocytic leukemia, status post chemotherapy, total body irradiation, and bone marrow transplant 3 years prior. On routine follow-up, axial contrast-enhanced CT shows several rounded hypodense masses in the left kidney (arrows).

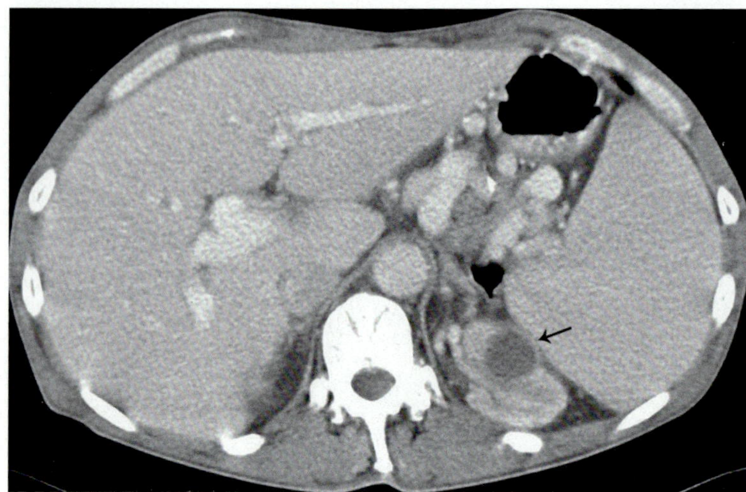

Figure 4.82 — Kidney, Aspergillus Fungal Infection. Axial contrast-enhanced CT slightly more inferiorly shows an additional rounded, hypodense mass in the left kidney (arrow).

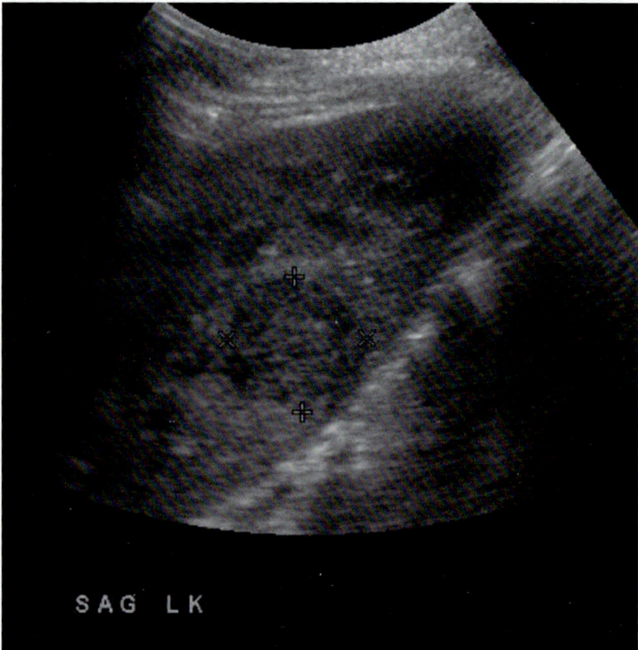

Figure 4.83 — Kidney, Aspergillus Fungal Infection. Sonographic image of the left kidney shows the heterogeneous renal mass. The appearance is nonspecific, but may represent infection. These lesions decreased in size 1 year later (not shown) following antifungal treatment.

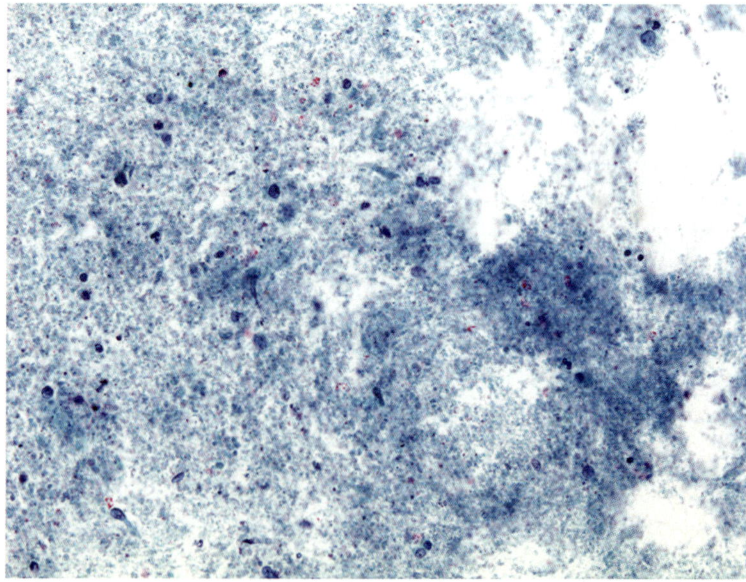

Figure 4.84 — Kidney, Aspergillus Fungal Infection. A field filled with granular debris is shown. An infectious cause is considered in the differential, but a neoplasm with extensive necrosis cannot be excluded. Material should be sent for culture if possible. (Papanicolaou stain, high power)

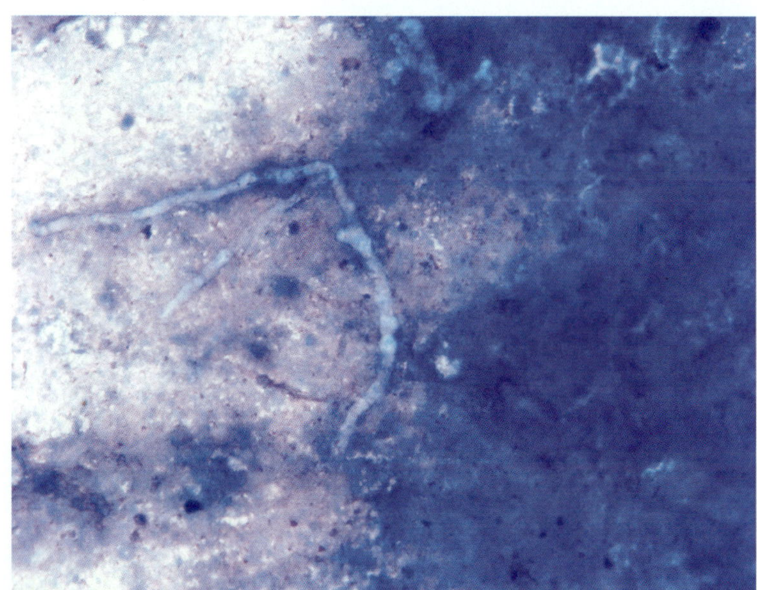

Figure 4.85 — Kidney, Aspergillus Fungal Infection. On Diff Quik stain, a pale outline of fungal hyphae is evident. *Aspergillus* is a filamentous fungus that possesses septate hyphae and is often encountered in the lung of transplant patients. A background of granular debris is present. (Diff Quik stain, high power)

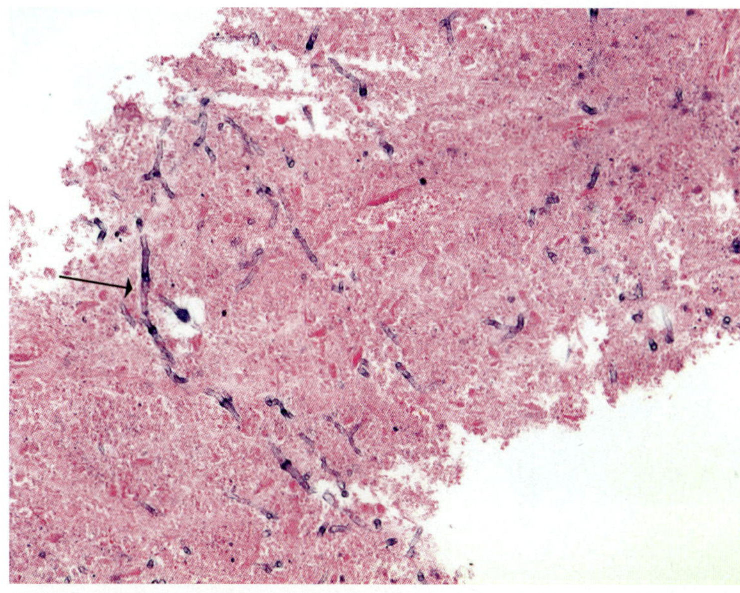

Figure 4.86 — Kidney, Aspergillus Fungal Infection (Cell Block). A cell block preparation shows numerous fungal forms (arrow) in a background of necrotic debris. Definitive classification of fungal organisms is not possible on histologic sections; thus, correlation with microbiology cultures is essential to guide therapy. (Hematoxylin and eosin stain, high power)

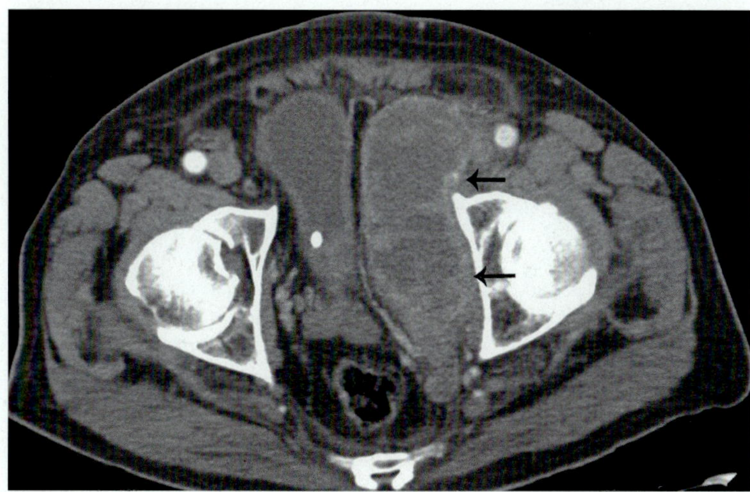

Figure 4.87 — Pelvic Sidewall, Metastatic Urothelial Carcinoma. Axial contrast-enhanced CT shows a large enhancing necrotic mass in the left pelvic sidewall (arrows). The patient had a history of urothelial carcinoma of the bladder.

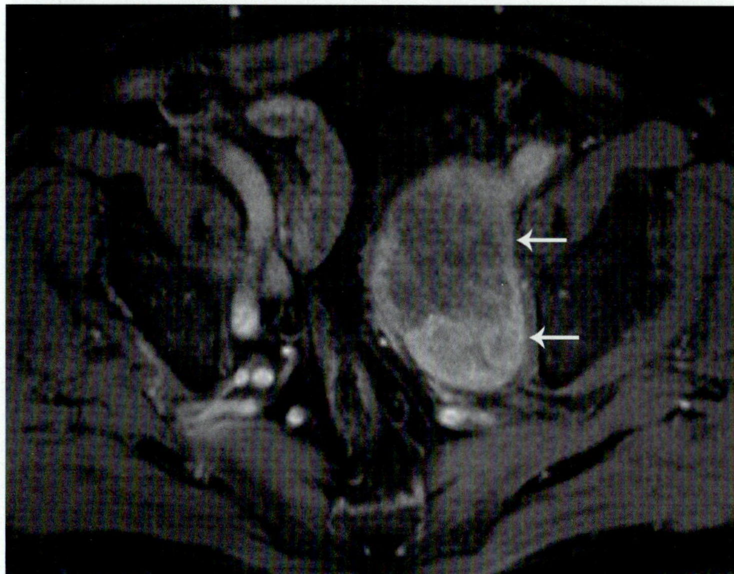

Figure 4.88 — Pelvic Sidewall, Metastatic Urothelial Carcinoma. Axial T1 fat-saturated post-contrast MR image confirms large, enhancing necrotic mass in the left pelvic sidewall (arrows).

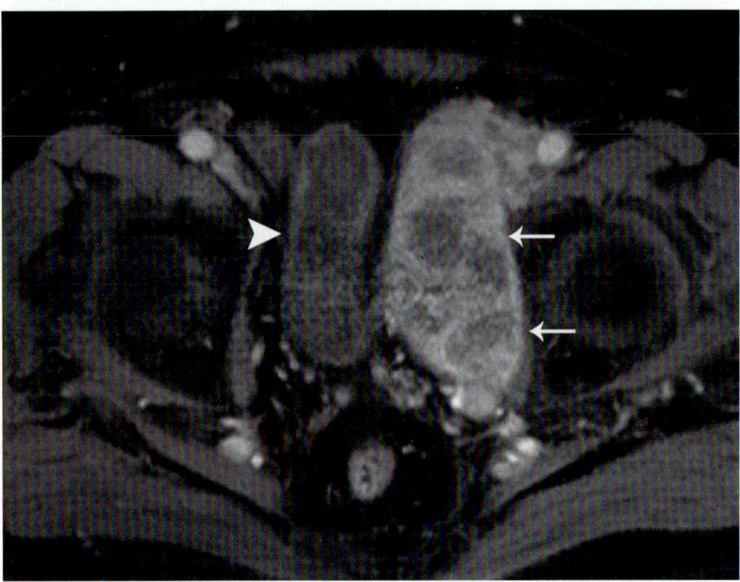

Figure 4.89 — Pelvic Sidewall, Metastatic Urothelial Carcinoma. Axial T1 fat-saturated postcontrast MR more inferiorly shows that the necrotic mass in the left pelvic sidewall (arrows) displaces the bladder (arrowhead).

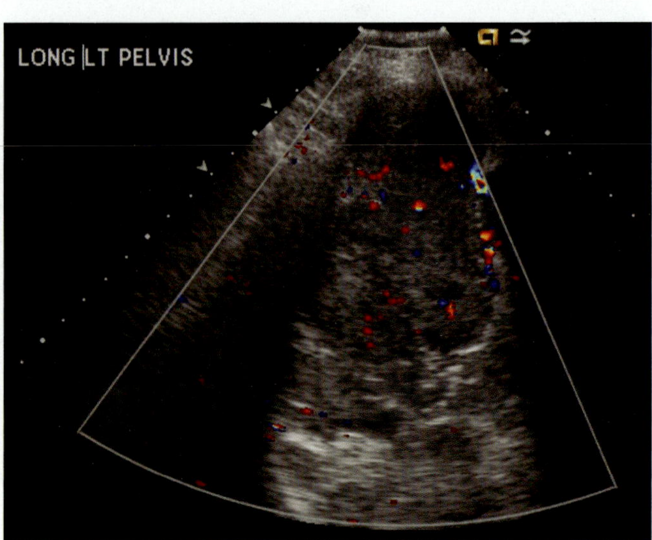

Figure 4.90 — Pelvic Sidewall, Metastatic Urothelial Carcinoma. Sonographic image with color Doppler at the time of ultrasound-guided biopsy shows the heterogeneous mass with internal vascularity in the left pelvis which was found to represent metastatic urothelial carcinoma.

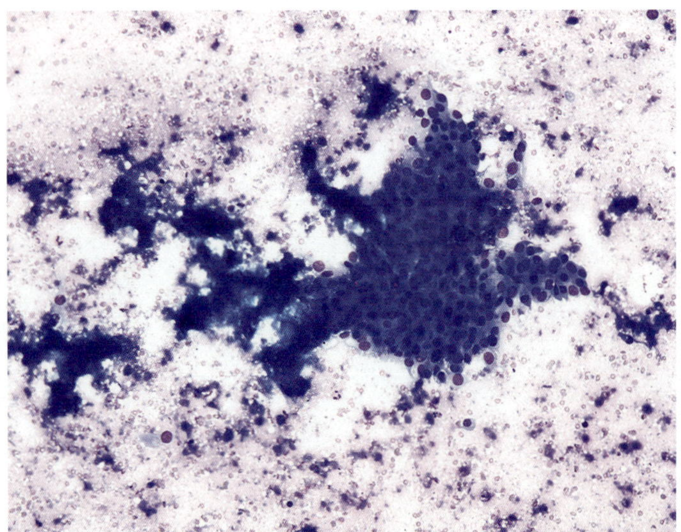

Figure 4.91 — Pelvic Sidewall, Metastatic Urothelial Carcinoma. A cohesive fragment of epithelial cells is present in a background of granular, acellular debris consistent with necrosis. This morphology is not specific; thus, material for immunostains is needed to determine a primary site in the absence of a history of malignancy. (Diff Quik stain, high power)

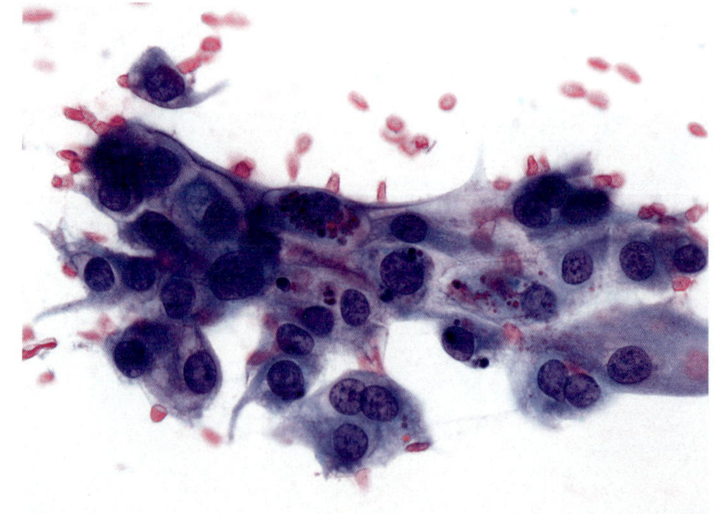

Figure 4.92 — Pelvic Sidewall, Metastatic Urothelial Carcinoma. These malignant cells show a moderate amount of cytoplasm, and round to oval nuclei with moderate anisonucleosis. In a male patient, urothelial, prostate, and gastrointestinal tract primaries would be considered in the differential. (Papanicolaou stain, high power)

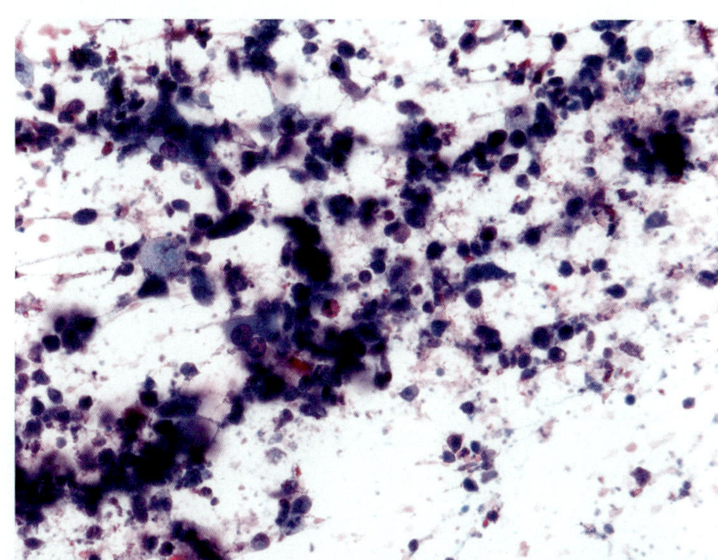

Figure 4.93 — Pelvic Sidewall, Metastatic Urothelial Carcinoma. Numerous single malignant cells with necrotic debris are seen. Abundant necrosis may obscure malignant cells and make definitive diagnosis difficult. (Papanicolaou stain, high power)

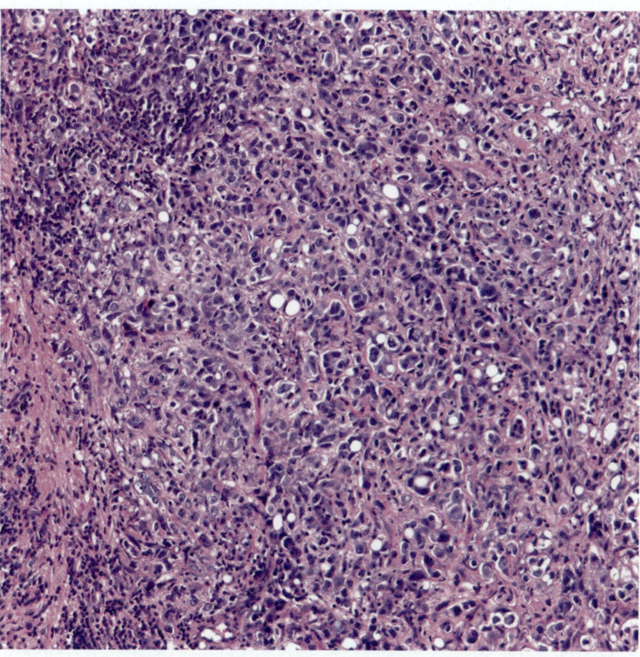

Figure 4.94 — Pelvic Sidewall, Metastatic Urothelial Carcinoma (Histology). Metastatic urothelial carcinoma with highly atypical urothelial cells with an infiltrative growth pattern. The nuclei are pleomorphic with prominent nucleoli. The patient has a history of urothelial carcinoma. (Hematoxylin and eosin stain, low power)

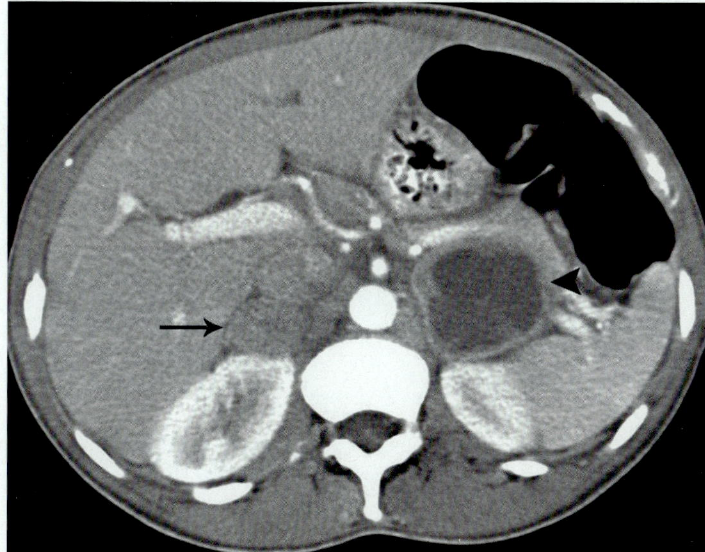

Figure 4.95 — Adrenal Gland, Pheochromocytoma. This 44-year-old female had a history of breast cancer and neurofibromatosis type 1. Axial contrast-enhanced CT demonstrates bilateral adrenal masses. The right adrenal mass is mostly solid (arrow) and the left adrenal gland mass is mostly cystic with solid areas (arrowhead).

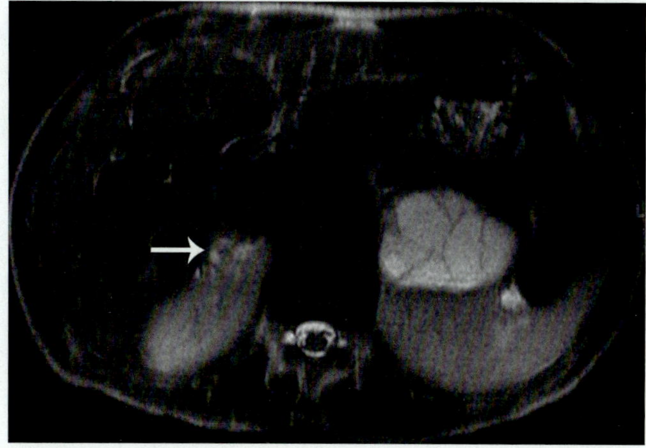

Figure 4.96 — Adrenal Gland, Pheochromocytoma. Axial single-shot fast-spin-echo (SSFSE) MR image confirms a heterogeneous, solid right adrenal mass (arrow) and mostly cystic left adrenal mass (arrowhead).

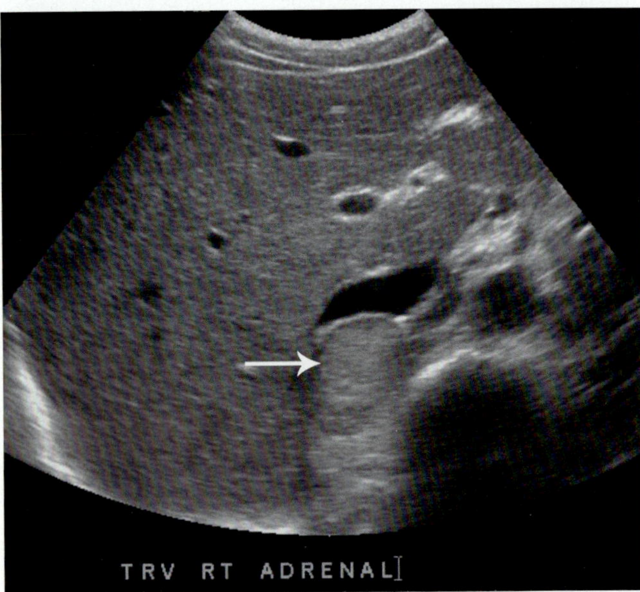

Figure 4.97 — Adrenal Gland, Pheochromocytoma. Sonographic image depicts the echogenic right adrenal mass (arrow). Patients with pheochromocytoma may present with extreme hypertension due to secretion of epinephrine and norepinephrine by the tumor.

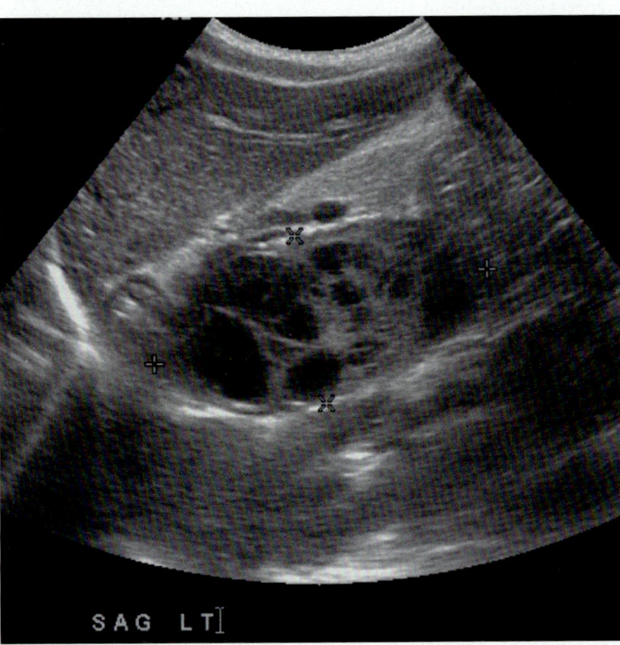

Figure 4.98 — Adrenal Gland, Pheochromocytoma. The solid and cystic left adrenal mass contains multiple thick septations. Pheochromocytomas can be solid or cystic and may contain calcifications.

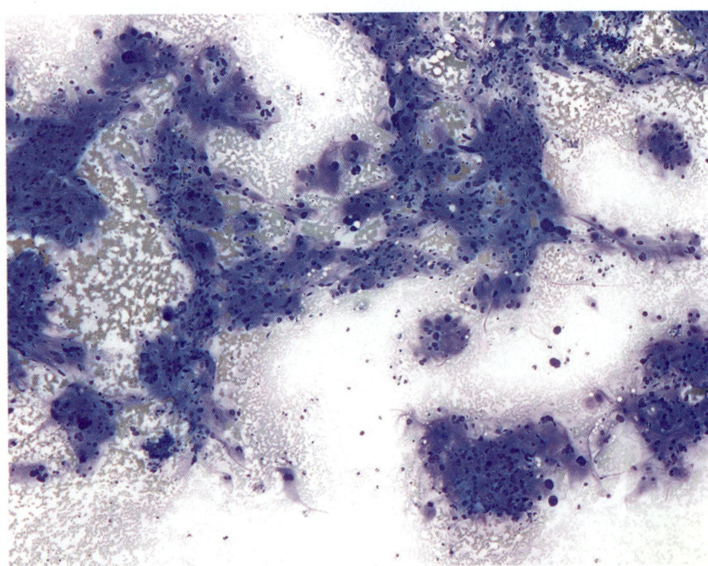

Figure 4.99 — Adrenal Gland, Pheochromocytoma. A cellular aspirate is shown with cohesive fragments of tumor cells. Even on low power, large nuclei are evident surrounded by voluminous cytoplasm. (Diff Quik stain, low power)

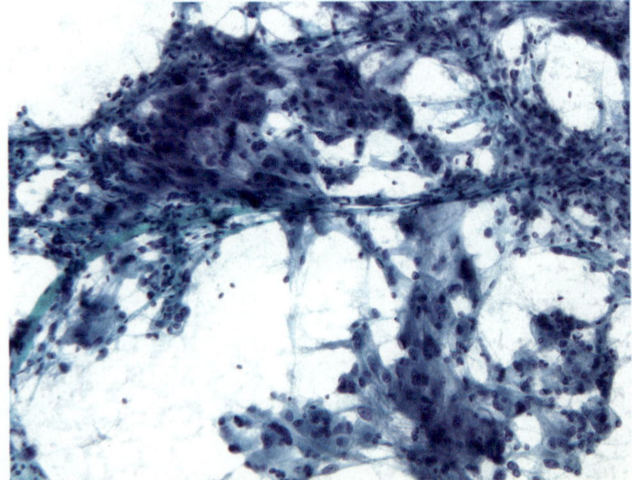

Figure 4.100 — Adrenal Gland, Pheochromocytoma. Delicate capillaries are seen surrounded by neoplastic cells with abundant cytoplasm and variably sized nuclei. Pheochromocytoma is known as the "ten percent" tumor as 10% are: bilateral, malignant, familial, extra-adrenal, and found in children. (Papanicolaou stain, high power)

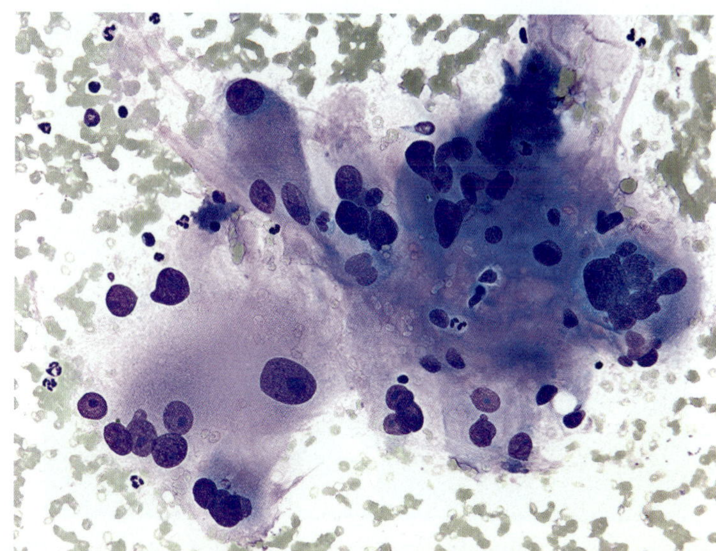

Figure 4.101 — Adrenal Gland, Pheochromocytoma. Marked nuclear pleomorphism is characteristic of pheochromocytoma, and is not an indicator of malignancy. Malignancy in a pheochromocytoma is only confirmed by the presence of metastatic lesions. (Diff Quik stain, high power)

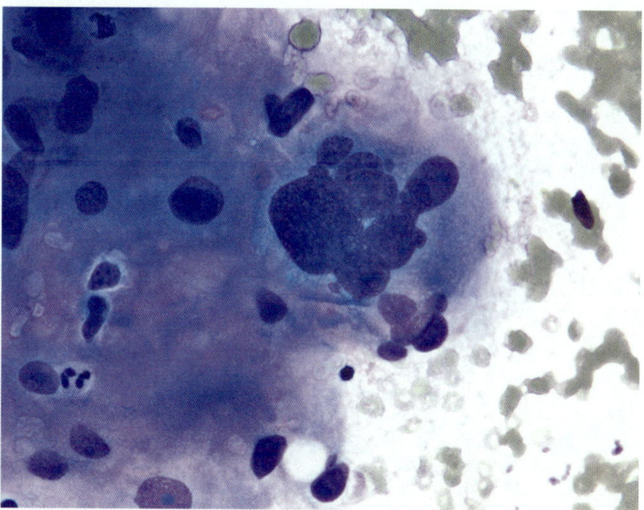

Figure 4.102 — Adrenal Gland, Pheochromocytoma. A bizarre tumor cell is shown consistent with pheochromocytoma. Urine and plasma catecholamines are elevated in patients with pheochromocytoma, and may aid in making the diagnosis. (Diff Quik stain, high power)

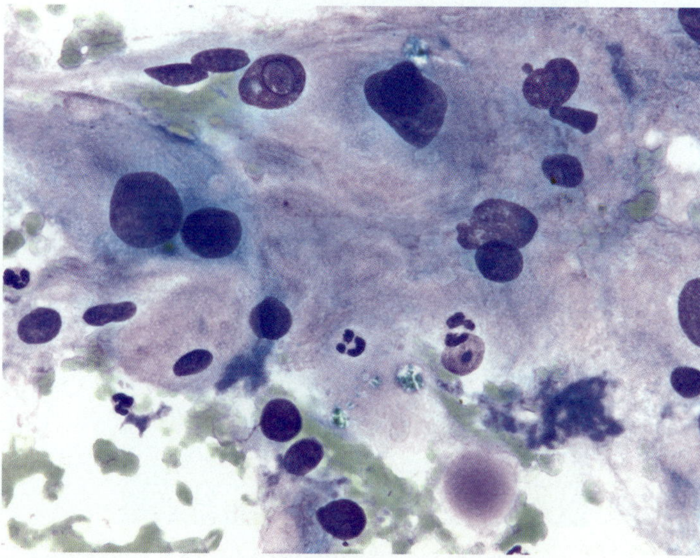

Figure 4.103 — Adrenal Gland, Pheochromocytoma. Anisonucleosis is evident in this group of tumor cells. There is abundant finely granular cytoplasm. The differential diagnosis includes adrenal cortical carcinoma, metastatic sarcomas, and poorly differentiated carcinoma. (Diff Quik stain, high power)

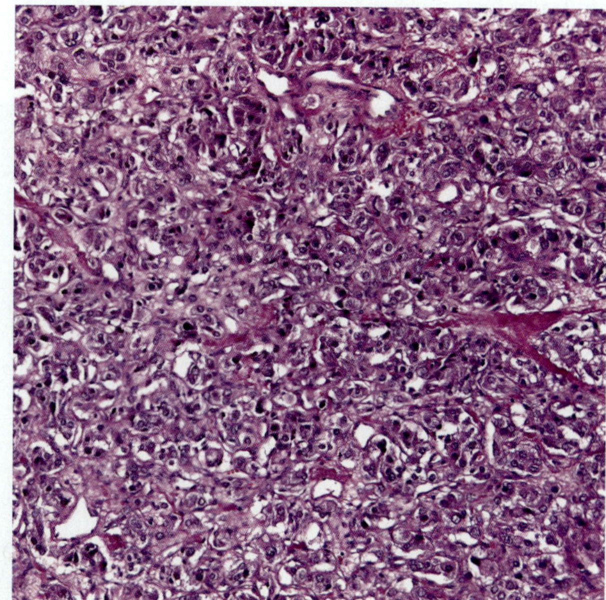

Figure 4.104 — Adrenal Gland, Pheochromocytoma. Pheochromocytomas originate from the adrenal medulla. The neoplastic cells can display a variety of growth patterns such as alveolar, trabecular, solid, or mixed patterns. An alveolar pattern of growth is illustrated here. There is a minimal stroma surrounding the nests of tumor cells. (Hematoxylin and eosin stain, low power)

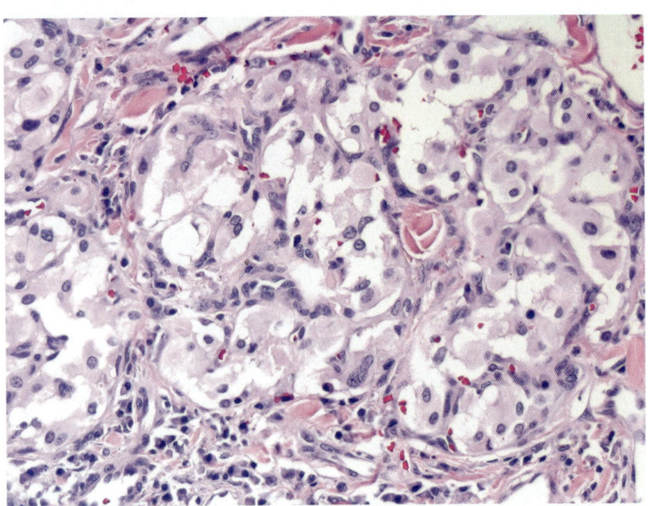

Figure 4.105 — Adrenal Gland, Pheochromocytoma. Tumor cells are arranged in clusters and nests surrounded by a rich and intricate vascular network (Zellballen pattern). The neoplastic cells have amphophilic cytoplasm and a polygonal shape. Histologic features associated with aggressive behavior include capsular invasion, vascular invasion, increase in mitoses, and necrosis. (Hematoxylin and eosin stain, high power)

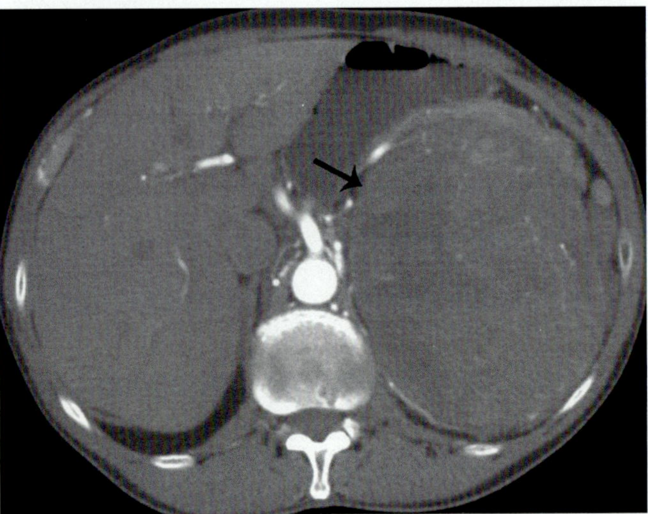

Figure 4.106 — Adrenal Gland, Adrenal Cortical Neoplasm. Axial contrast-enhanced CT in the arterial phase shows a large heterogeneous mass in the left upper quadrant (arrow).

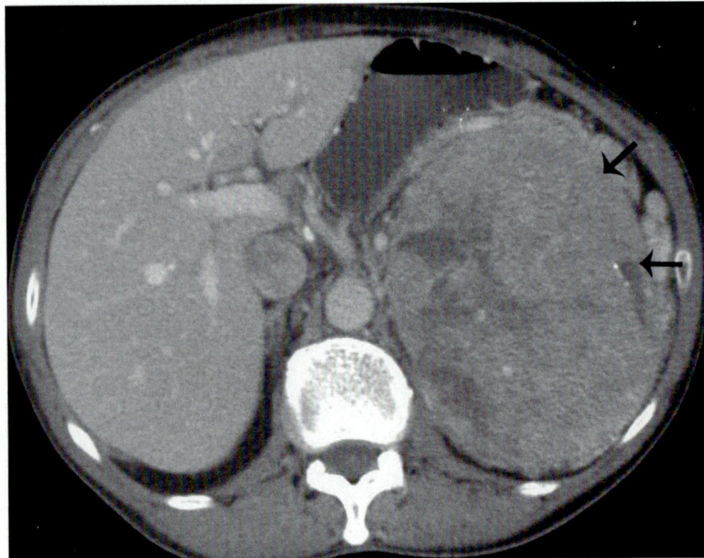

Figure 4.107 — Adrenal Gland, Adrenal Cortical Neoplasm. Axial contrast-enhanced CT in the venous phase shows multiple enhancing soft tissue components and several small low-density areas within the mass (arrows).

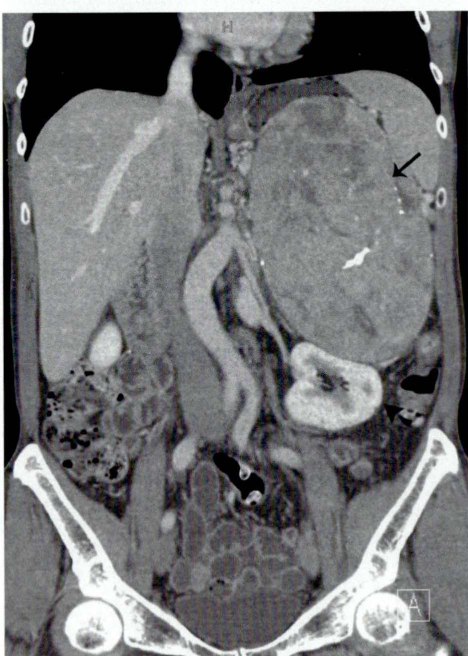

Figure 4.108 — Adrenal Gland, Adrenal Cortical Neoplasm. Coronal contrast-enhanced CT in the venous phase shows the extent of the mass in the left adrenal gland (arrow) which displaces the left kidney inferiorly (arrowhead). The mass contains coarse calcifications. Adrenal cortical neoplasms are often large and heterogeneous.

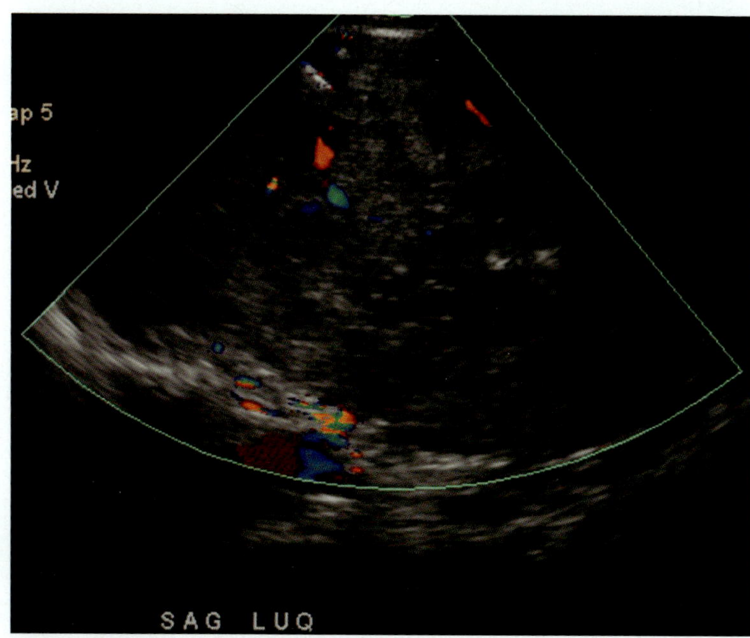

Figure 4.109 — Adrenal Gland, Adrenal Cortical Neoplasm. Sonographic image with color Doppler at the time of ultrasound-guided biopsy shows the heterogeneous, hypoechoic left upper quadrant mass with internal vascularity.

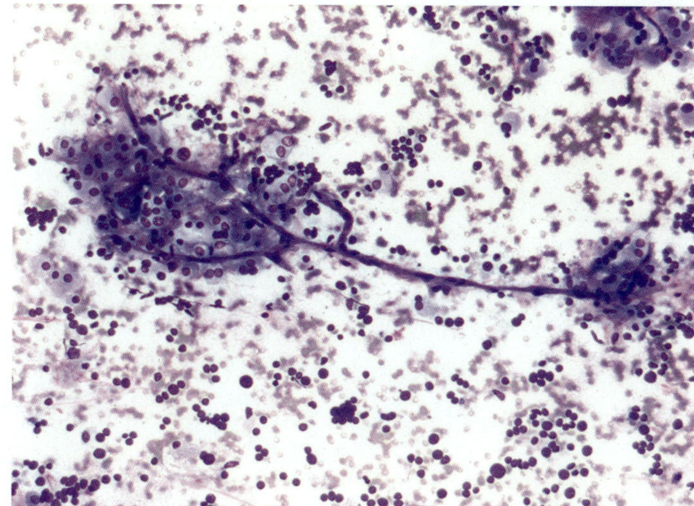

Figure 4.111 — Adrenal Gland, Adrenal Cortical Neoplasm. A delicate vascular structure is present, connecting two groups of epithelial cells with numerous bare nuclei present in the background. Malignant histopathologic features include increased mitotic rate, large tumor size and weight, and vascular and capsular invasion. (Diff Quik stain, high power)

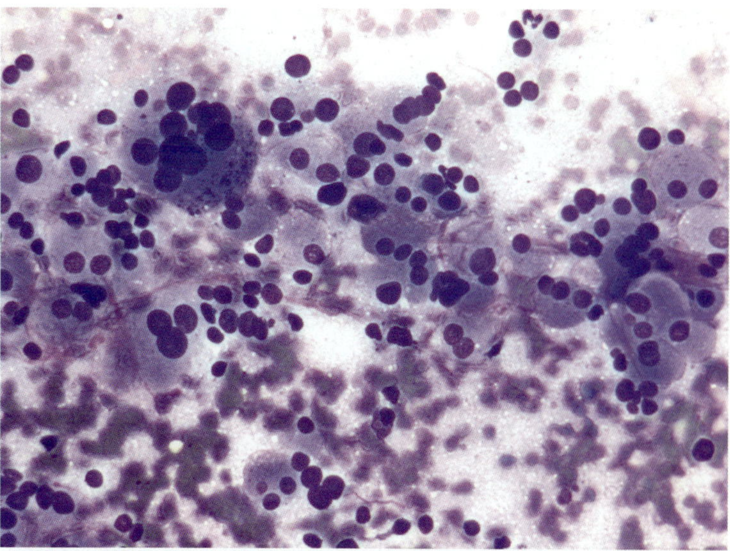

Figure 4.110 — Adrenal Gland, Adrenal Cortical Neoplasm. A cellular aspirate consisting of loosely cohesive epithelioid cells is shown. The tumor cells have abundant cytoplasm and small- to medium-sized round nuclei. A large population of naked nuclei is also evident. (Diff Quik stain, medium power)

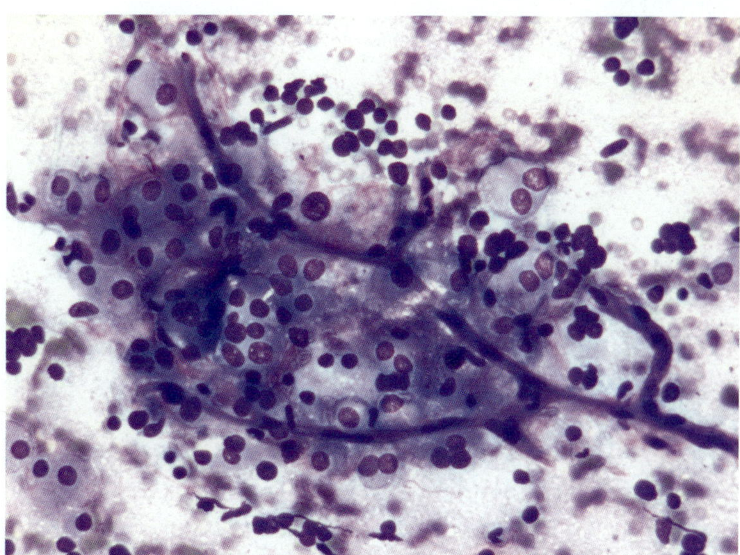

Figure 4.112 — Adrenal Gland, Adrenal Cortical Neoplasm. Tumor cells with abundant cytoplasm and occasional binucleation are present. (Diff Quik stain, high power)

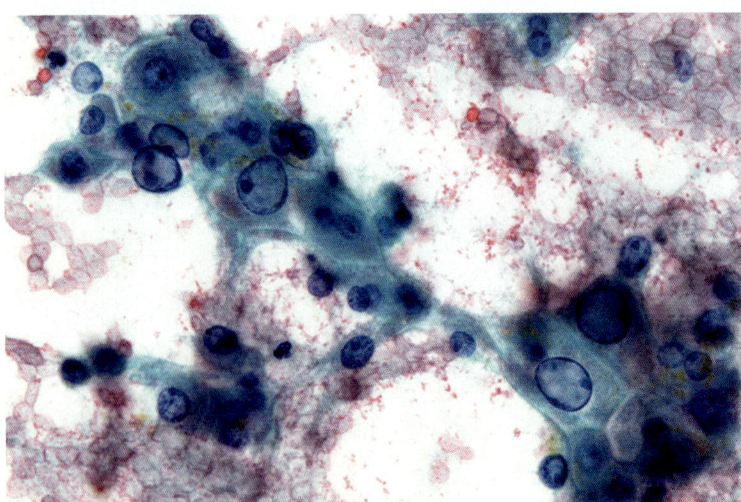

Figure 4.113 — Adrenal Gland, Adrenal Cortical Neoplasm. The neoplastic cells appear to have abundant granular cytoplasm. This tumor had oncocytic morphology, both cytologically and histologically. Occasional prominent nucleoli are seen as well as cytoplasmic pigmentation. (Papanicolaou stain, high power)

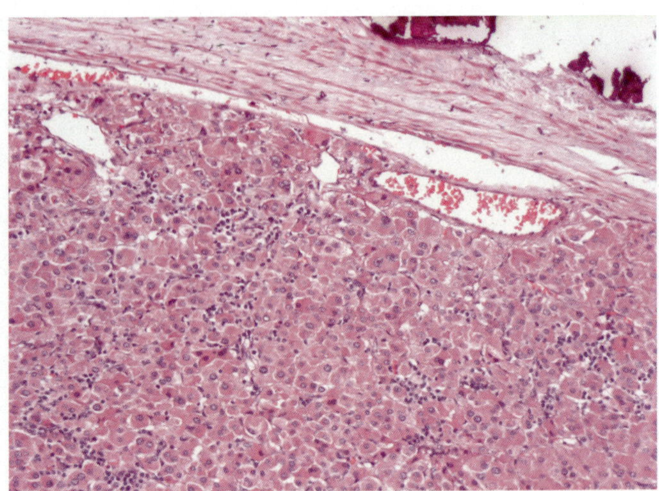

Figure 4.114 — Adrenal Gland, Adrenal Cortical Neoplasm (Histology). The neoplastic cells show oncocytic features with abundant eosinophilic cytoplasm and round, uniform nuclei. Despite the very large size of this neoplasm, it appeared entirely encapsulated and completely excised upon resection; thus, the lesion was termed "adrenal cortical neoplasm of indeterminant malignant potential." (Hematoxylin and eosin stain, high power)

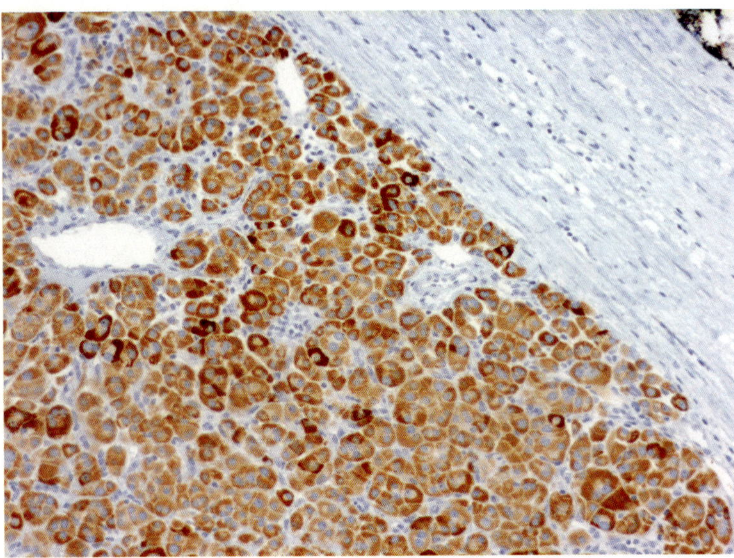

Figure 4.115 — Adrenal Gland, Adrenal Cortical Neoplasm (Histology). An immunostain for Melan-A was strongly and diffusely positive in the resected tumor consistent with adrenal cortical origin. Immunostains for Cytokeratin (AE1/3), EMA, and S-100 protein were negative and a Ki67 shows a low proliferative rate (less than 1%). (Melan-A stain, high power)

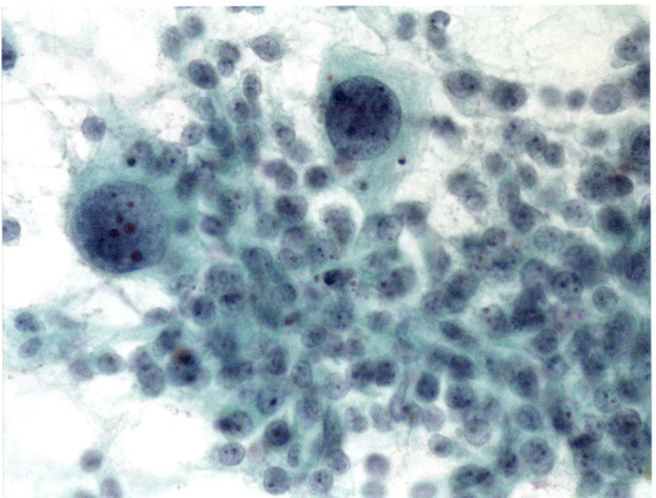

Figure 4.116 — Adrenal Gland, Adrenal Cortical Carcinoma. Pleomorphic cell population, composed predominantly of epithelioid cells and interspersed giant cell. Malignant cells have prominent single or multiple nucleoli. The diagnosis of adrenal cortical carcinoma is supported by tumor size (greater than 5 cm), tumor weight (greater than 100 g), increased nuclear atypia, presence of lymph-vascular invasion, and high mitotic rate (>5/50HPF). (Papanicolaou stain, medium power)

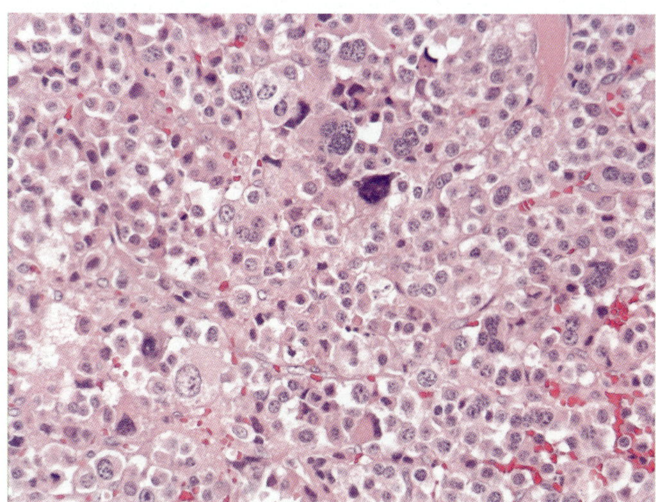

Figure 4.117 — Adrenal Gland, Adrenal Cortical Carcinoma (Histology). The tumor is composed of sheets of polygonal-shaped eosinophilic cells with well-defined cell borders. Several of the tumor cells have enlarged nuclei with prominent nucleoli. The neoplastic cells of adrenal cortical neoplasm stain positive for Melan-A and synaptophysin, but are negative for chromogranin or HMB45. (Hematoxylin and eosin stain, high power)

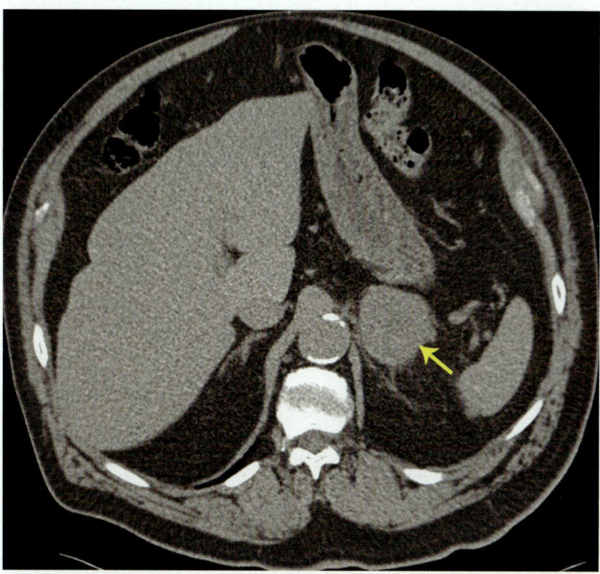

Figure 4.118 — Adrenal Gland, Metastatic Melanoma. This 80-year-old man had a history of prostate cancer, squamous cell carcinoma of the head and neck, and a history of melanoma involving neck lymph nodes 8 years prior. A chest CT was ordered for chest pain. Axial noncontrast CT shows a lobulated mass in the left adrenal gland (arrow).

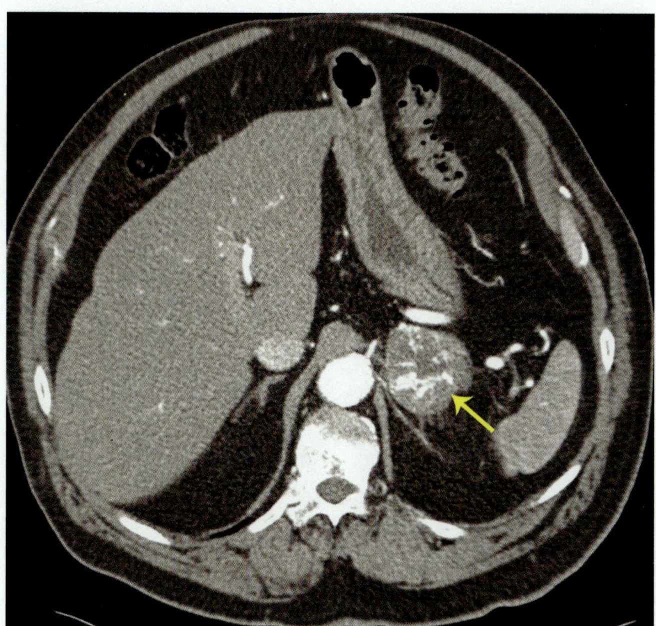

Figure 4.119 — Adrenal Gland, Metastatic Melanoma. Axial contrast-enhanced CT in the arterial phase shows the left adrenal mass with marked central vascularity (arrow).

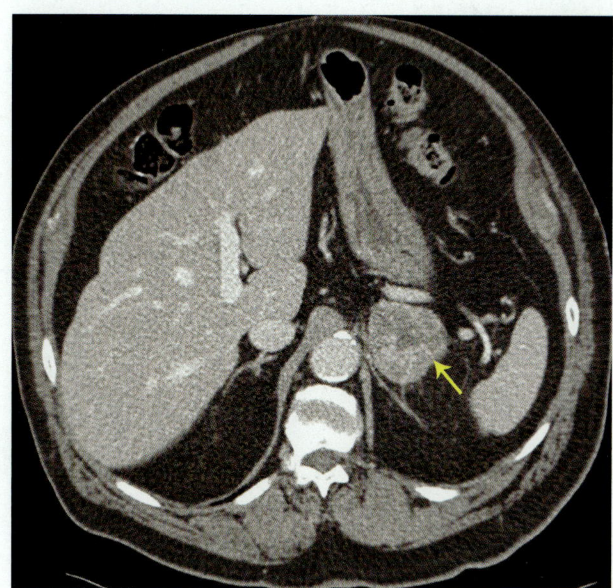

Figure 4.120 — Adrenal Gland, Metastatic Melanoma. Axial contrast-enhanced CT in the venous phase is shown. There is mild de-enhancement of the mass in the venous phase (arrow).

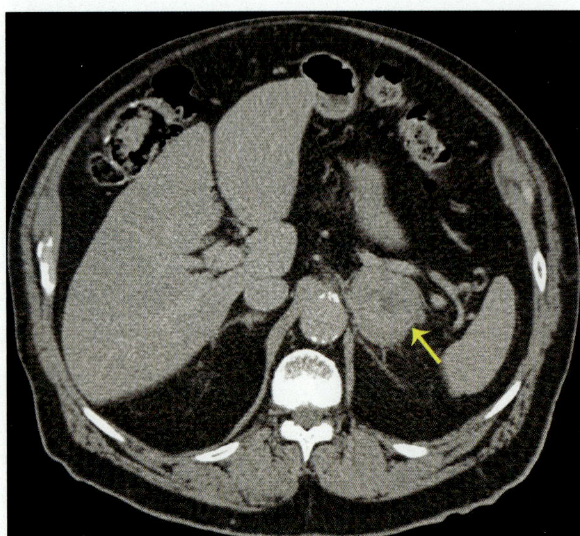

Figure 4.121 — Adrenal Gland, Metastatic Melanoma. Axial contrast-enhanced CT in the delayed phase demonstrates that there is further de-enhancement of the heterogeneous left adrenal mass in the delayed phase (arrow). The appearance is nonspecific, but was found to represent metastatic malignant melanoma. Metastases are the most common malignant lesion of the adrenal glands. Common primary tumors include the lung and breast.

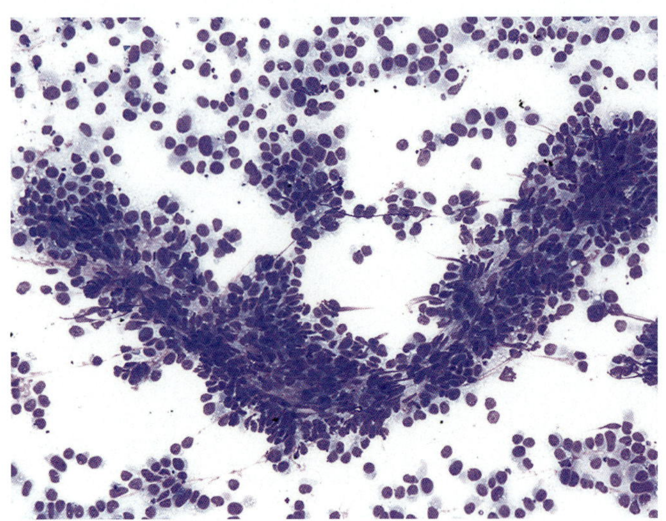

Figure 4.122 — Adrenal Gland, Metastatic Melanoma. A fragment of tumor cells surrounding a fibrovascular center is shown with numerous single dispersed cells in the background. Cells have eccentric nuclei with a plasmacytoid appearance. Metastases to the adrenal gland, particularly from the lung, are not uncommon. (Diff Quik stain, medium power)

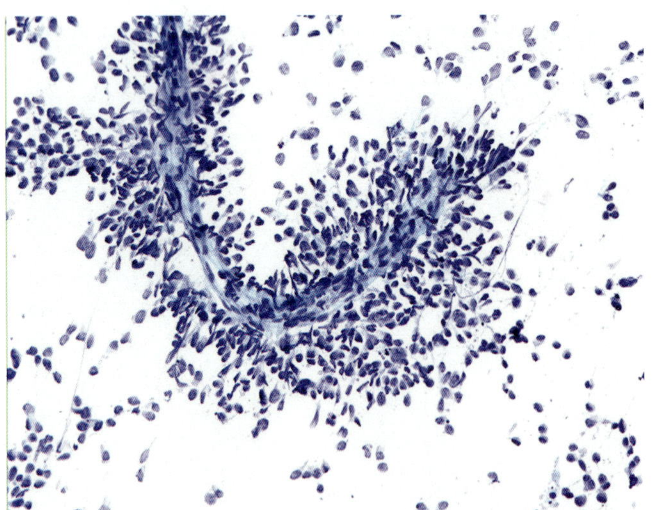

Figure 4.123 — Adrenal Gland, Metastatic Melanoma. A small vessel runs through the center of this tumor fragment. Individual cells appear loosely cohesive surrounding the fragment and are also present singly. The differential diagnosis includes adrenal cortical neoplasm, metastatic carcinoma, and melanoma. (Papanicolaou stain, medium power)

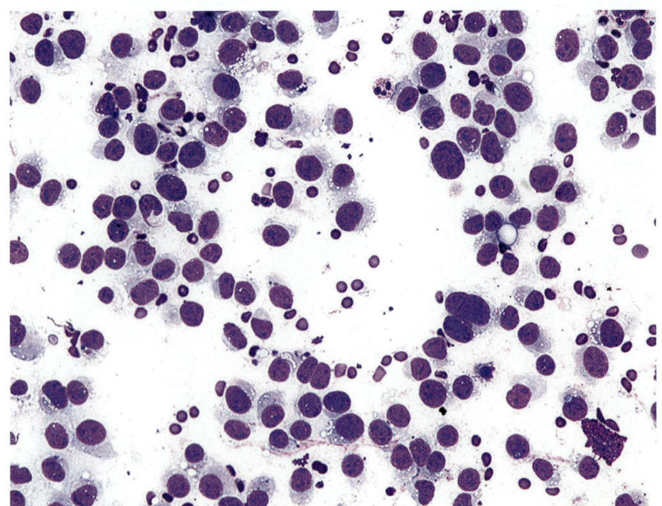

Figure 4.124 — Adrenal Gland, Metastatic Melanoma. On high power, the single cells show a plasmacytoid morphology with round to oval nuclei and a monotonous appearance. A panel of immunostains should be ordered as both adrenal cortical tissue and melanoma are positive for Melan-A. S-100 protein, HMB-45, and inhibin help distinguish the two. (Diff Quik stain, medium power)

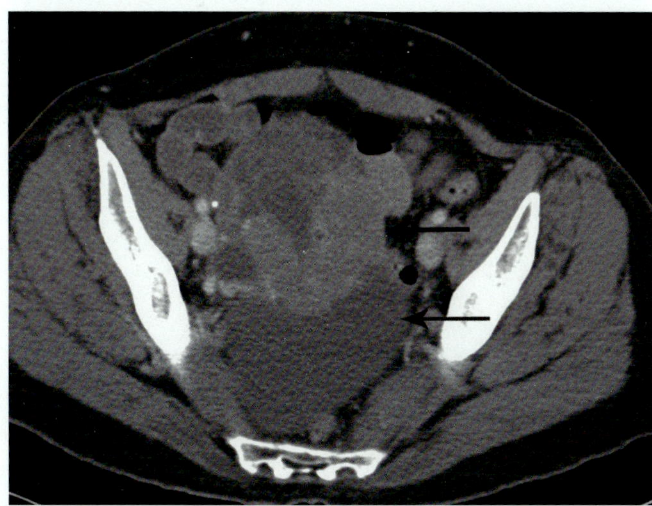

Figure 4.125 — Ovary, Brenner Tumor. This 52-year-old woman presented with abdominal pain. Axial contrast-enhanced CT shows a solid and cystic mass in the pelvis (arrows).

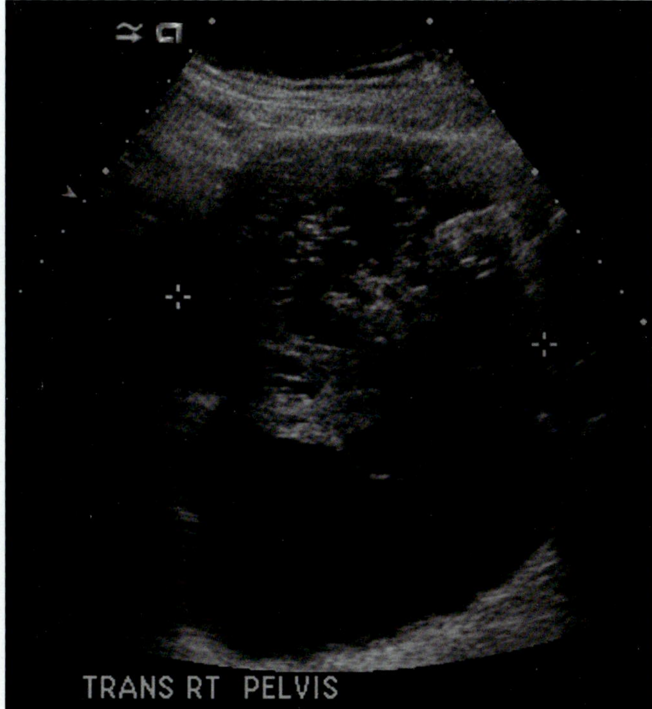

Figure 4.127 — Ovary, Brenner Tumor. Sonographic image confirms heterogeneous solid and cystic mass in the pelvis. Brenner tumors are uncommon, representing 1–2% of all ovarian tumors.

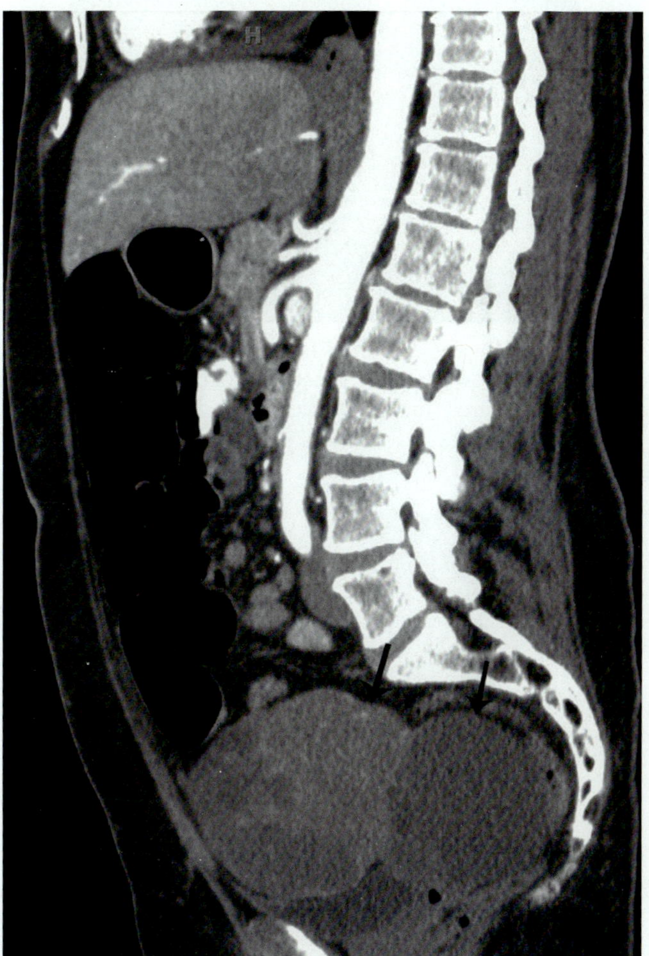

Figure 4.126 — Ovary, Brenner Tumor. Sagittal contrast-enhanced CT shows the solid and cystic mass in the pelvis (arrows) which is superior to the bladder. Brenner tumors are rare, mostly benign tumors that can be solid and cystic; however, this appearance is nonspecific.

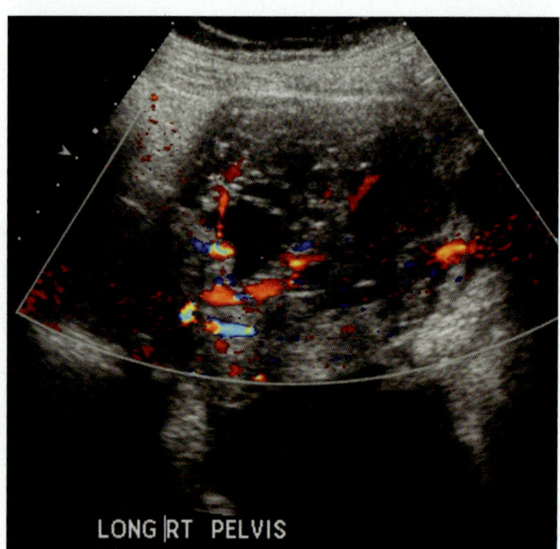

Figure 4.128 — Ovary, Brenner Tumor. The mass shows internal vascularity with color Doppler. Most Brenner tumors are unilateral and they are very rarely malignant (less than 5%).

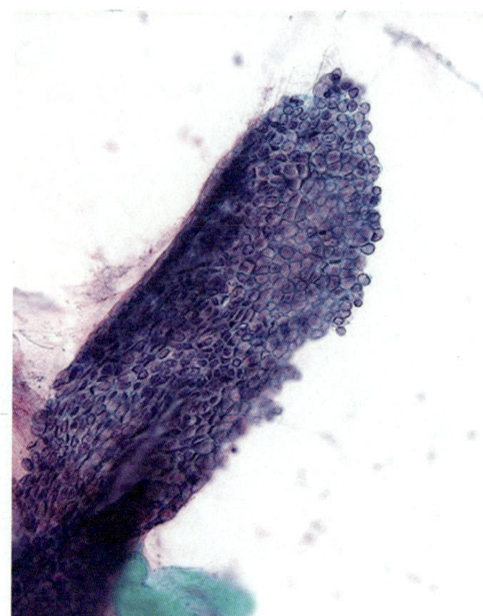

Figure 4.129 — Ovary, Brenner Tumor. The aspirate smears from this lesion showed predominantly mucinous type epithelium. The nuclei were bland and uniform, suggesting a low-grade mucinous lesion. (Papanicolaou stain, high power)

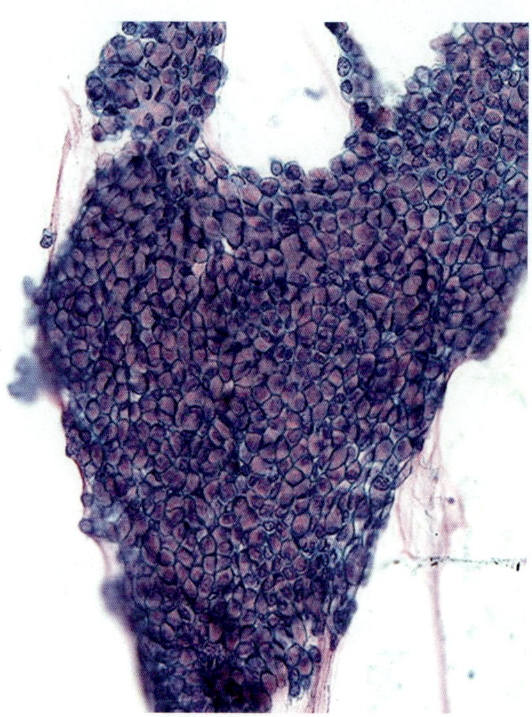

Figure 4.130 — Ovary, Brenner Tumor. The presence of only mucinous epithelium led to an FNA impression consistent with a low-grade mucinous neoplasm. This represented sampling of the cystic area of the mass. (Papanicolaou stain, high power)

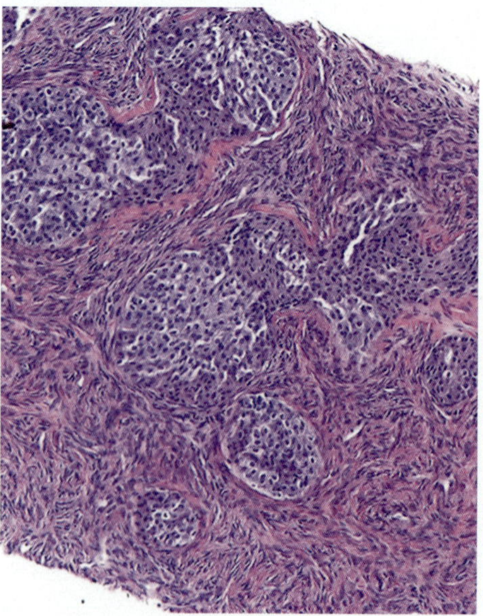

Figure 4.131 — Ovary, Brenner Tumor (Core Biopsy). A core biopsy was also obtained and showed two distinct components to the mass, a Brenner tumor with a mucinous cystic component. Brenner tumors are composed of transitional-type epithelium, and are positive for cytokeratins and EMA. (Hematoxylin and eosin stain, medium power)

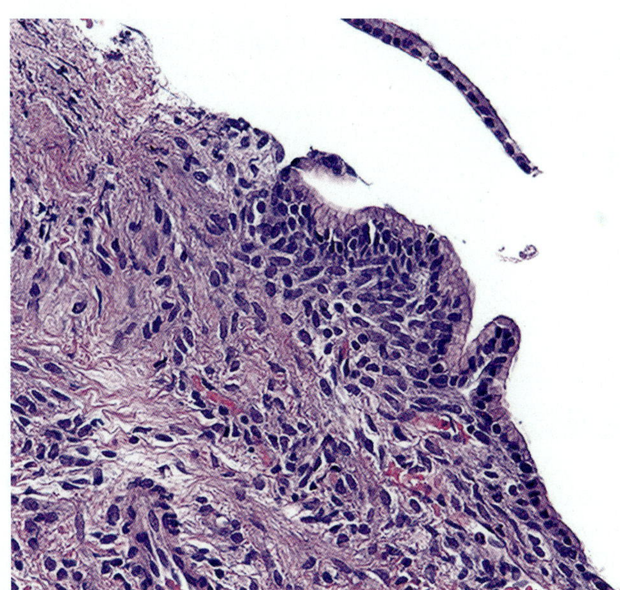

Figure 4.132 — Ovary, Brenner Tumor (Core Biopsy). The cystic component, sampled by FNA, is seen here with bland nuclei and cytoplasmic mucin. Mucinous cystic change may be prominent in Brenner tumors. (Hematoxylin and eosin stain, high power)

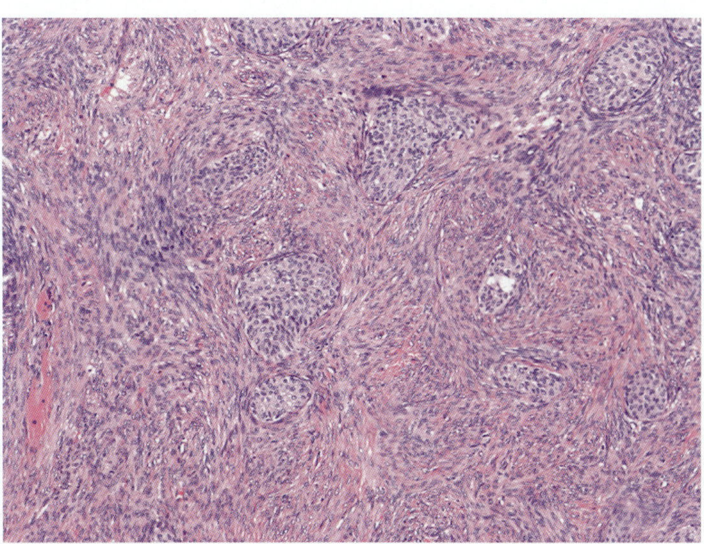

Figure 4.133 — Ovary, Brenner Tumor (Histology). Benign Brenner tumors comprise 1–2% of all ovarian neoplasms. The neoplasm shows solid epithelial nests within a stroma which is composed of spindle-shaped cells. (Hematoxylin and eosin stain, low power)

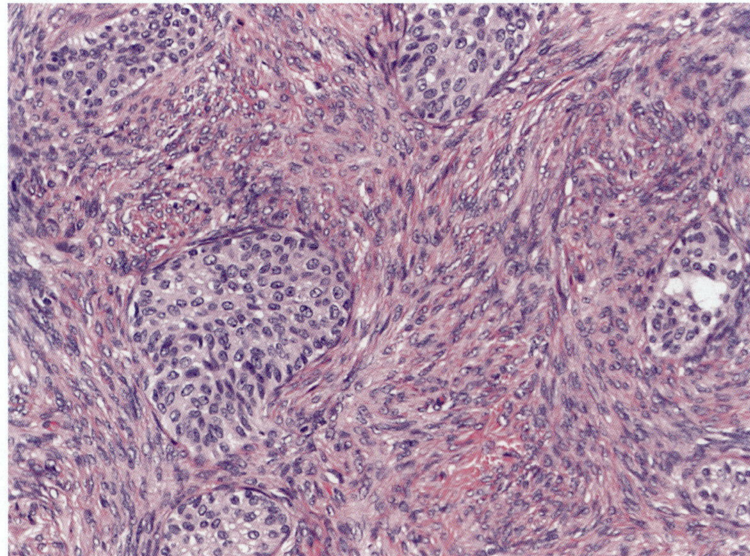

Figure 4.134 — Ovary, Brenner Tumor (Histology). These squamoid nests are reminiscent of a urothelial proliferation. The background stroma is composed of bland spindle-shaped cells with minimal cytological atypia and no mitoses. (Hematoxylin and eosin stain, medium power)

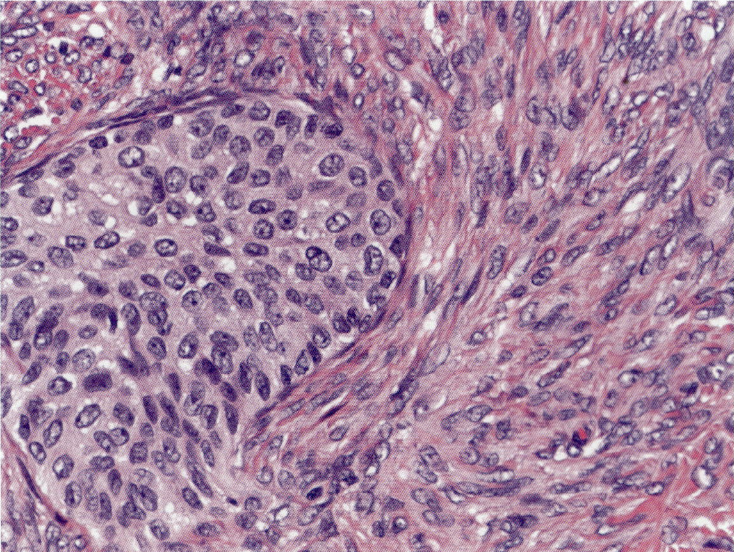

Figure 4.135 — Ovary, Brenner Tumor (Histology). The epithelial cells within the nests have a squamoid morphology. The cells are eosinophilic, with round to oval nuclei with small nucleoli. Occasional nuclei have grooves, giving them a "coffee-bean" appearance. (Hematoxylin and eosin stain, high power)

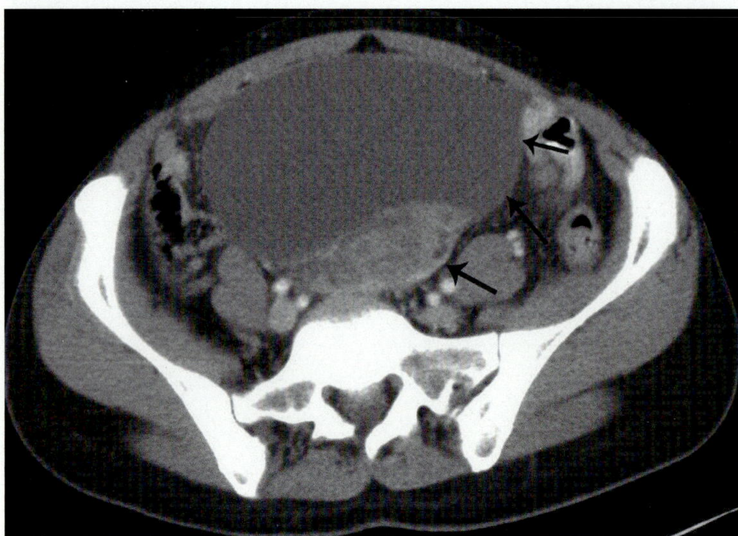

Figure 4.136 — Ovary, High-Grade Serous Carcinoma. A 41-year-old woman presented with abdominal pain. Axial contrast-enhanced CT shows a solid and cystic mass in the pelvis (arrows).

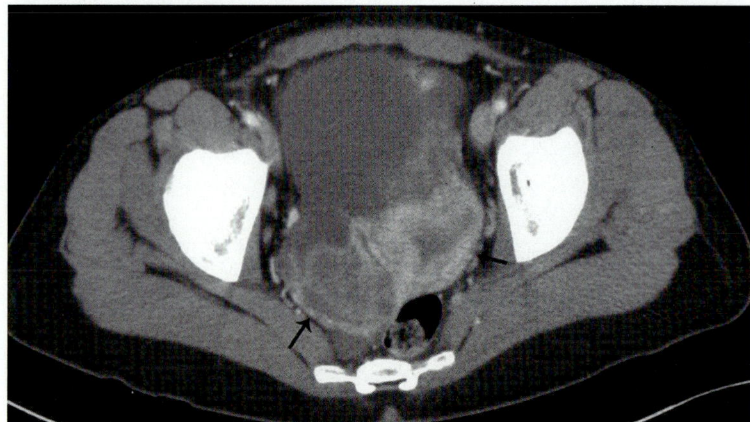

Figure 4.137 — Ovary, High-Grade Serous Carcinoma. Axial contrast-enhanced CT slightly more inferiorly shows bilateral solid and cystic adnexal masses (arrows). The presence of large solid, enhancing components in an adnexal mass is highly suggestive of malignancy.

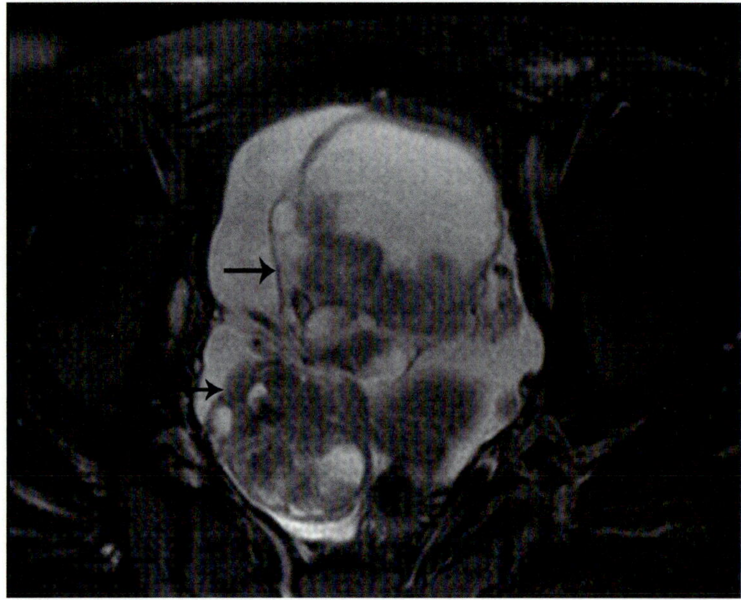

Figure 4.138 — Ovary, High-Grade Serous Carcinoma. Axial T2 fat-saturated MR image confirms the solid and cystic masses in the pelvis (arrows). There is also a small amount of ascites.

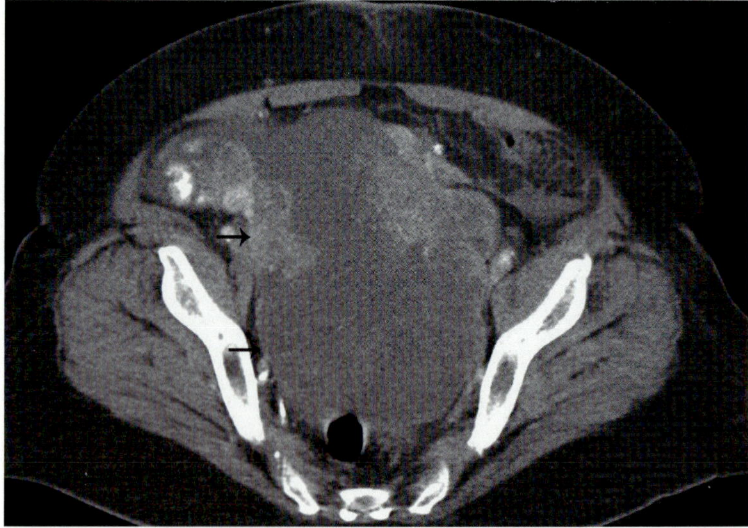

Figure 4.139 — Ovary, High-Grade Serous Carcinoma. Axial contrast-enhanced CT in a different patient shows a similar-appearing pelvic mass with extensive areas of soft tissue nodularity (arrows). Ovarian serous carcinomas are commonly cystic with varying degrees of solid component.

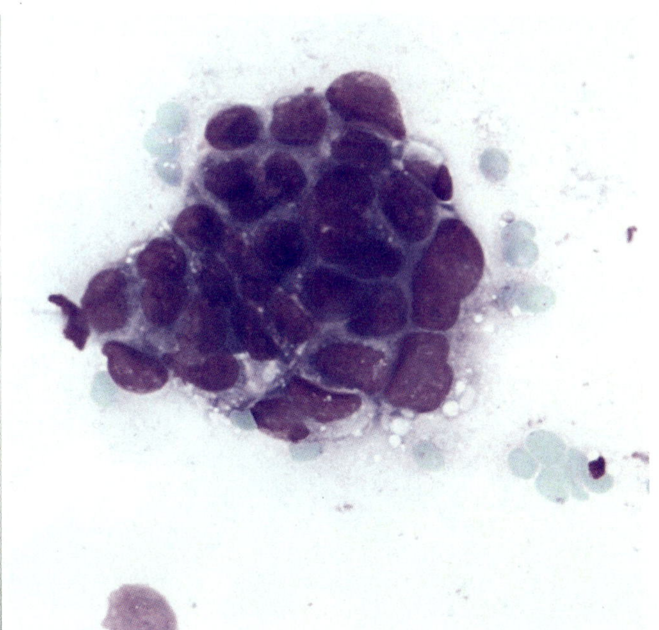

Figure 4.140 — Ovary, High-Grade Serous Carcinoma. A fragment of malignant epithelium is present showing high nuclear-to-cytoplasmic ratios and nuclear hyperchromasia. Ovarian tumors are not often biopsied due to the risk of rupture and tumor seeding. (Diff Quik stain, high power)

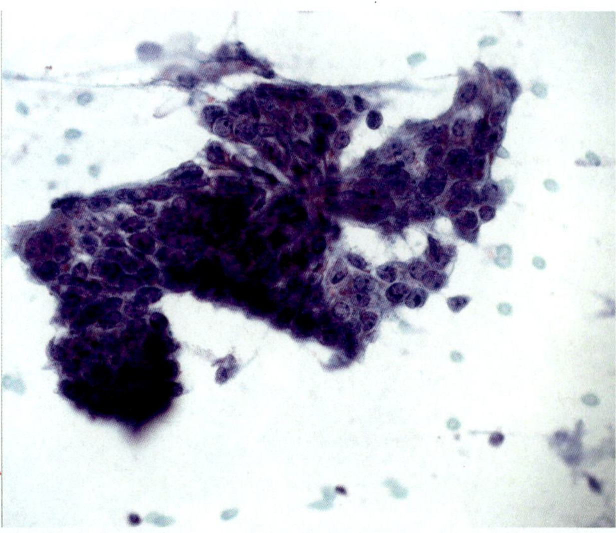

Figure 4.141 — Ovary, High-Grade Serous Carcinoma. This sheet of malignant epithelial cells shows anisonucleosis and prominent nucleoli. Pelvic lesions may be aspirated if there is a question of gastrointestinal versus gynecologic origin, or if there is a possibility of extensive metastases from another site. (Papanicolaou stain, high power)

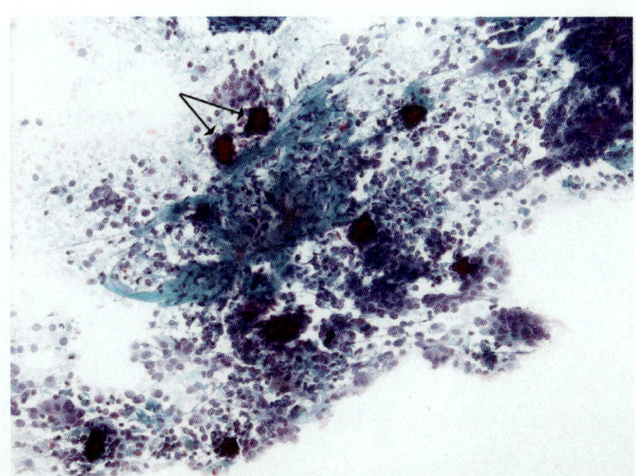

Figure 4.142 — Ovary, High-Grade Serous Carcinoma. Loosely cohesive fragments of malignant cells are admixed with numerous single cells. Psammoma bodies, characteristic of high-grade serous carcinoma, are scattered throughout (arrows). Immunostains confirmed that the tumor was positive for WT1, CK7, and PAX8. (Papanicolaou stain, high power)

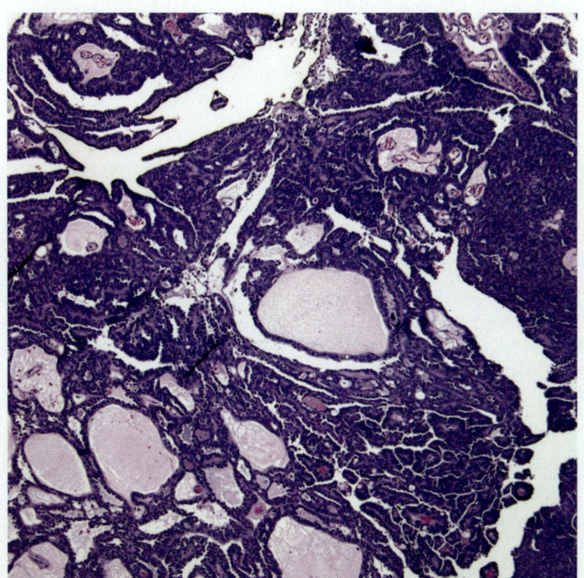

Figure 4.143 — Ovary, High-Grade Serous Carcinoma (Histology). Ovarian serous carcinoma is the most common ovarian epithelial malignancy. This tumor shows a papillary growth pattern with irregular slit-like spaces and high-grade nuclear features. (Hematoxylin and eosin stain, low power)

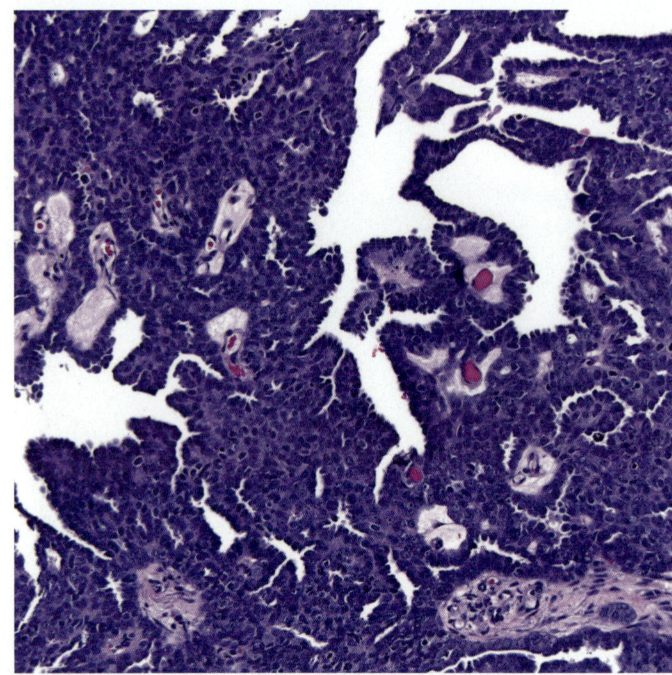

Figure 4.144 — Ovary, High-Grade Serous Carcinoma (Histology). A proliferation of malignant cells showing a papillary growth pattern is illustrated. There is high nuclear-to-cytoplasmic ratio and significant nuclear pleomorphism with enlarged round to oval nuclei, frequent mitoses and hyperchromasia. (Hematoxylin and eosin stain, medium power)

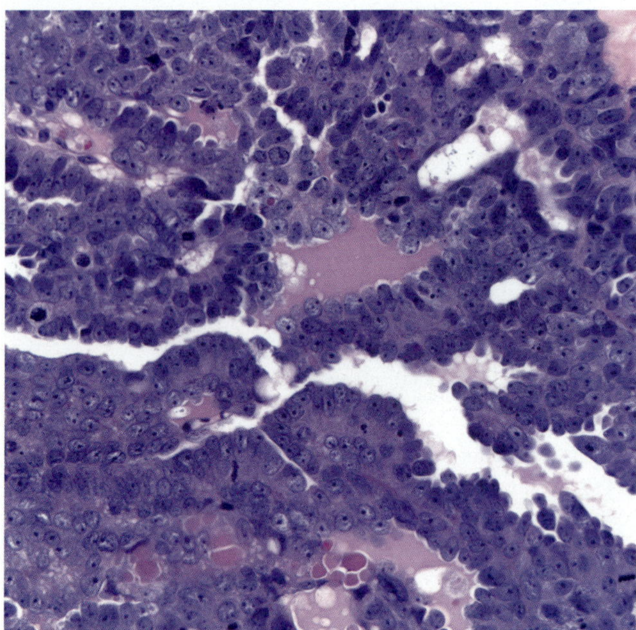

Figure 4.145 — Ovary, High-Grade Serous Carcinoma (Histology). At high power, marked nuclear atypia is evident including nuclear enlargement, hyperchromasia, and prominent nucleoli. Mitoses are readily identified. (Hematoxylin and eosin stain, high power)

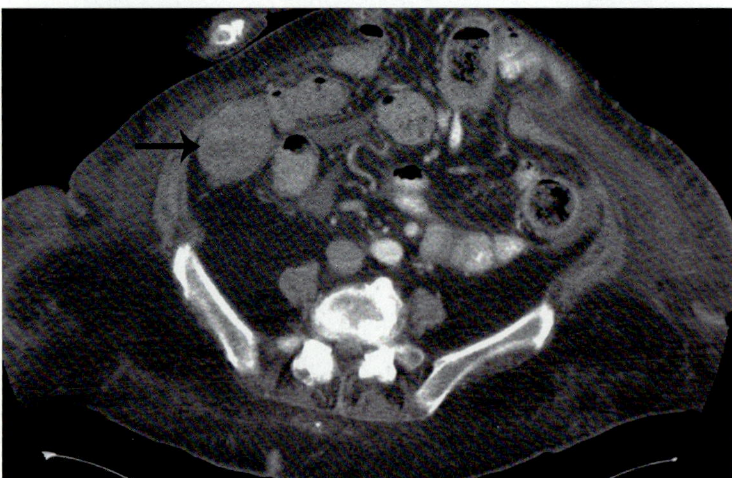

Figure 4.146 — Omentum, Metastatic Adult Granulosa Cell Tumor. Axial contrast-enhanced CT demonstrates an omental nodule in the right lower quadrant (arrow).

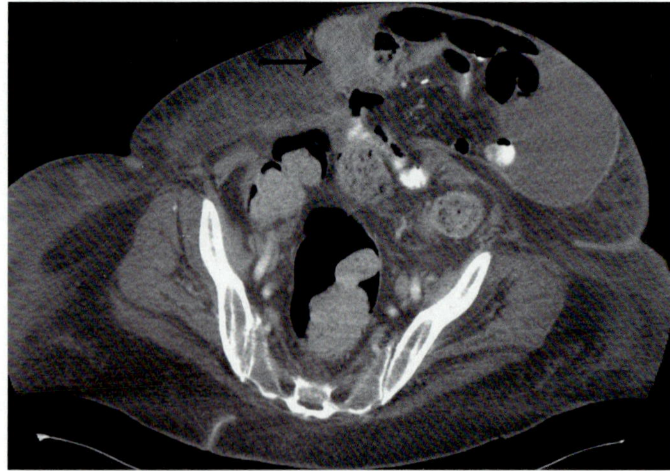

Figure 4.147 — Omentum, Metastatic Adult Granulosa Cell Tumor. Axial contrast-enhanced CT demonstrates an additional omental nodule in the right lower quadrant (arrow). The patient has a history of granulosa cell tumor of the ovary and these nodules are suspicious for omental implants.

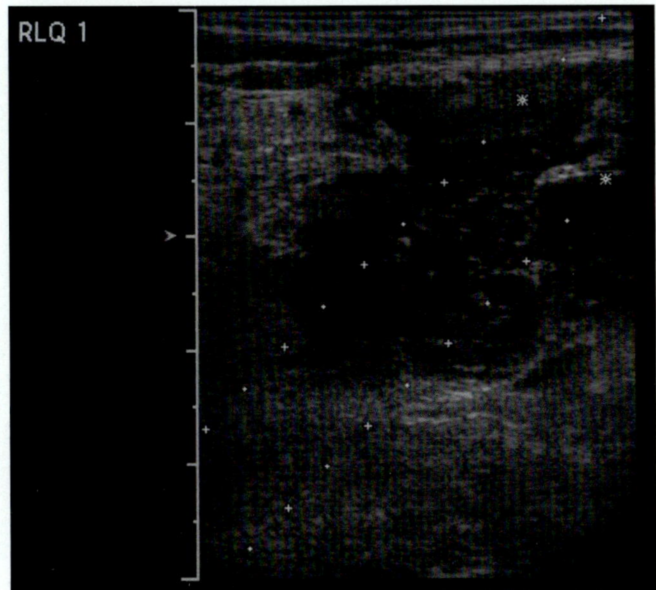

Figure 4.148 — Omentum, Metastatic Adult Granulosa Cell Tumor. Sonographic image at the time of ultrasound-guided biopsy shows a hypoechoic mass in the right lower quadrant. Granulosa cell tumors secrete estrogens; thus, patients may present with menstrual irregularities or endometrial hyperplasia or carcinoma.

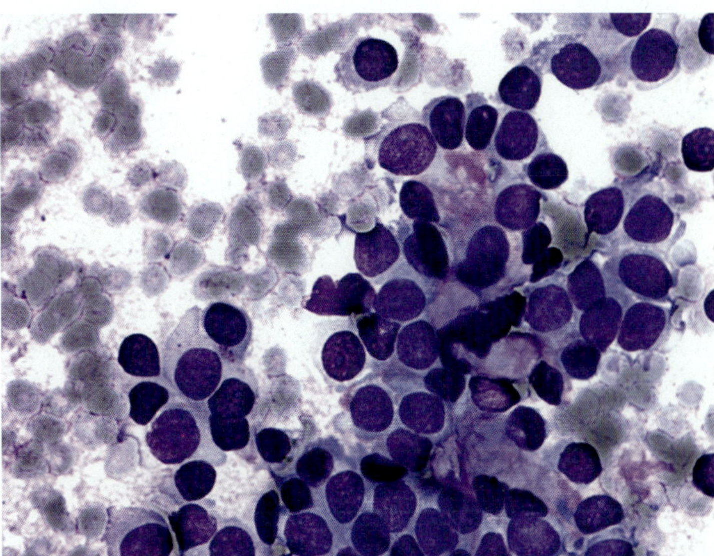

Figure 4.149 — Omentum, Metastatic Adult Granulosa Cell Tumor. This fragment of epithelioid cells shows rosette formations with a small amount of fibrillary material in the center. The nuclei are intermediate sized with round to oval nuclei and slight nuclear membrane irregularities. (Diff Quik stain, medium power)

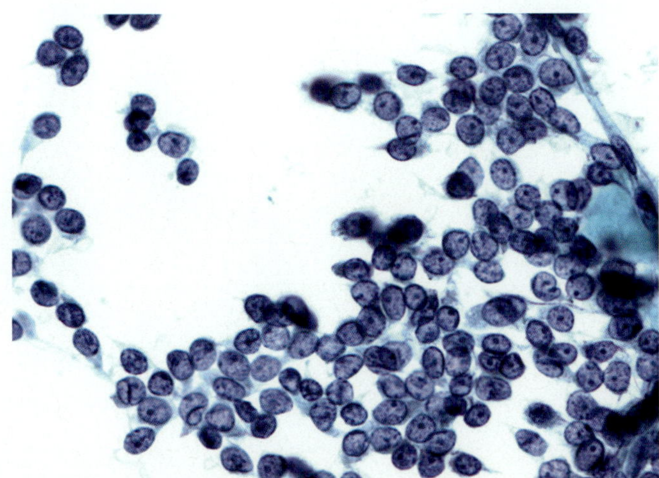

Figure 4.150 — Omentum, Metastatic Adult Granulosa Cell Tumor. These tumor cells show the classic "coffee bean" nuclear shape with focal nucleoli and prominent nuclear membranes. Granulosa cell tumor typically follows an indolent course but can recur, typically 4–6 years following primary resection. (Papanicolaou stain, high power)

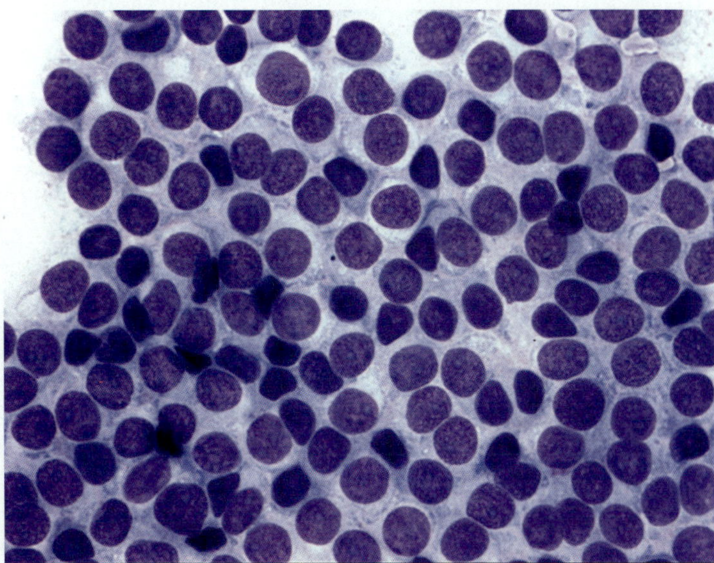

Figure 4.151 — Omentum, Metastatic Adult Granulosa Cell Tumor. This sheet of tumor cells shows uniform spacing with bland, regular nuclei. Sampling of benign mesothelial cells should be considered in the differential diagnosis given the bland appearance of the neoplastic cells. (Diff Quik stain, high power)

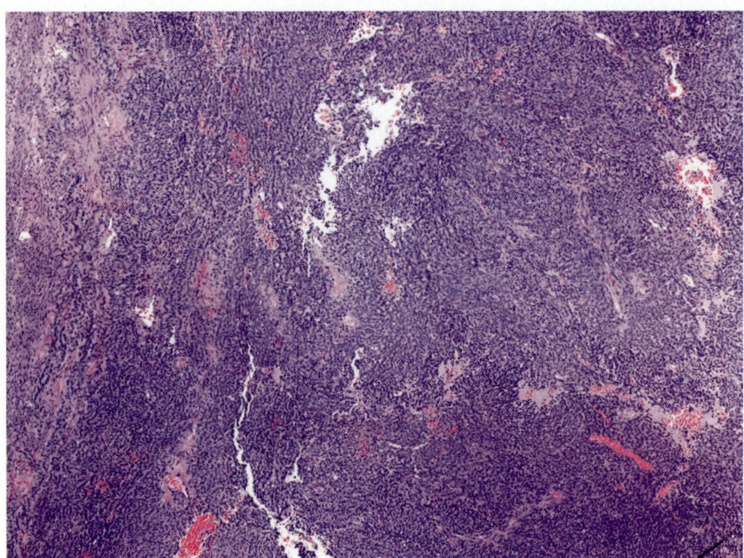

Figure 4.152 — Omentum, Metastatic Adult Granulosa Cell Tumor (Histology). Adult type granulosa cell tumors occur in women of reproductive age and in postmenopausal women. This tumor shows solid sheets of tumor cells with a scant stromal component. Focal areas of hemorrhage are seen. Note the presence of Call–Exner bodies which are small follicle-like structures filled with pink material. (Hematoxylin and eosin stain, low power)

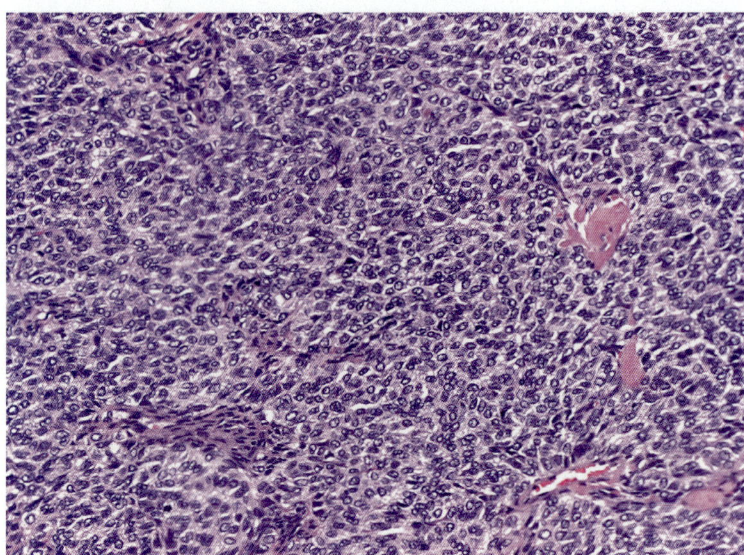

Figure 4.153 — Omentum, Metastatic Adult Granulosa Cell Tumor (Histology). Solid sheets of neoplastic cells show scant, pale cytoplasm, and round to oval nuclei with a longitudinal nuclear groove imparting a "coffee bean" appearance. The stroma is scant with the occasional presence of Call–Exner bodies. (Hematoxylin and eosin stain, medium power)

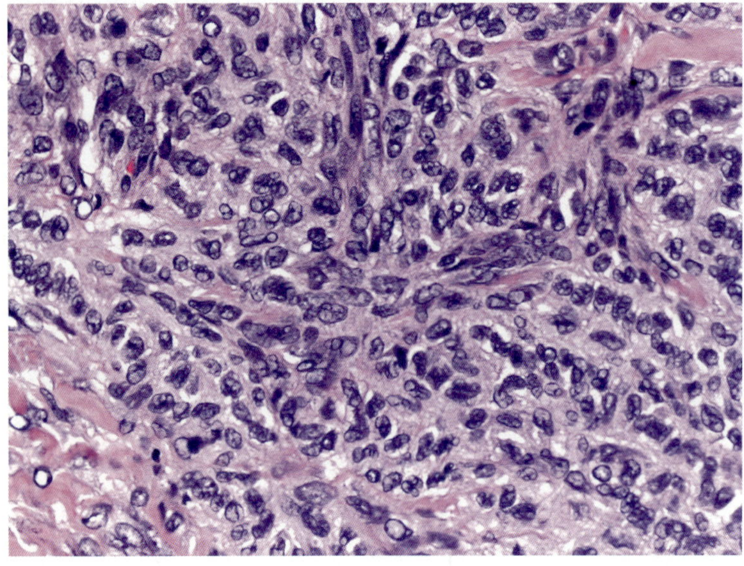

Figure 4.154 — Omentum, Metastatic Adult Granulosa Cell Tumor (Histology). Nests of cells are shown containing cells with high nuclear-to-cytoplasmic ratio. Nuclei are oval-shaped with irregular nuclear contours and rare nucleoli. Occasional nuclear grooves are present. (Hematoxylin and eosin stain, high power)

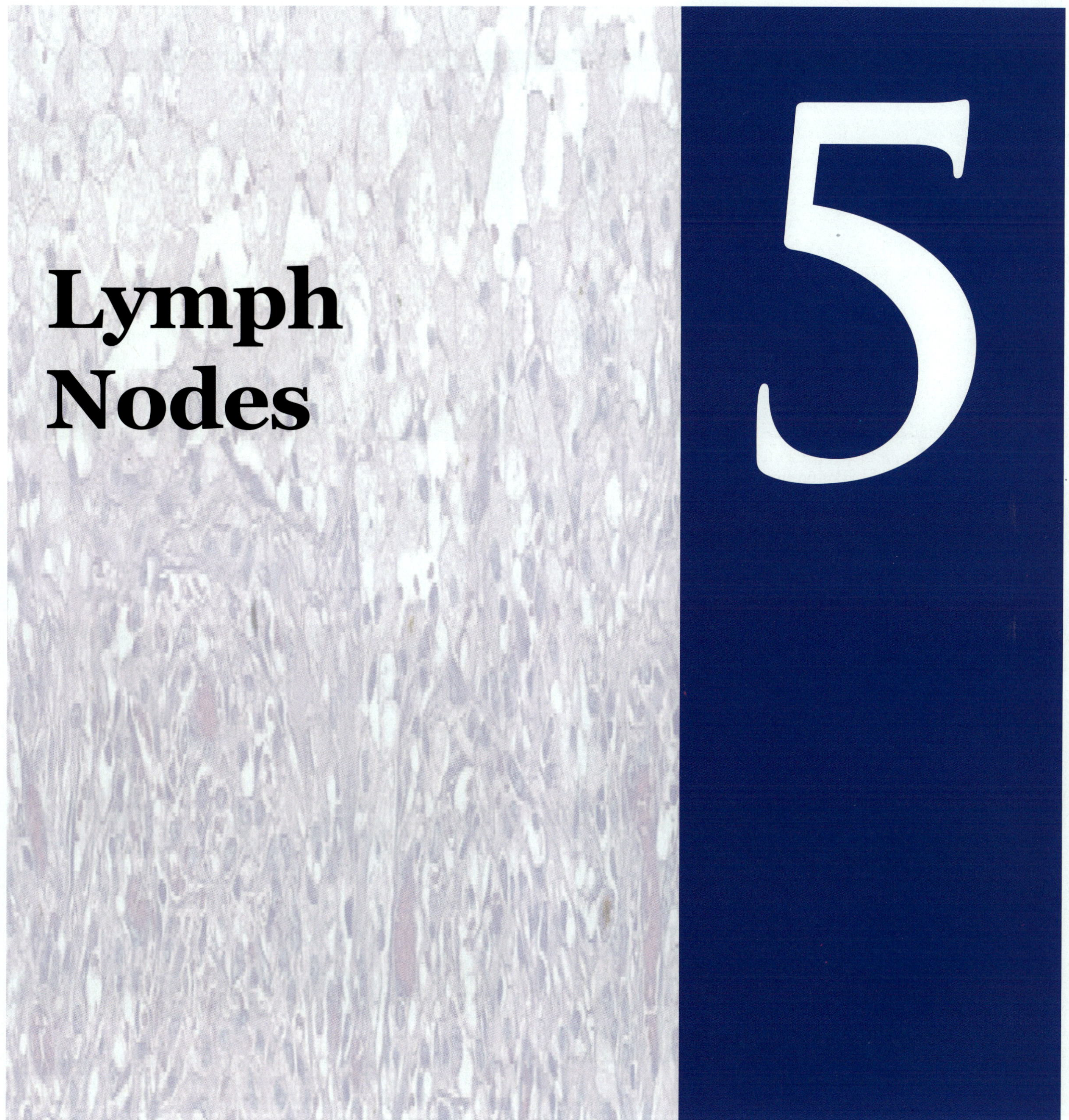

5

Lymph Nodes

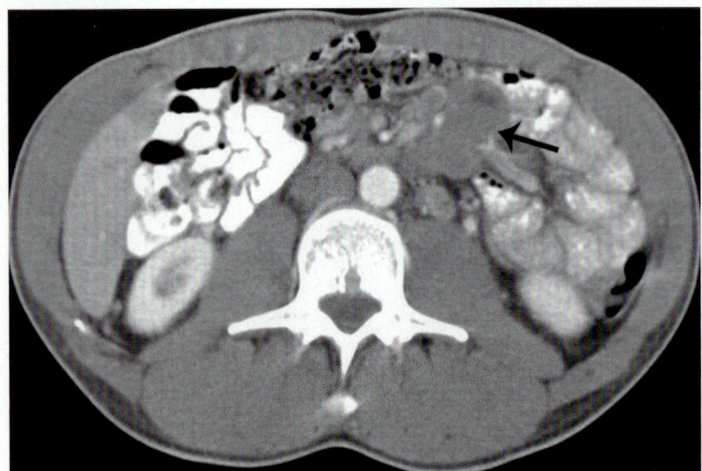

FIGURE 5.1 — Lymph Node, Mesenteric, Mycobacterial Infection. This 32-year-old HIV-positive man with a CD4 count of 82 presented with new swelling of lymph nodes and pain at multiple sites. Axial contrast-enhanced CT image demonstrates extensive mesenteric adenopathy (arrow). Included in the differential diagnosis is lymphoma and *Mycobacterium* infection.

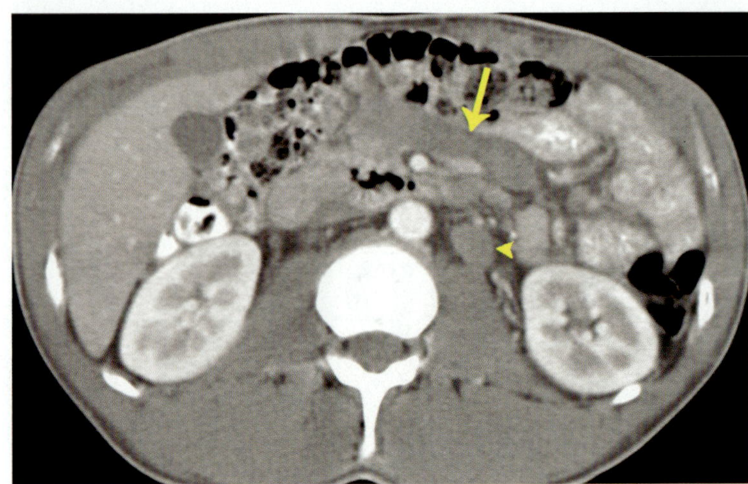

FIGURE 5.2 — Lymph Node, Mesenteric, Mycobacterial Infection. Axial contrast-enhanced CT shows that the adenopathy extends more inferiorly into the mesentery (arrow) and also involves the retroperitoneum (arrowhead).

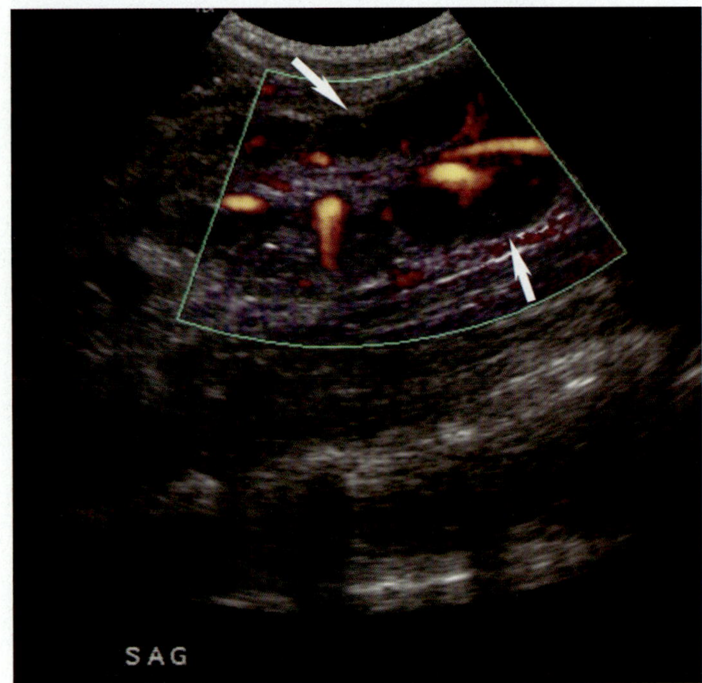

FIGURE 5.3 — Lymph Node, Mesenteric, Mycobacterial Infection. Sonographic image with power Doppler in a different patient shows marked abdominal adenopathy (arrows).

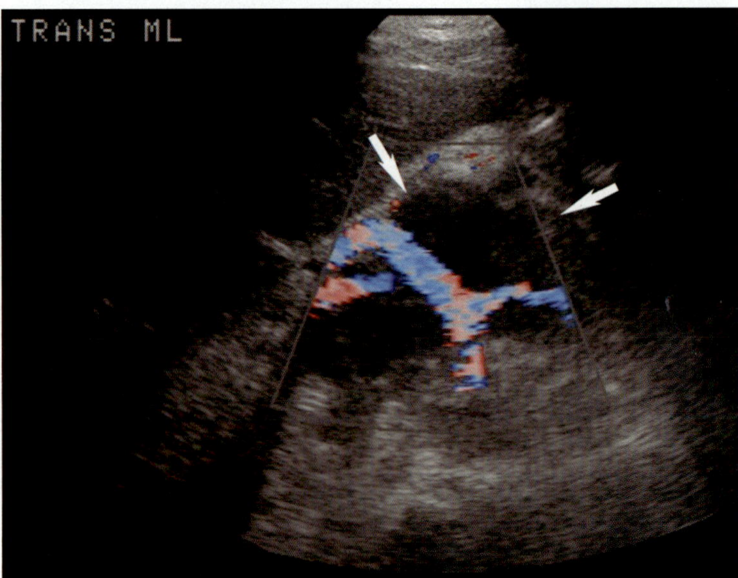

FIGURE 5.4 — Lymph Node, Mesenteric, Mycobacterial Infection. Sonographic image with color Doppler in a different patient shows enlarged hypoechoic abdominal lymph nodes (arrows). Included in the differential diagnosis are lymphoma and *Mycobacterium* infection.

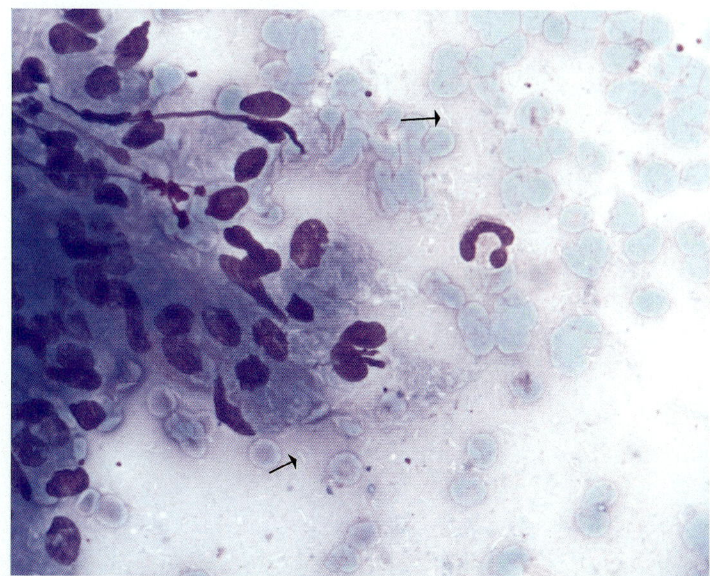

FIGURE 5.5 — Lymph Node, Mesenteric, Mycobacterial Infection. A group of macrophages forming a loose granuloma is present in the left portion of the field. The macrophages show negative images or "ghosts" of mycobacterial organisms. The outline of these organisms can also be seen floating freely in the background (arrows). (Diff Quik stain, medium power)

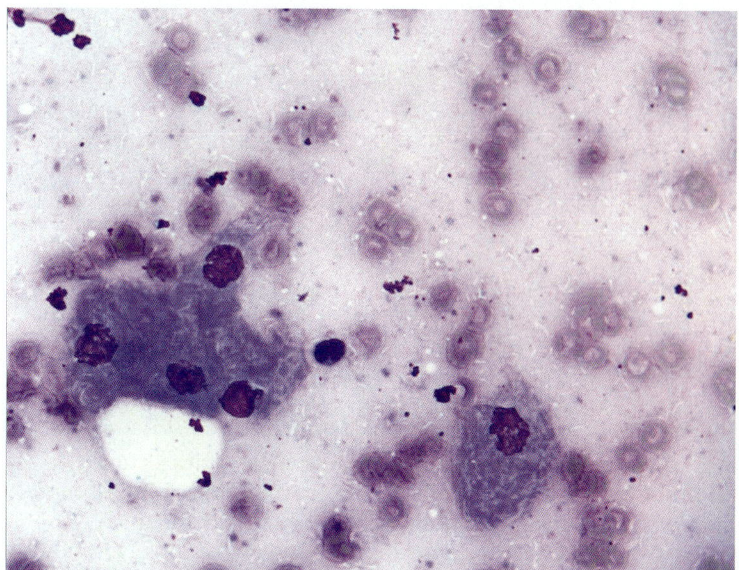

FIGURE 5.6 — Lymph Node, Mesenteric, Mycobacterial Infection. This patient had a history of poorly controlled HIV/AIDS, and a prior abdominal *Mycobacterium avium-intracellulare* (MAI) infection. The mesenteric lymph nodes enlarged despite microbial therapy; thus, an FNA was requested to rule out another process. There are numerous mycobacterial organisms filling these macrophages and present in the background. (Diff Quik stain, high power)

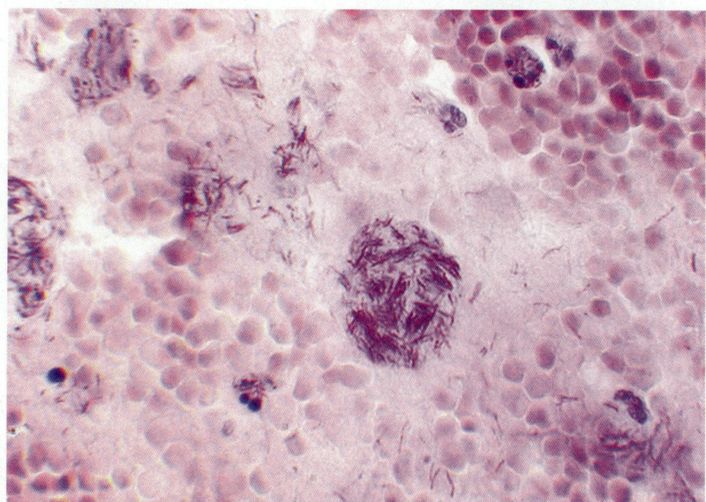

FIGURE 5.7 — Lymph Node, Mesenteric, Mycobacterial Infection. A stain for acid fast bacilli highlights numerous thin, delicate rod-like organisms. The organisms are often plentiful in MAI infection in contrast to *Mycobacterium tuberculosis*, in which organisms are typically scant. (Ziehl–Neelsen stain, high power)

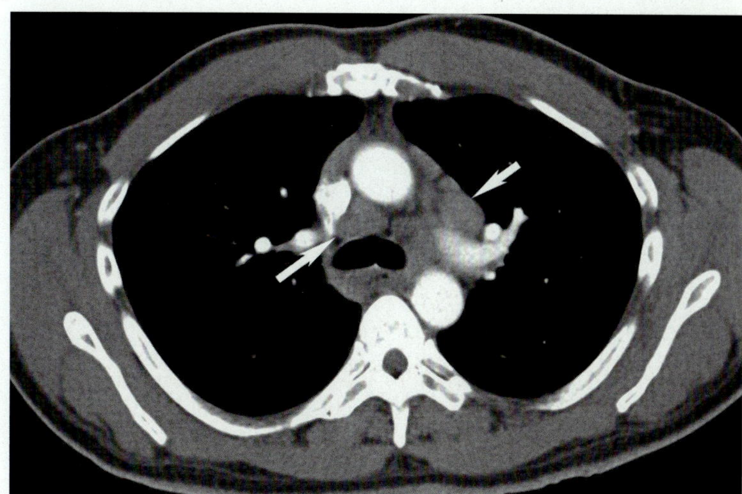

FIGURE 5.8 — Lymph Node, Mediastinal, Noncaseating Granulomatous Inflammation. Axial contrast-enhanced CT shows extensive mediastinal adenopathy (arrows).

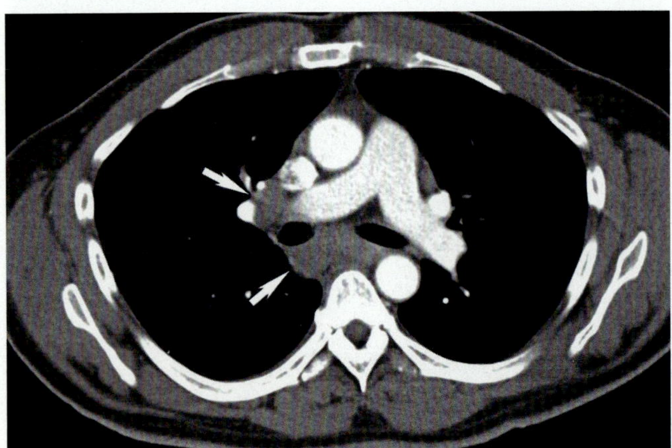

FIGURE 5.9 — Lymph Node, Mediastinal, Noncaseating Granulomatous Inflammation. Axial contrast-enhanced CT more inferiorly confirms extent of mediastinal and hilar adenopathy (arrows). Differential diagnosis includes sarcoidosis and lymphoma; however, bilaterally symmetric hilar and mediastinal lymph node involvement is suggestive of sarcoidosis.

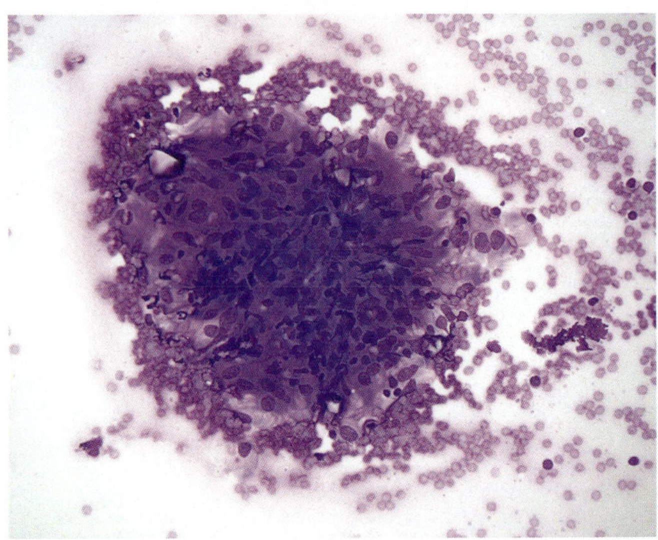

FIGURE 5.10 — Lymph Node, Mediastinal, Noncaseating Granulomatous Inflammation. An aggregate of densely packed epithelioid histiocytes forming a granuloma is shown. The histiocytes have oval- to kidney-bean-shaped nuclei and abundant pale cytoplasm. Few lymphocytes are scattered within the granuloma. (Diff Quik stain, medium power)

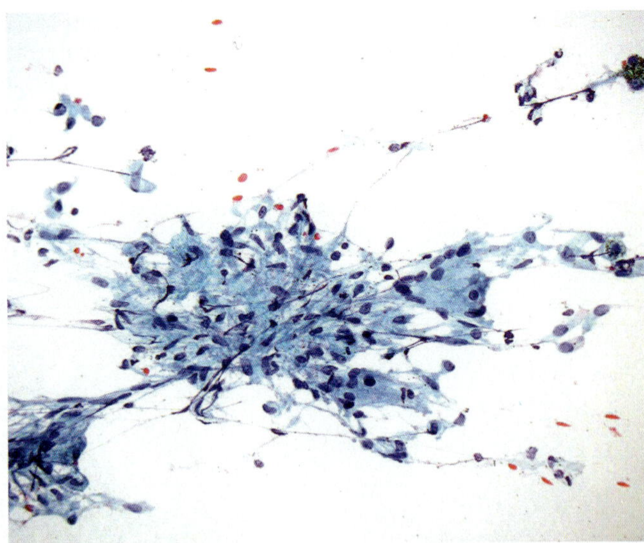

FIGURE 5.11 — Lymph Node, Mediastinal, Noncaseating Granulomatous Inflammation. Numerous epithelioid histiocytes are present with voluminous cytoplasm and ill-defined cell borders. A multinucleated giant cell is present. There is no necrosis or acute inflammation present in the background; thus, the granulomatous inflammation is termed noncaseating. If infectious and neoplastic causes are ruled out, these findings are consistent with sarcoidosis. (Papanicolaou stain, medium power)

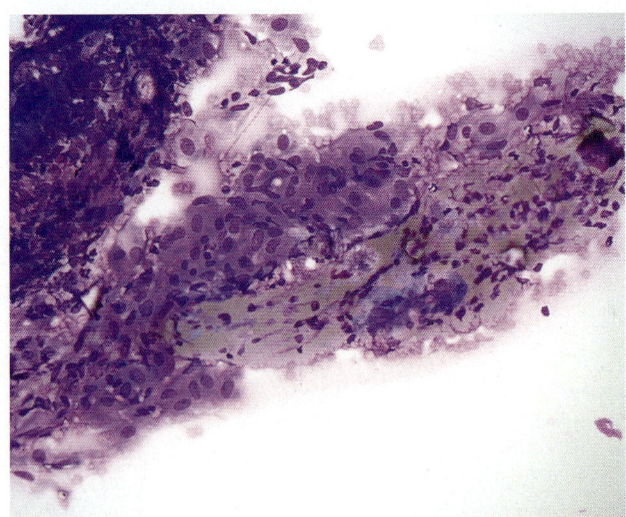

FIGURE 5.12 — Lymph Node, Mediastinal, Noncaseating Granulomatous Inflammation. The epithelioid appearance of these histiocytes can prompt consideration of an epithelial neoplasm, but the low nuclear-to-cytoplasmic ratio and bland nuclei support a benign diagnosis. Correlation with clinical and radiologic appearance is important as granulomatous inflammation can occur within or adjacent to malignancies. (Diff Quik stain, high power)

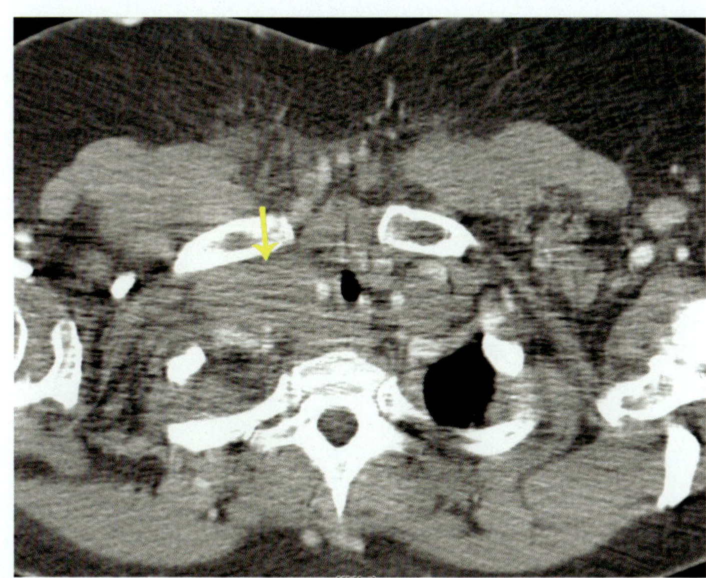

FIGURE 5.13 — Lymph Node, Neck, Hodgkin Lymphoma. Axial contrast-enhanced CT shows bilateral supraclavicular adenopathy, right (arrow) greater than left.

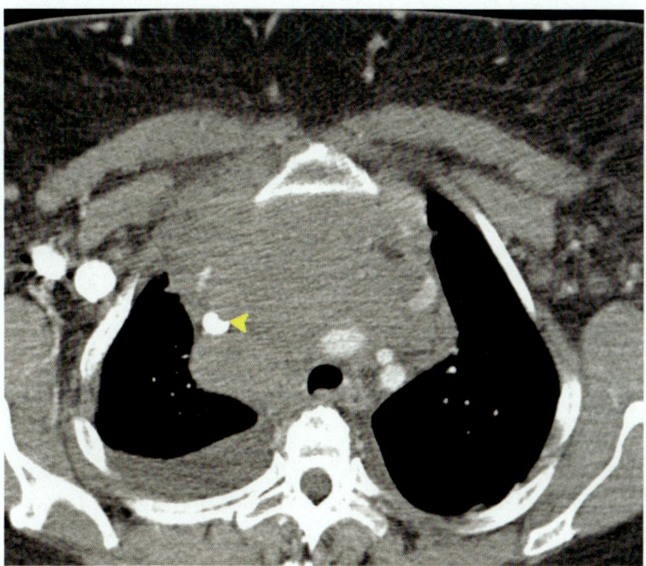

FIGURE 5.14 — Lymph Node, Neck, Hodgkin Lymphoma. Axial contrast-enhanced CT shows that conglomerate adenopathy extends inferiorly into the anterior mediastinum, severely narrowing the SVC (arrowhead). The mediastinal mass is encasing the vessels.

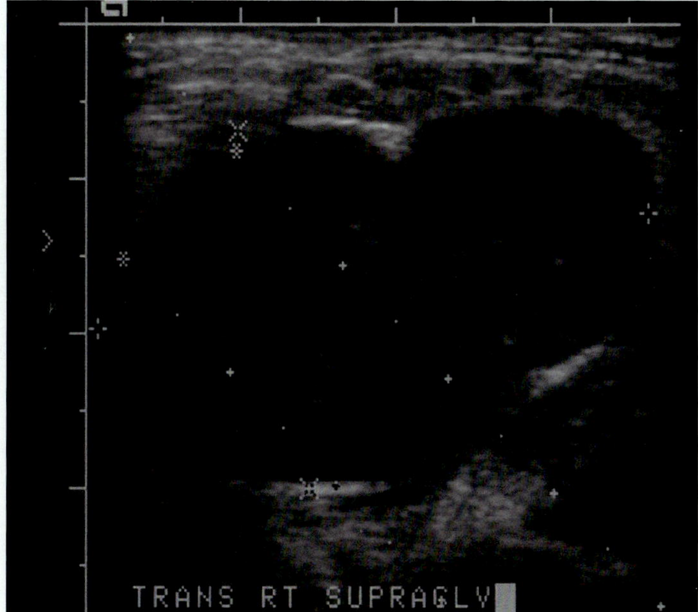

FIGURE 5.15 — Lymph Node, Neck, Hodgkin Lymphoma. Sonographic image at the time of ultrasound-guided biopsy shows enlarged, hypoechoic right supraclavicular adenopathy. Hodgkin lymphoma was found on biopsy of this lymph node.

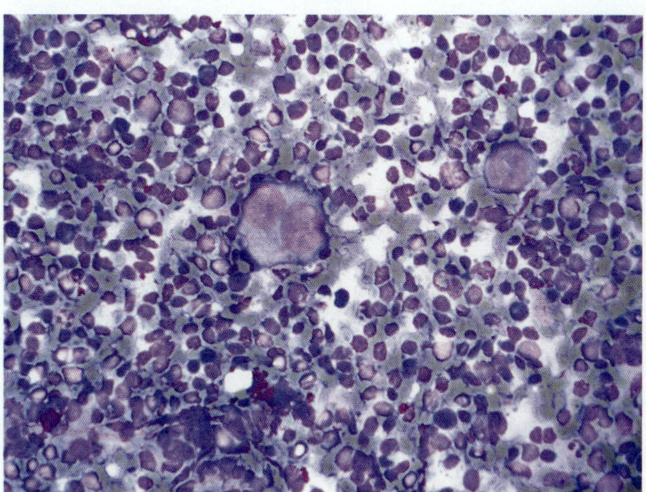

FIGURE 5.16 — Lymph Node, Neck, Hodgkin Lymphoma. This patient had a history of mixed cellularity Hodgkin lymphoma and a recurrence was suspected clinically. The aspirate demonstrated numerous markedly enlarged cells in a background of mixed inflammatory cells, predominantly lymphocytes. One of the large cells shown here shows a classic Reed–Sternberg morphology with binucleation and large nucleoli. (Diff Quik stain, medium power)

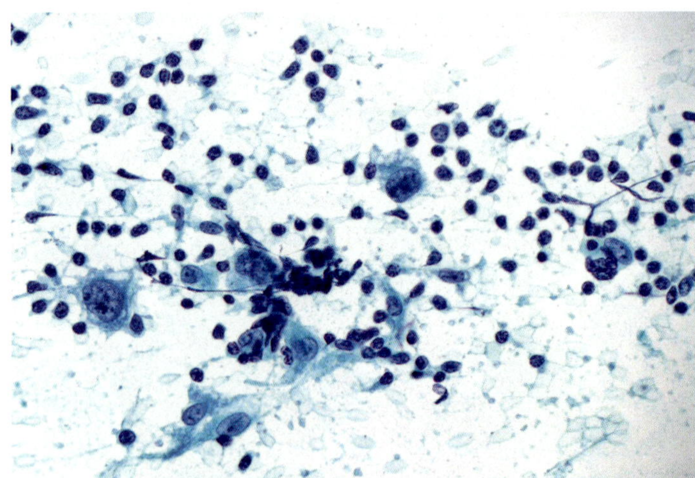

FIGURE 5.17 — Lymph Node, Neck, Hodgkin Lymphoma. Scattered large cells with variably sized nucleoli and abundant cytoplasm are admixed with numerous small lymphocytes. If possible, material should be obtained for cell block or core biopsy in order to perform confirmatory immunostains. (Papanicolaou stain, medium power)

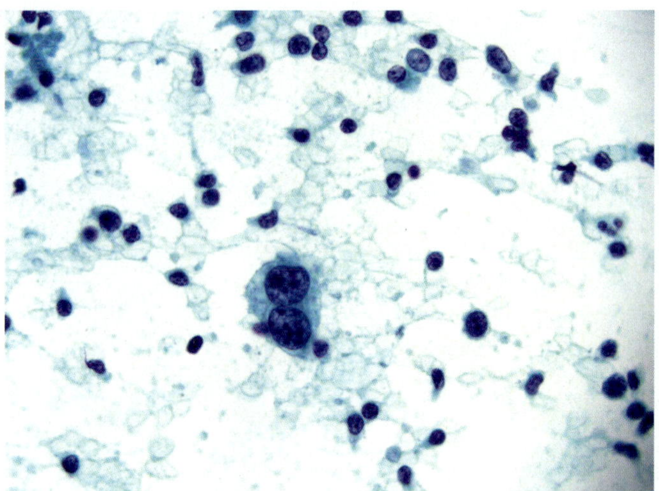

FIGURE 5.18 — Lymph Node, Neck, Hodgkin Lymphoma. A large binucleated cell is present in the center of the field. Reed–Sternberg-type cells may be encountered in other hematopoietic neoplasms, including anaplastic large cell lymphoma and small lymphocytic lymphoma, which should be considered in the differential, particularly in a primary diagnosis. (Papanicolaou stain, high power)

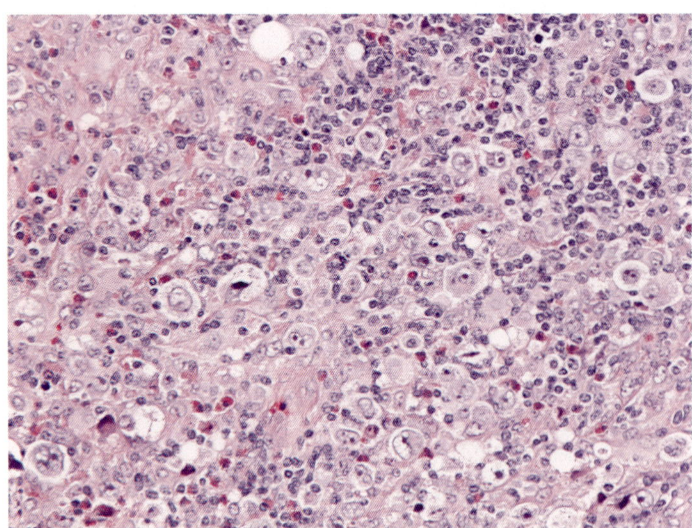

FIGURE 5.19 — Lymph Node, Neck, Hodgkin Lymphoma (Histology). The normal architecture of this lymph node is completely disrupted. The cellularity is composed of mixed inflammation surrounding scattered, large, atypical cells consistent with Reed–Sternberg cells and numerous eosinophils. Cervical lymph nodes are a common site for Hodgkin lymphoma. (Hematoxylin and eosin stain, medium power)

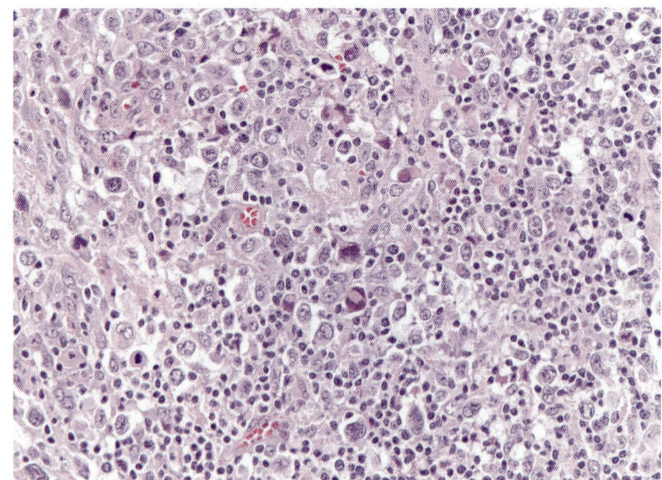

FIGURE 5.20 — Lymph Node, Neck, Hodgkin Lymphoma (Histology). The large, atypical cells are quite evident in this case, showing prominent nucleoli. Reed–Sternberg cells may be mononucleated or binucleated. The background is typically composed of polymorphous lymphocytes, plasma cells and eosinophils (not shown in this case), characteristic of Hodgkin lymphoma. (Hematoxylin and eosin stain, medium power)

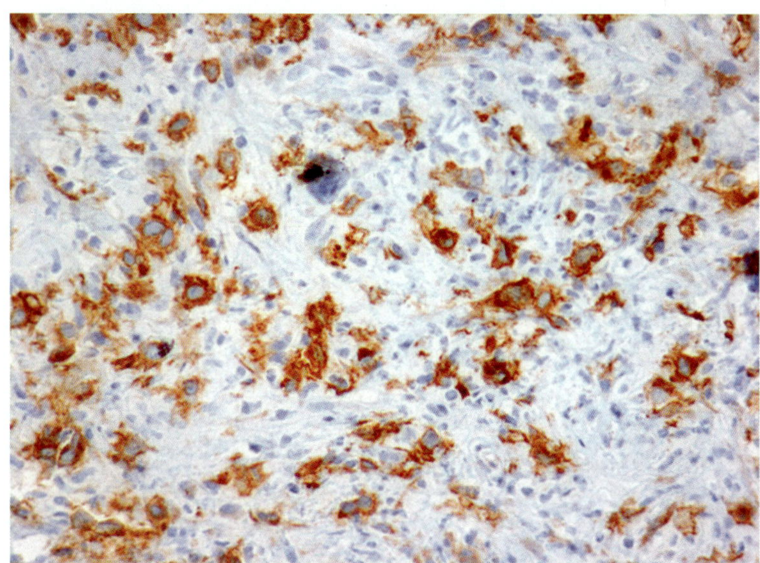

FIGURE 5.21 — Lymph Node, Neck, Hodgkin Lymphoma (Histology). A CD30 immunostain highlights the Reed–Sternberg cells. CD30 is not specific, and anaplastic large cell lymphoma should be ruled out with negative EMA staining, as it was in this case, as well as positive CD15. (CD30 immunostain, high power)

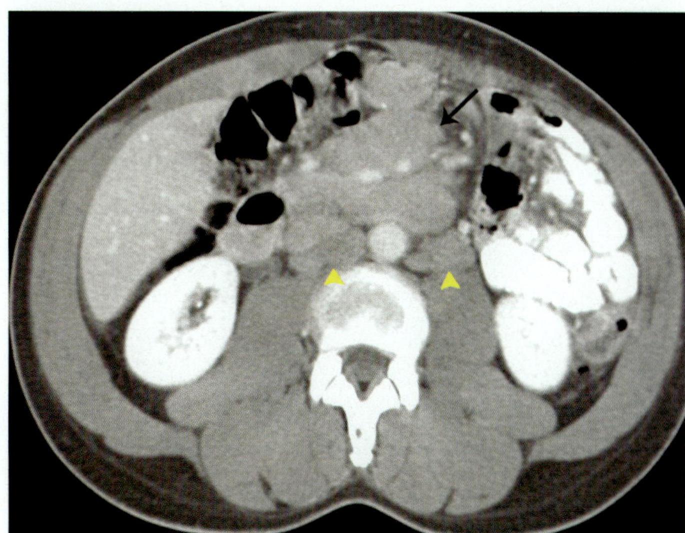

FIGURE 5.22 — Lymph Node, Abdominal, Follicular Lymphoma. Axial contrast-enhanced CT shows a large mesenteric mass (arrow) encasing mesenteric vessels. There is also mild retroperitoneal adenopathy (arrowheads).

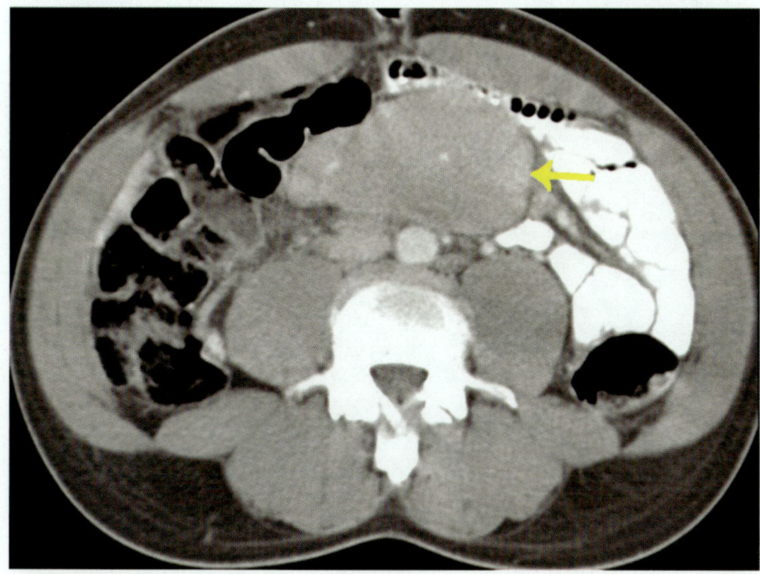

FIGURE 5.23 — Lymph Node, Abdominal, Follicular Lymphoma. Axial contrast-enhanced CT image slightly more inferiorly shows the large mesenteric mass, which is due to conglomerate adenopathy (arrow).

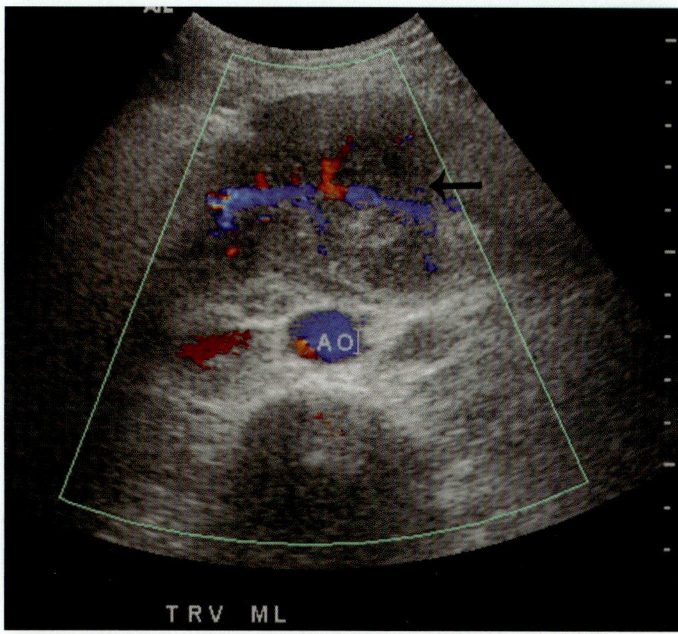

FIGURE 5.24 — Lymph Node, Abdominal, Follicular Lymphoma. Sonographic image at the time of ultrasound-guided biopsy confirms a hypoechoic mass (arrow) encasing mesenteric vessels.

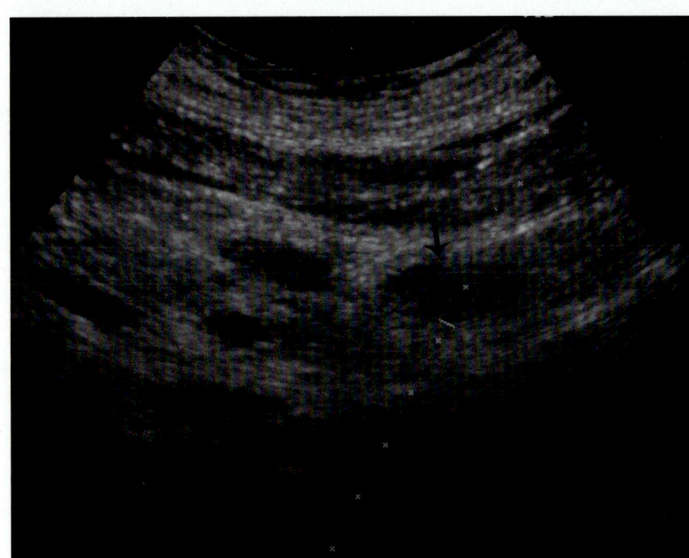

FIGURE 5.25 — Lymph Node, Abdominal, Follicular Lymphoma. This patient presented with abdominal and retroperitoneal adenopathy. Sonographic image in a different patient shows several hypoechoic enlarged abdominal lymph nodes, one of which was targeted for biopsy (arrow).

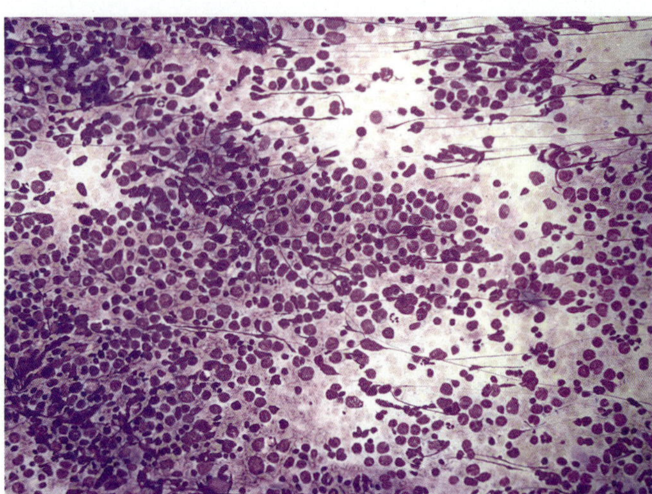

FIGURE 5.26 — Lymph Node, Abdominal, Follicular Lymphoma. This aspirate smear shows abundant cellularity consisting of numerous single dispersed cells. Long strands of cytoplasm are seen smeared across the field representing crush artifact from these delicate cells. The majority of the cells are intermediate sized with round to slightly irregular nuclear shape and scant cytoplasm. (Diff Quik stain, medium power)

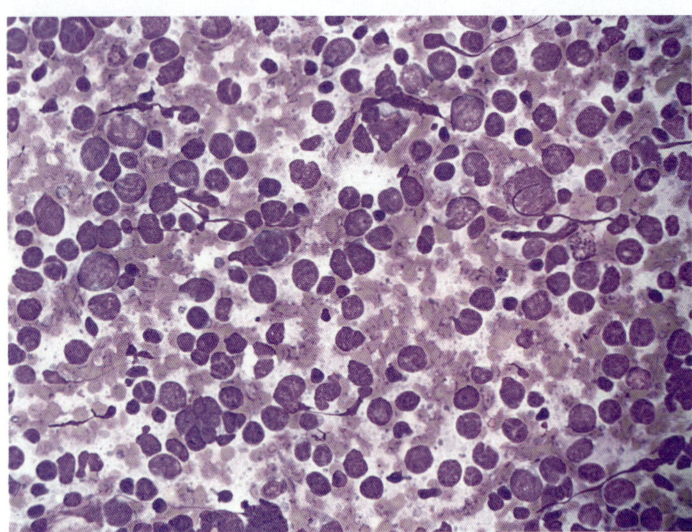

FIGURE 5.27 — Lymph Node, Abdominal, Follicular Lymphoma. A population of monotonous medium-sized lymphocytes with rare larger forms is present. Material should be obtained for immunophenotyping (flow cytometry), which should show CD10 positivity with high bcl2. (Diff Quik stain, high power)

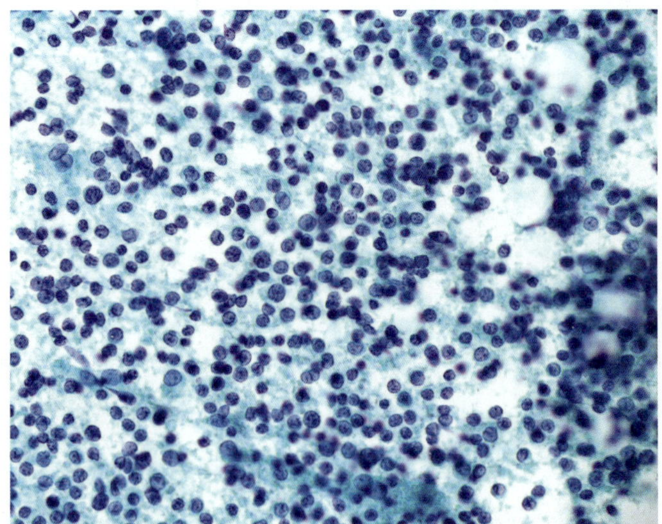

FIGURE 5.28 — Lymph Node, Abdominal, Follicular Lymphoma. Follicular lymphoma is the most common of all non-Hodgkin lymphomas. The clinical course is generally indolent, but transformation to a large B-cell lymphoma occurs in 20–30% of patients. These neoplastic lymphocytes appear small to intermediate size and have cleaved nuclei. (Papanicolaou stain, high power)

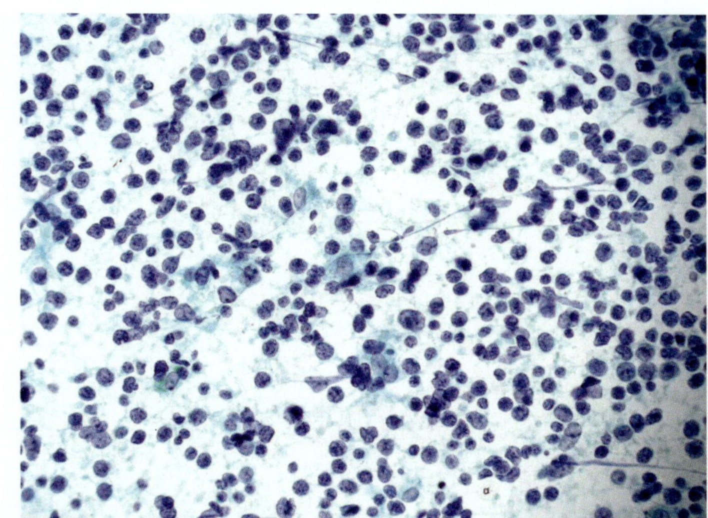

FIGURE 5.29 — Lymph Node, Abdominal, Follicular Lymphoma. The predominant population is medium-sized lymphoid cells with scant cytoplasm and cleaved nuclei. Rare larger centroblasts are present. Tissue studies (large core biopsies or excisional biopsies) are often needed to diagnose follicular lymphoma, as architectural features are important factors in tumor grading. (Papanicolaou stain, high power)

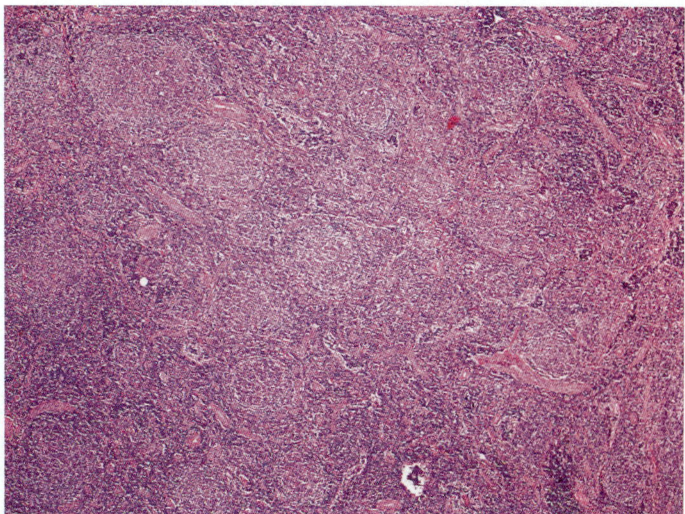

FIGURE 5.30 — Lymph Node, Abdominal, Follicular Lymphoma (Histology). The normal lymph node architecture is effaced by a proliferation of crowded, back-to-back follicles. The primary differential diagnosis in this case is follicular hyperplasia, which would show greater interfollicular space and follicular polarity, which is not seen here. (Hematoxylin and eosin stain, low power)

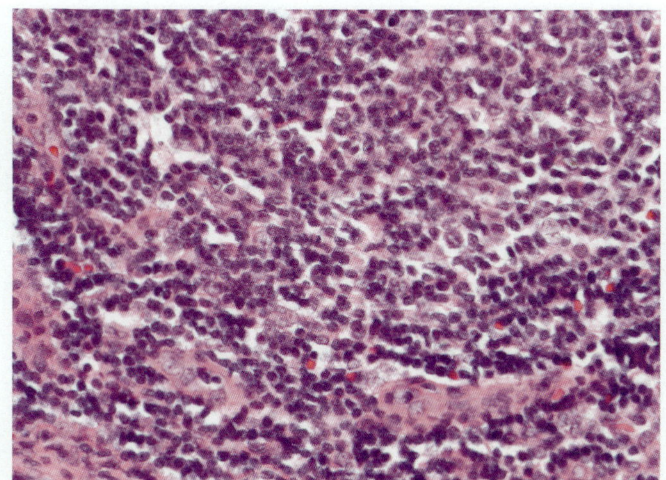

FIGURE 5.31 — Lymph Node, Abdominal, Follicular Lymphoma (Histology). A monotonous population of small lymphocytes is present. There is an absence of tingible body macrophages. Flow cytometric analysis demonstrated a lambda-restricted lymphoid population expressing CD20, CD19, CD22, and CD10. (Hematoxylin and eosin stain, high power)

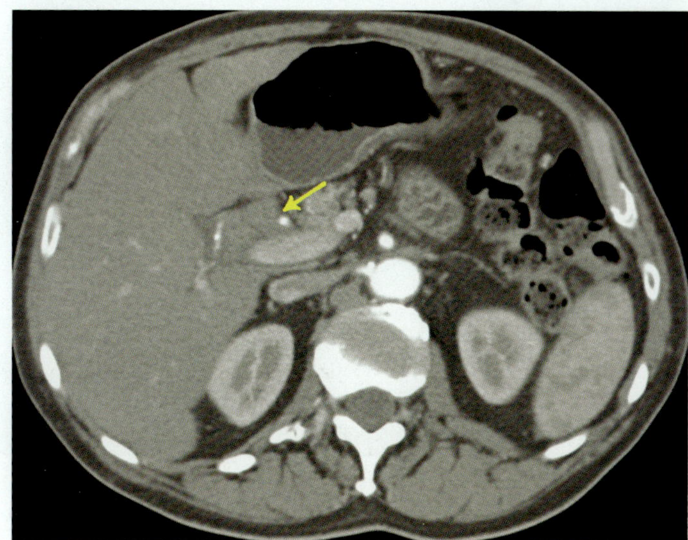

FIGURE 5.32 — Lymph Node, Peripancreatic, Burkitt Lymphoma. Axial contrast-enhanced CT shows a soft tissue mass in the porta hepatis encasing the hepatic artery (arrow). The mass is near, but separate from, the pancreatic head.

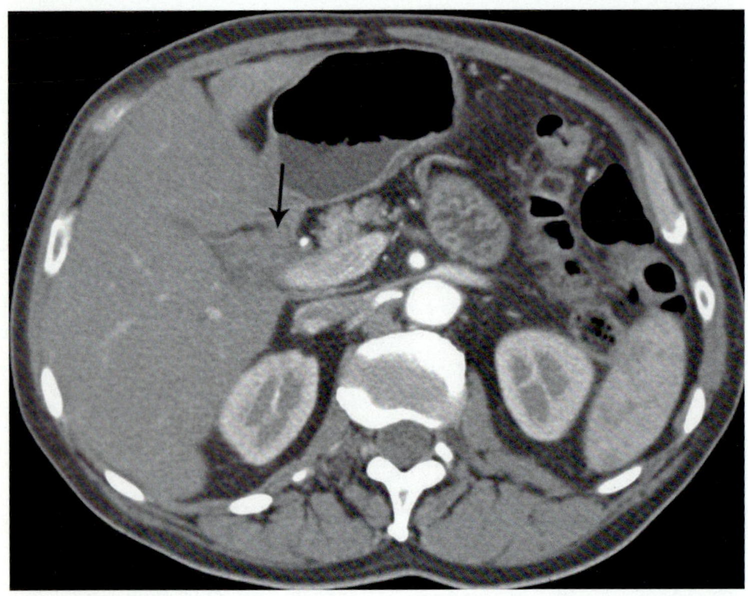

FIGURE 5.33 — Lymph Node, Peripancreatic, Burkitt Lymphoma. Axial contrast-enhanced CT more inferiorly shows further extension of the mass in the porta hepatis (arrow). The mass extrinsically compresses the common bile duct.

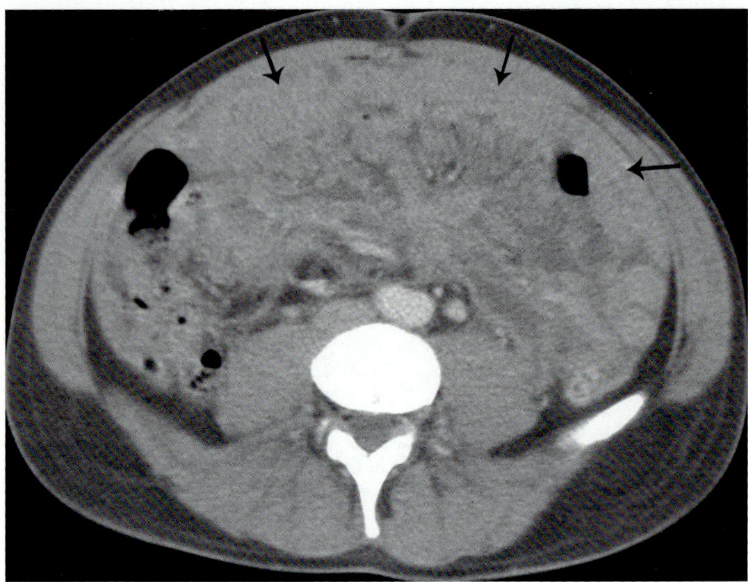

FIGURE 5.34 — Omentum and Lymph Nodes, Abdominal, Burkitt Lymphoma. Axial contrast-enhanced CT shows extensive omental thickening and nodularity (arrows).

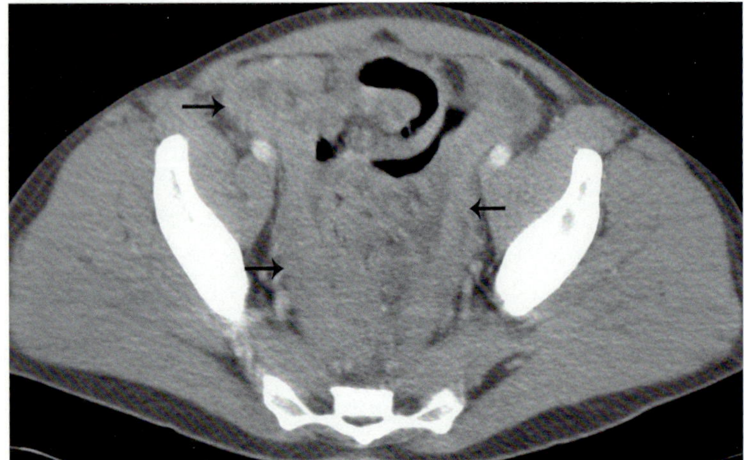

FIGURE 5.35 — Omentum and Lymph Nodes, Abdominal, Burkitt Lymphoma. Axial contrast-enhanced CT more inferiorly in the pelvis shows extensive thickening of the peritoneal lining (arrows) and a small amount of ascites. Although this was found to represent an abdominal Burkitt-like lymphoma, metastatic disease and primary peritoneal carcinomatosis are included in the differential diagnosis.

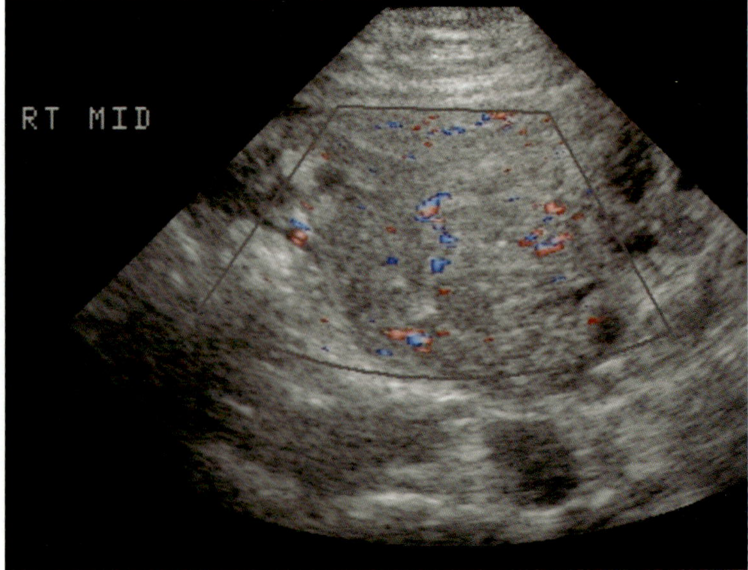

FIGURE 5.36 — Omentum and Lymph Nodes, Abdominal, Burkitt Lymphoma. Sonographic image also shows the omental mass with internal vascularity.

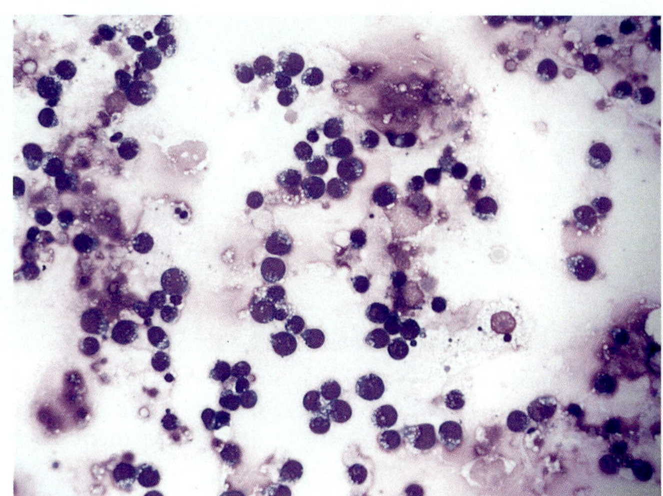

FIGURE 5.37 — Lymph Node, Peripancreatic, Burkitt Lymphoma. Numerous large single cells are shown with high nuclear-to-cytoplasmic ratio, hyperchromatic nuclei, and a thin rim of basophilic cytoplasm. Vacuoles are seen in the cytoplasm of most cells, characteristic of Burkitt lymphoma, although not specific. (Diff Quik stain, medium power)

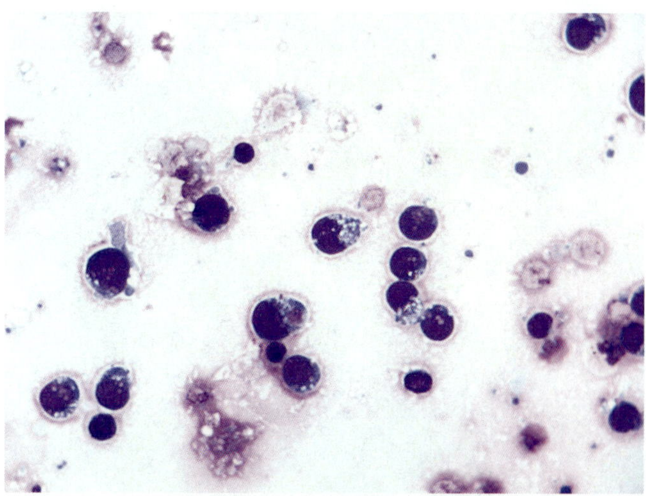

FIGURE 5.38 — Lymph Node, Peripancreatic, Burkitt Lymphoma. Burkitt lymphoma is a high-grade B-cell lymphoma and may be endemic (EBV-related), sporadic (children and young adults), or immunodeficiency related. All tumor types are related to translocations involving c-myc. Large lymphoid cells with vacuolated cytoplasm are present. (Diff Quik stain, medium power)

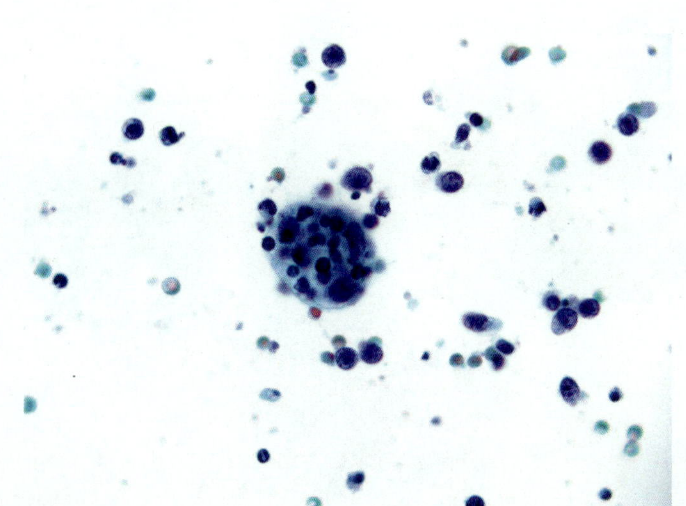

FIGURE 5.39 — Lymph Node, Peripancreatic, Burkitt Lymphoma. A large tingible body macrophage containing abundant cellular debris is present in the center of the field. Due to the high proliferative rate, numerous mitotic figures, apoptotic bodies, and tingible body macrophages are encountered. (Papanicolaou stain, high power)

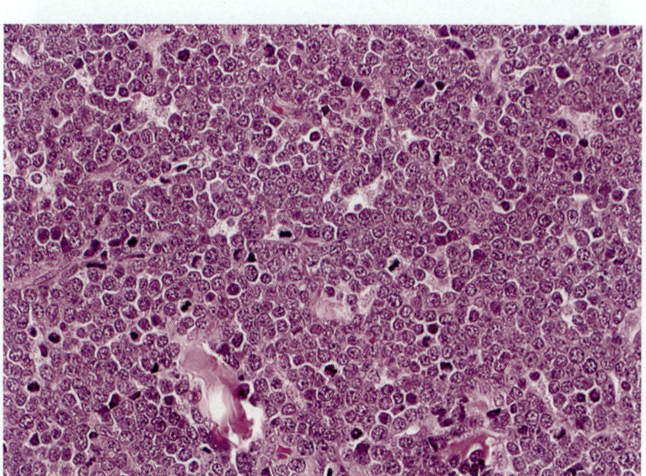

FIGURE 5.40 — Lymph Node, Peripancreatic, Burkitt Lymphoma (Histology). On histologic section, large neoplastic lymphocytes are admixed with numerous apoptotic bodies and areas of necrosis. There are numerous mitotic figures seen. The admixture of numerous lymphocytes and tingible body macrophages imparts a "starry sky" appearance at low power (not shown). (Hematoxylin and eosin stain, low power)

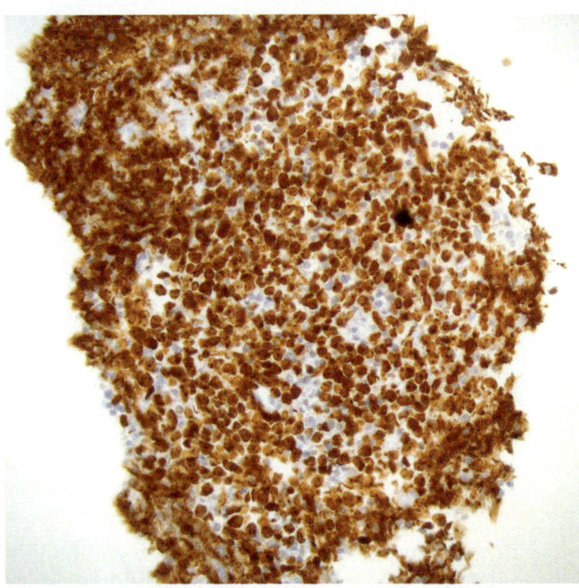

FIGURE 5.41 — Lymph Node, Peripancreatic, Burkitt Lymphoma. This Ki67 immunostain highlights the very high proliferative rate characteristic of Burkitt lymphoma. Almost every neoplastic nucleus is positive. (Ki67 immunostain, high power)

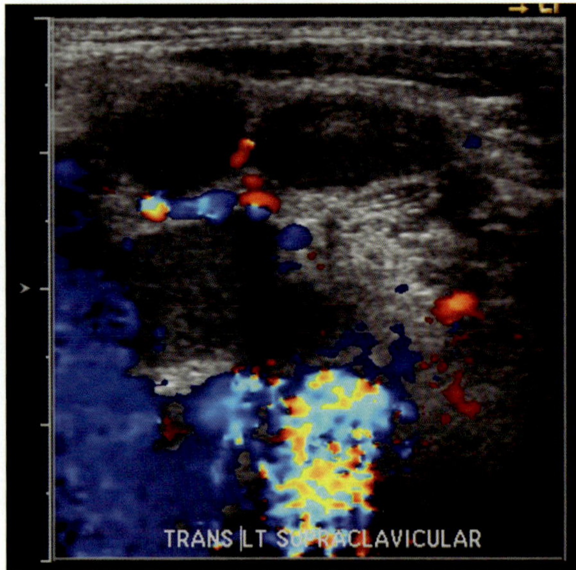

FIGURE 5.43 — Lymph Node, Left Supraclavicular, Metastatic Mammary Carcinoma. Sonographic image confirms enlarged hypoechoic left supraclavicular lymph nodes. This node was targeted for biopsy and found to represent metastatic mammary cancer.

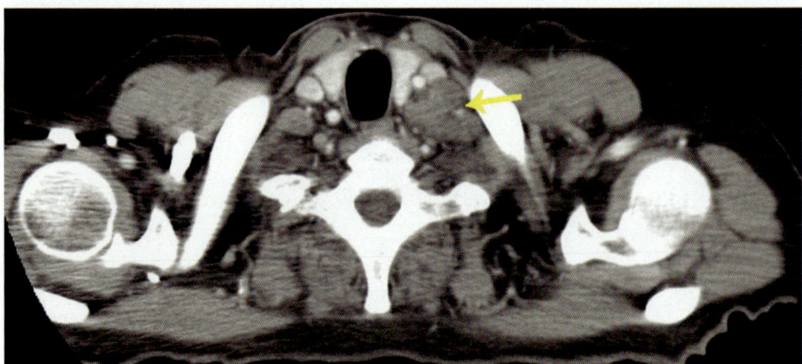

FIGURE 5.42 — Lymph Node, Left Supraclavicular, Metastatic Mammary Carcinoma. Axial contrast-enhanced CT in the left neck shows left supraclavicular adenopathy (arrow). The patient has a history of breast cancer.

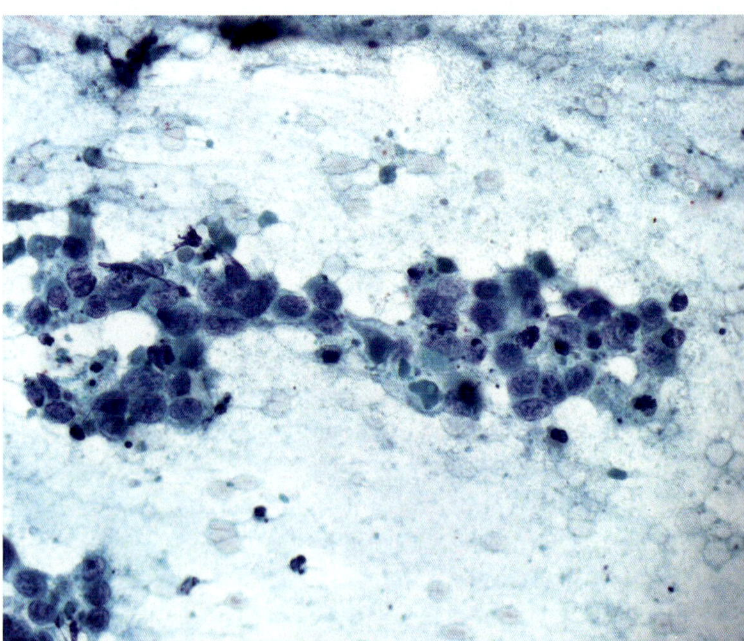

FIGURE 5.44 — Lymph Node, Left Supraclavicular, Metastatic Mammary Carcinoma. This patient had a history of ductal carcinoma of the breast. These epithelial cells form a cohesive fragment and show high nuclear-to-cytoplasmic ratios and nuclear hyperchromasia. Crude glandular formations are present in the right portion of the field. (Papanicolaou stain, high power)

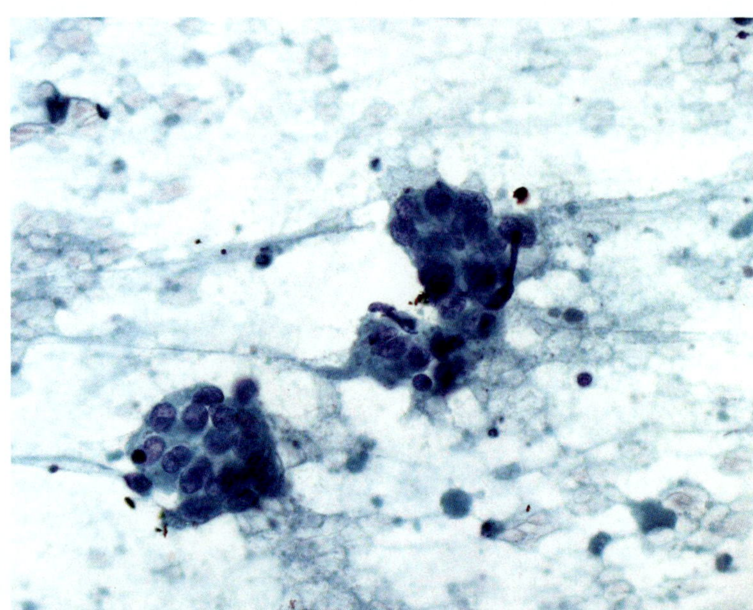

FIGURE 5.45 — Lymph Node, Left Supraclavicular, Metastatic Mammary Carcinoma. Two fragments of malignant glandular epithelium consistent with ductal carcinoma are present. The morphology is not specific, however, and immunostains may be required to definitively determine a primary site. (Papanicolaou stain, high power)

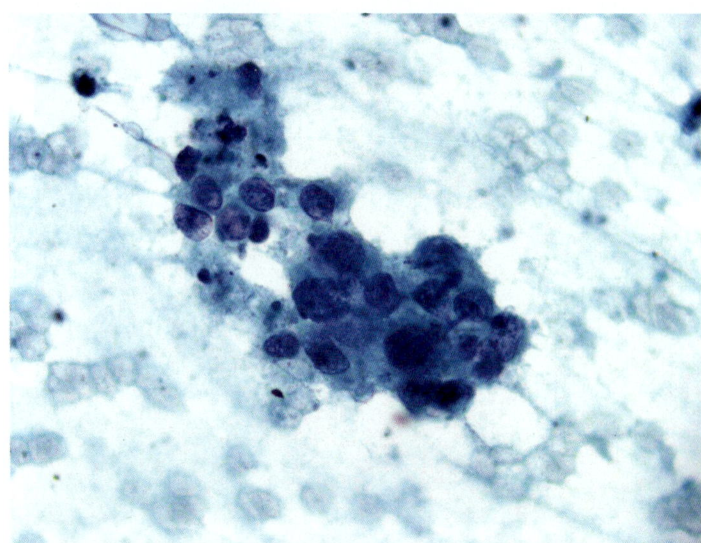

FIGURE 5.46 — Lymph Node, Left Supraclavicular, Metastatic Mammary Carcinoma. Marked nuclear atypia is evident and the tumor is forming glandular structures. Treating clinicians may request that immunostains for estrogen receptor, progesterone receptor, and Her2/Neu be performed on metastatic lesions in order to guide therapy for recurrent disease. (Papanicolaou stain, high power)

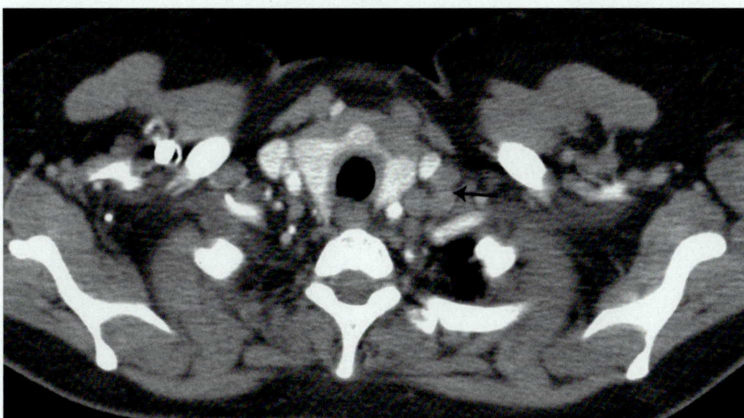

FIGURE 5.47 — Lymph Node, Left Supraclavicular, Metastatic Ovarian Carcinoma. Axial contrast-enhanced CT shows left supraclavicular adenoapathy (arrow). "Virchow's node" is a lymph node in the left supraclavicular area, which is a frequent metastatic site for intra-abdominal carcinoma, including carcinoma of the stomach and ovary.

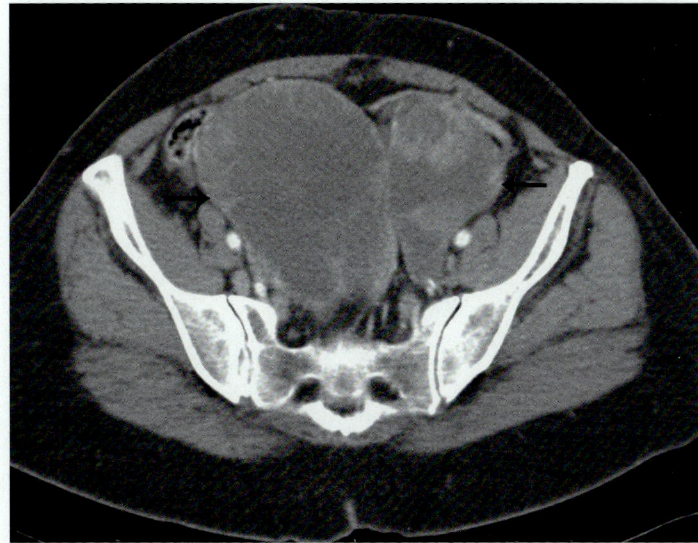

FIGURE 5.48 — Lymph Node, Left Supraclavicular, Metastatic Ovarian Carcinoma. Axial contrast-enhanced CT in the same patient also shows bilateral solid and cystic ovarian masses (arrows) consistent with ovarian cancer.

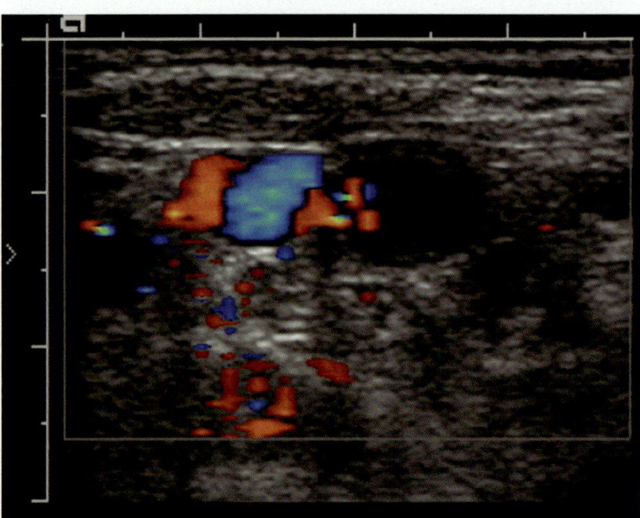

FIGURE 5.49 — Lymph Node, Left Supraclavicular, Metastatic Ovarian Carcinoma. Sonographic image confirms hypoechoic, left supraclavicular lymph node with some internal vascularity. This node was targeted for biopsy and found to represent metastatic ovarian cancer.

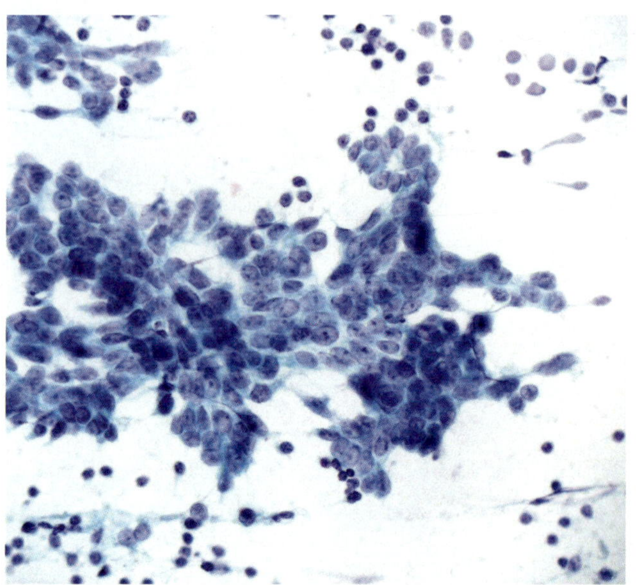

FIGURE 5.50 — Lymph Node, Left Supraclavicular, Metastatic Ovarian Carcinoma. A fragment of malignant epithelium is present in a background of lymphocytes. The cells show increased nuclear-to-cytoplasmic ratio and occasional nucleoli. The appearance is not specific and could represent a metastasis from many organ sites. (Papanicolaou stain, medium power)

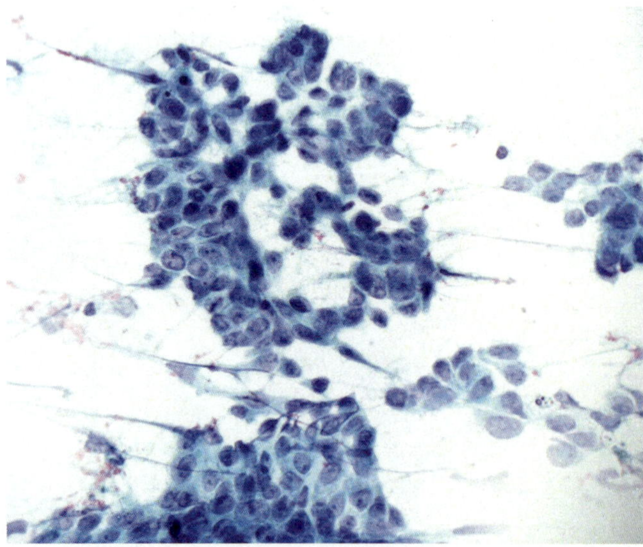

FIGURE 5.51 — Lymph Node, Left Supraclavicular, Metastatic Ovarian Carcinoma. Multiple cohesive tumor fragments are present indicating an epithelial malignancy. Poorly differentiated carcinoma of lung, breast, or ovarian origin would be top considerations for this sample. (Papanicolaou stain, medium power)

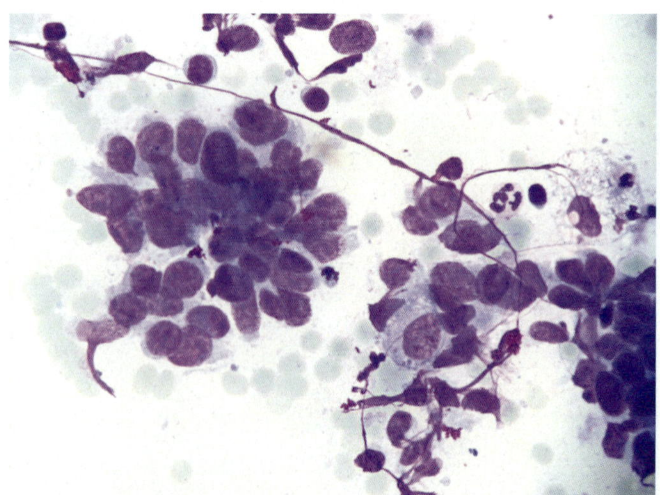

FIGURE 5.52 — Lymph Node, Left Supraclavicular, Metastatic Ovarian Carcinoma. This sheet of malignant epithelium shows no architectural clues to determine a site of origin. Prominent nucleoli present in this fragment raise the possibility of malignant melanoma. Material should be obtained for cell block or core biopsy to perform immunostains. (Diff Quik stain, high power)

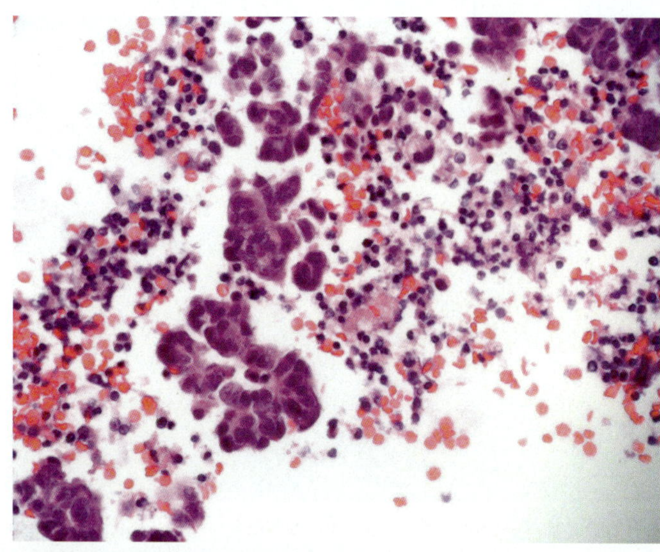

FIGURE 5.53 — Lymph Node, Left Supraclavicular, Metastatic Ovarian Carcinoma. Multiple fragments of tumor cells are present in the cell block preparation. Core biopsy may be difficult to obtain in the supraclavicular area due to the close proximity to large vessels and other structures. (Hematoxylin and eosin stain, high power)

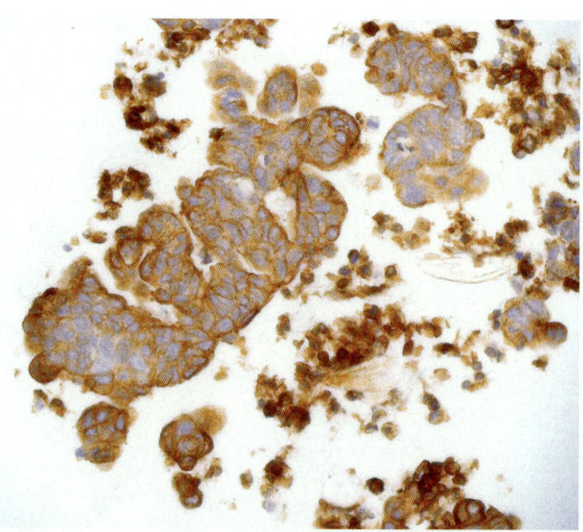

FIGURE 5.54 — Lymph Node, Left Supraclavicular, Metastatic Ovarian Carcinoma. A Cytokeratin 7 immunostain is positive in the tumor cells indicating an epithelial origin. This stain does not distinguish between lung, breast, and ovarian tumors, so additional immunostains were required. (Cytokeratin 7 immunostain, high power)

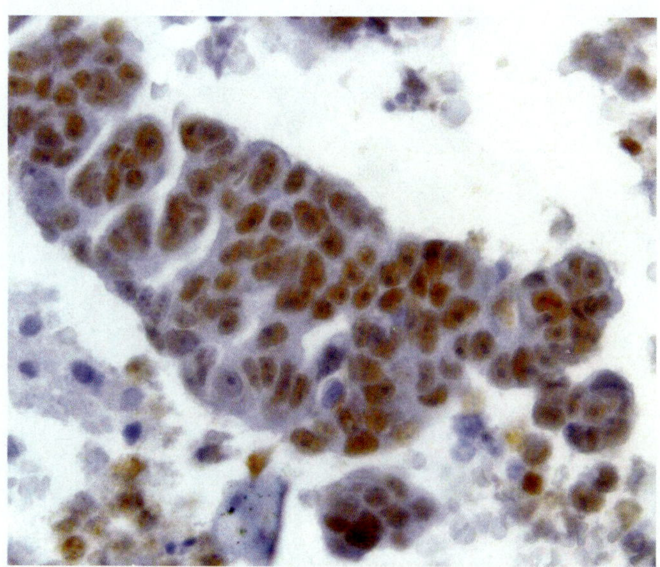

FIGURE 5.55 — Lymph Node, Left Supraclavicular, Metastatic Ovarian Carcinoma. A WT1 immunostain shows strong staining in tumor cell nuclei. This finding is consistent with a metastatic serous ovarian carcinoma. (WT1 immunostain, high power)

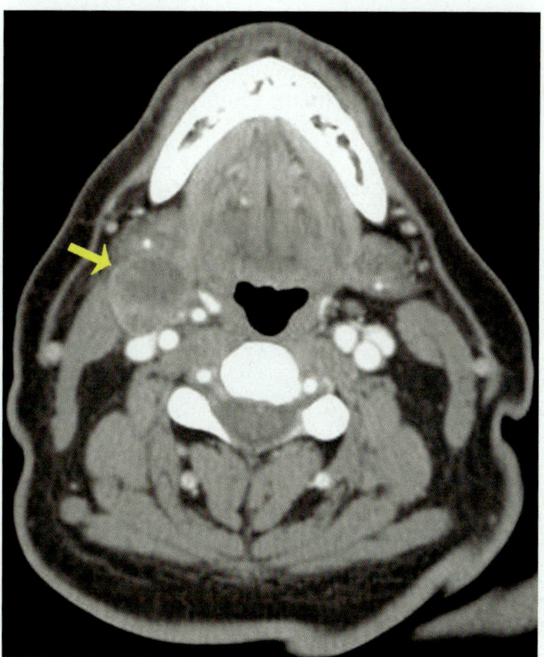

FIGURE 5.56 — Lymph Node, Left Neck, Metastatic Squamous Cell Carcinoma. Axial contrast-enhanced CT of the neck shows an enhancing enlarged lymph node with central necrosis in the right neck, level IIA (arrow).

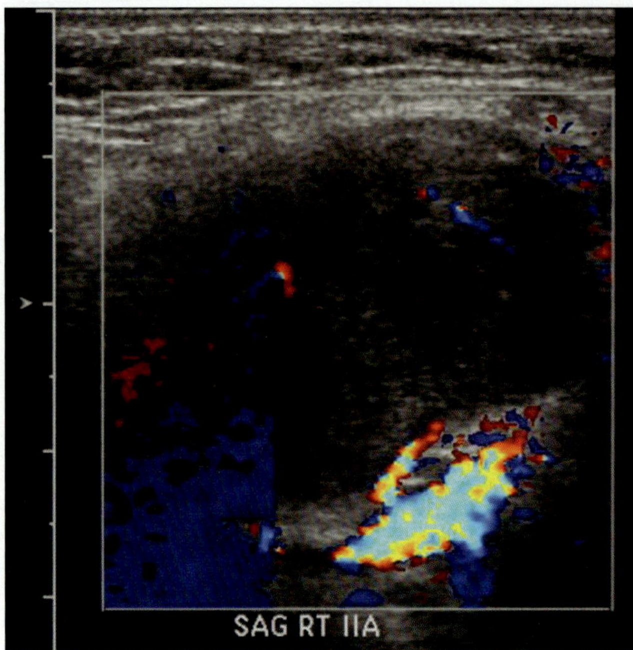

FIGURE 5.57 — Lymph Node, Left Neck, Metastatic Squamous Cell Carcinoma. Sonographic image with color Doppler confirms enlarged, hypoechoic lymph node in right level IIA. Biopsy was positive for squamous cell carcinoma. Although presumed to be of head and neck origin, the primary tumor could not be found.

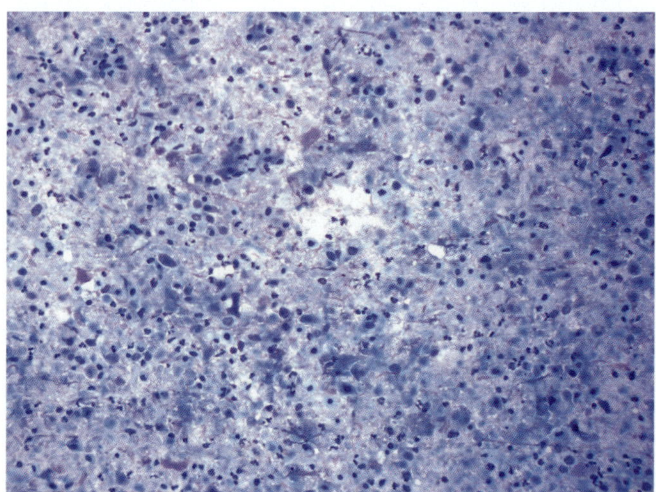

FIGURE 5.58 — Lymph Node, Left Neck, Metastatic Squamous Cell Carcinoma. The background of this aspirate is a sea of anucleated squamous cells and keratin debris showing the "robin's egg" blue color characteristic of squamous cells on Diff Quik stain. The nucleated cells show hyperchromatic, dense nuclei concerning for malignancy. (Diff Quik stain, medium power)

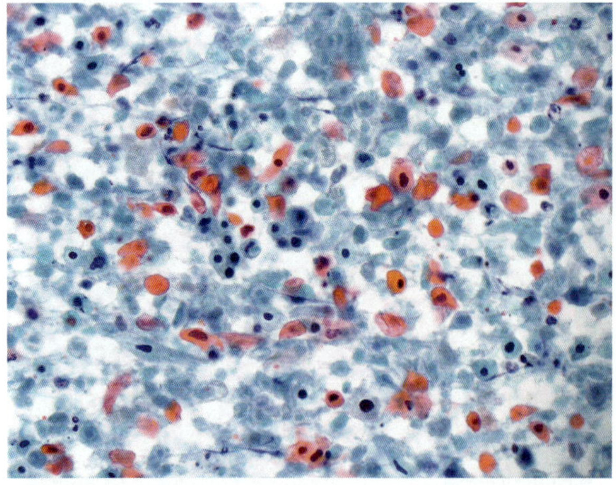

FIGURE 5.59 — Lymph Node, Left Neck, Metastatic Squamous Cell Carcinoma. At high power, the nucleated squamous cells are clearly malignant, showing dark, pyknotic nuclei with irregular nuclear shapes. Keratinized cells appear bright orange on Papanicolaou stain. (Papanicolaou stain, medium power)

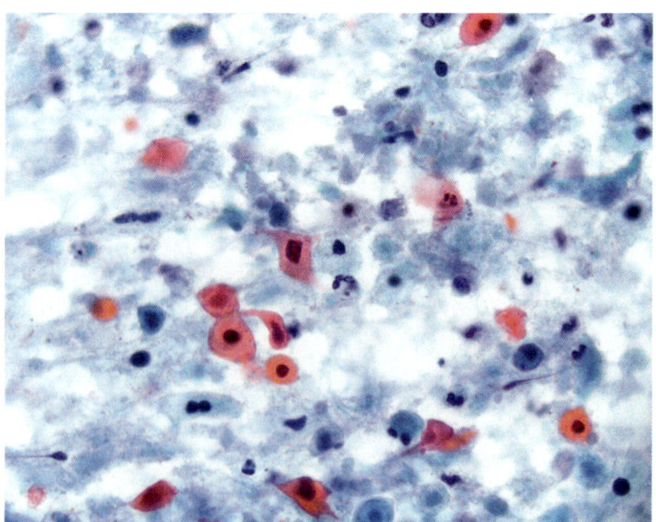

FIGURE 5.60 — Lymph Node, Left Neck, Metastatic Squamous Cell Carcinoma. The abundant granular and keratinaceous debris in the background corresponds to the cystic appearance seen radiographically. Necrosis is quite common in metastatic squamous cell carcinoma and viable tumor cells may be scarce. (Papanicolaou stain, high power)

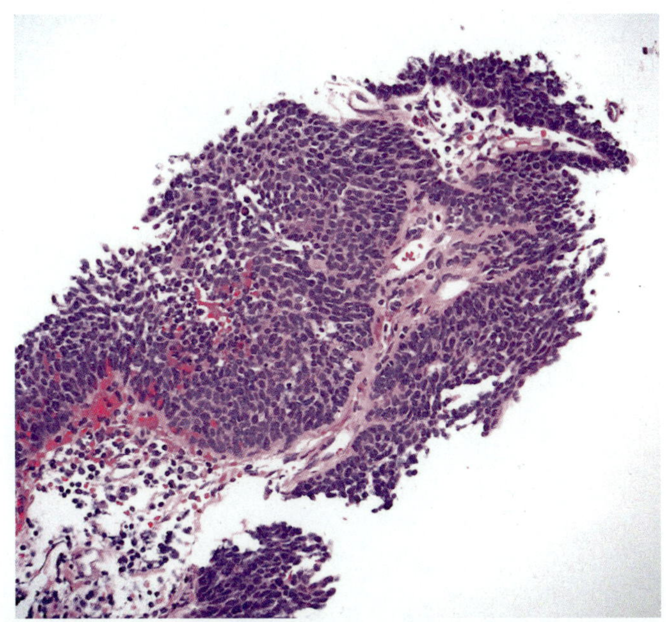

FIGURE 5.61 — Lymph Node, Left Neck, Metastatic Squamous Cell Carcinoma (Core Biopsy). A core biopsy shows malignant epithelium with a nuclear crowing and high nuclear-to-cytoplasmic ratio. Squamous cell carcinoma detected in the neck without a known primary (as in this case) almost always represents metastasis from an oropharyngeal primary. (Hematoxylin and eosin stain, high power)

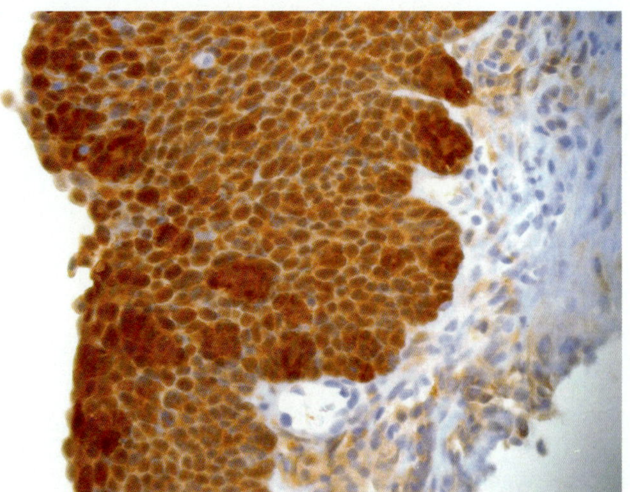

FIGURE 5.62 — Lymph Node, Left Neck, Metastatic Squamous Cell Carcinoma (Core Biopsy). The majority of oropharyngeal squamous cell carcinomas are related to high-risk types of human papillomavirus (HPV). In fact, HPV positivity in a neck metastasis strongly points to the oropharynx as the site of tumor origin. An immunostain for p16 is a surrogate marker for the presence of high-risk HPV, and is almost always diffusely positive in HPV-related squamous cell carcinomas. (p16 immunostain, high power)

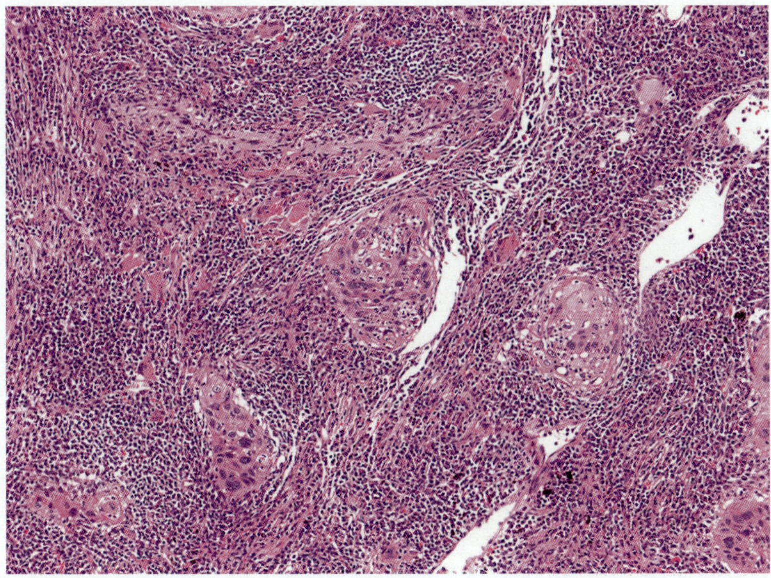

FIGURE 5.63 — Lymph Node, Left Neck, Metastatic Squamous Cell Carcinoma (Histology). Nests of metastatic squamous cell carcinoma, originating in the head and neck region, are seen infiltrating into a left neck lymph node. Note the prominent keratinization in the nests. (Hematoxylin and eosin stain, low power)

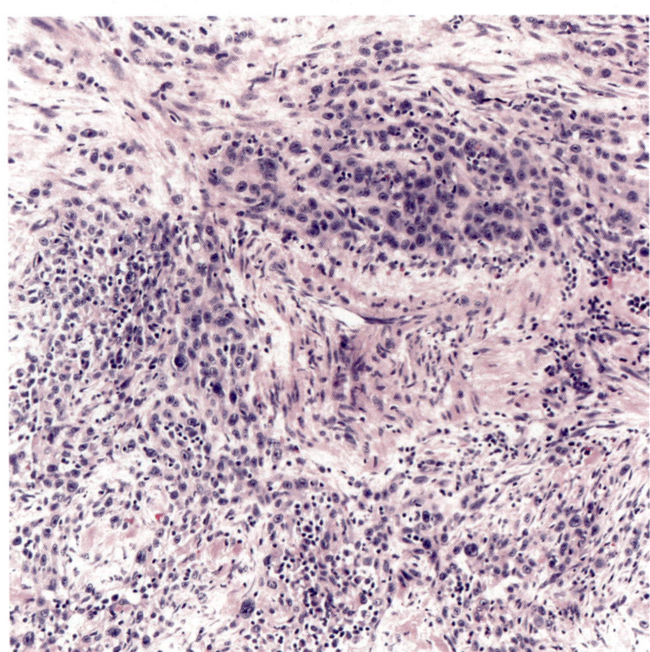

FIGURE 5.64 — Lymph Node, Left Neck, Metastatic Squamous Cell Carcinoma (Histology). Metastatic squamous cell carcinoma, poorly differentiated, with clusters and single neoplastic cells with marked cytological atypia, including pleomorphism and irregular nuclear outlines with prominent nucleoli. (Hematoxylin and eosin stain, medium power)

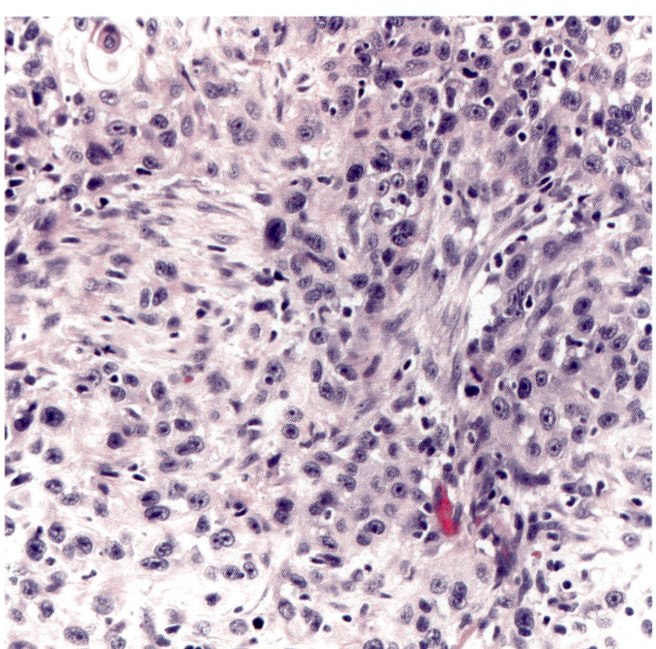

FIGURE 5.65 — Lymph Node, Left Neck, Metastatic Squamous Cell Carcinoma (Histology). Metastatic squamous cell carcinoma, poorly differentiated, with highly atypical neoplastic cells is shown infiltrating into a lymph node. Note the significant cytological atypia with prominent nucleoli. (Hematoxylin and eosin stain, high power)

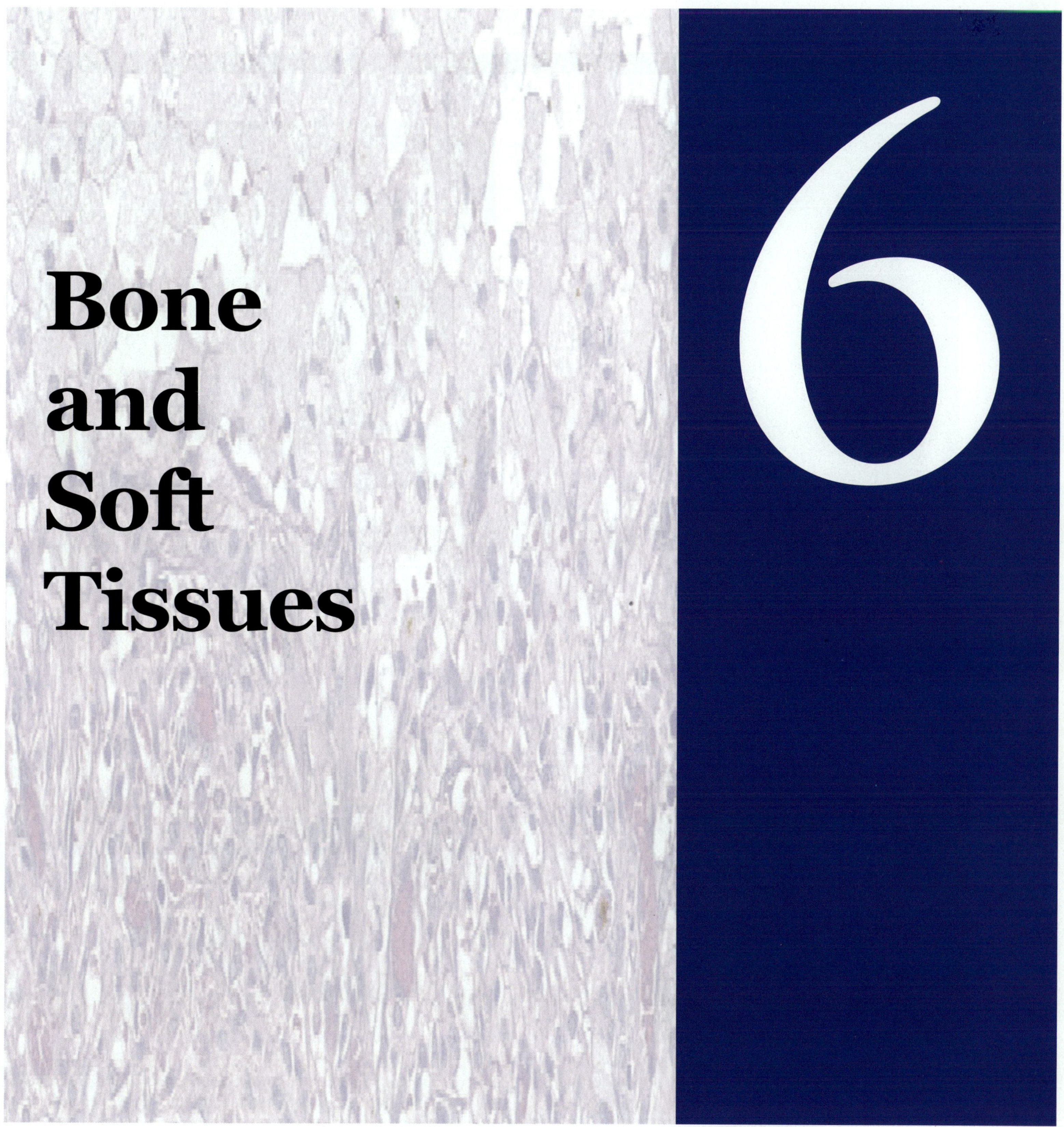

Bone and Soft Tissues

6

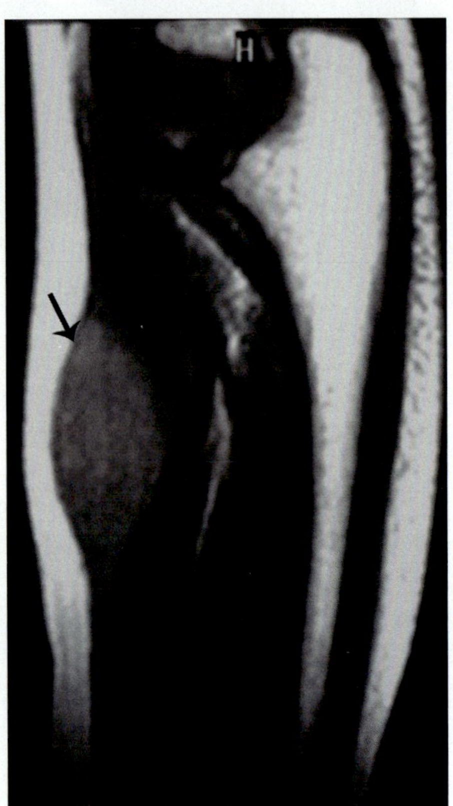

FIGURE 6.1 — Soft Tissue, Left Forearm, Granular Cell Tumor. This patient complained of arm pain and had no history of trauma. Sagittal T1-weighted MR image shows a well-defined, hypoechoic mass in the left forearm (arrow).

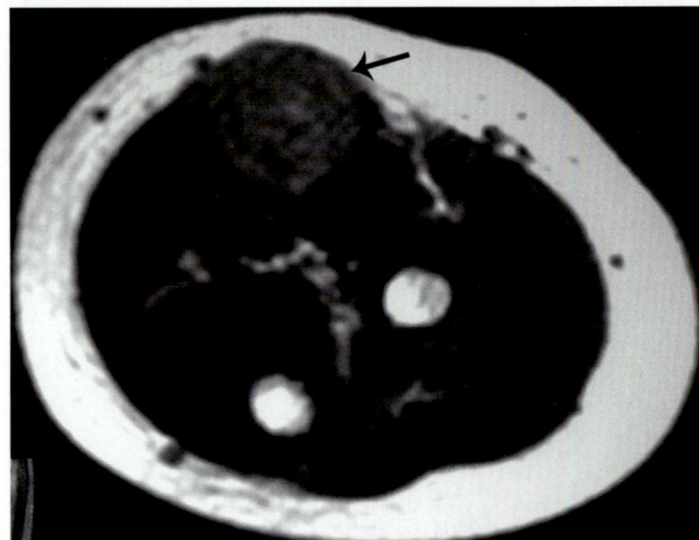

FIGURE 6.2 — Soft Tissue, Left Forearm, Granular Cell Tumor. Axial T1-weighted MR image confirms well-defined, hypoechoic mass (arrow) in the left forearm. Granular cell tumors are usually small and are generally benign when less than 4 cm in size.

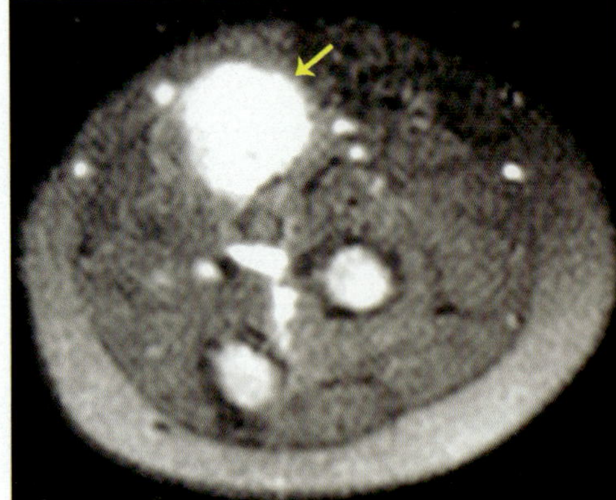

FIGURE 6.3 — Soft Tissue, Left Forearm, Granular Cell Tumor. Axial T2-weighted MR image shows the mass is hyperintense on this sequence (arrow). Granular cell tumors are rarely diagnosed prospectively based on imaging characteristics.

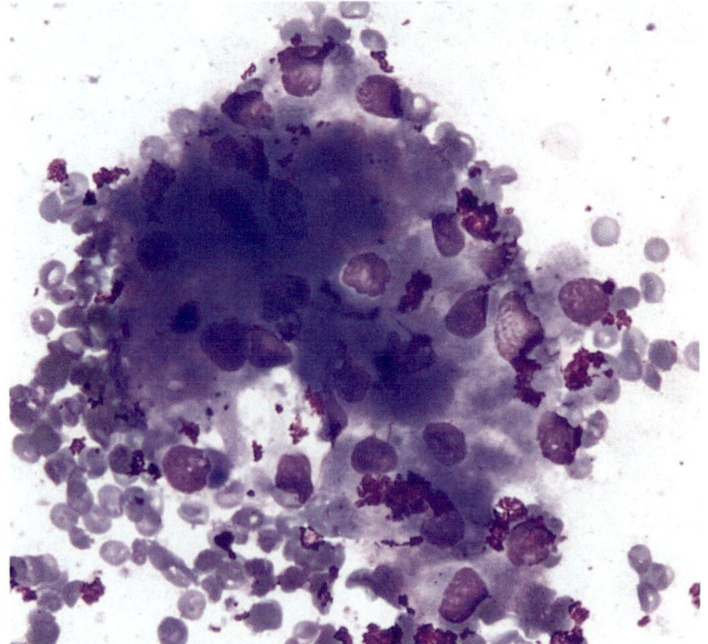

FIGURE 6.4 — Soft Tissue, Left Forearm, Granular Cell Tumor. This cohesive fragment of cells shows abundant cytoplasm with oval to slightly irregular nuclear shapes. Cell borders are ill defined. (Diff Quik stain, high power)

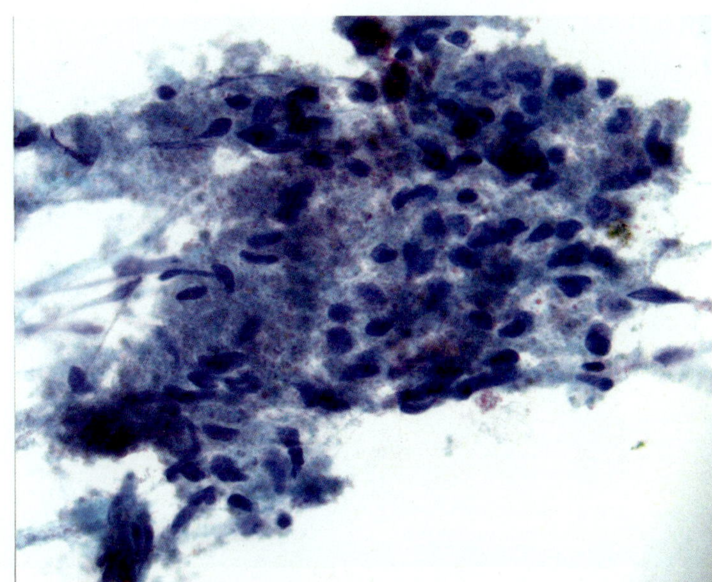

FIGURE 6.5 — Soft Tissue, Left Forearm, Granular Cell Tumor. On Papanicolaou-stained material, the granularity of the cytoplasm is much more evident. If the characteristic granularity is present, the cytologic differential diagnosis is limited, but includes alveolar soft parts sarcoma, which is quite rare. (Papanicolaou stain, high power)

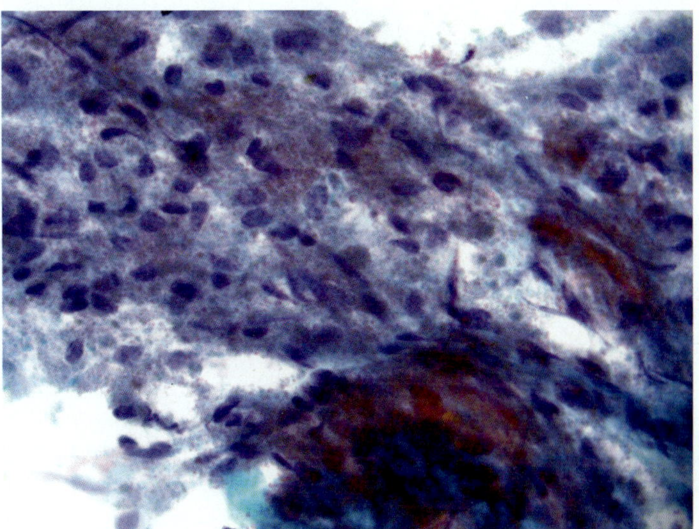

FIGURE 6.6 — Soft Tissue, Left Forearm, Granular Cell Tumor. The neoplastic cells show abundant granular cytoplasm and oval- to spindle-shaped nuclei. The tongue is the most common site for granular cell tumors, although they can occur anywhere, including the breast and soft tissues. (Papanicolaou stain, high power)

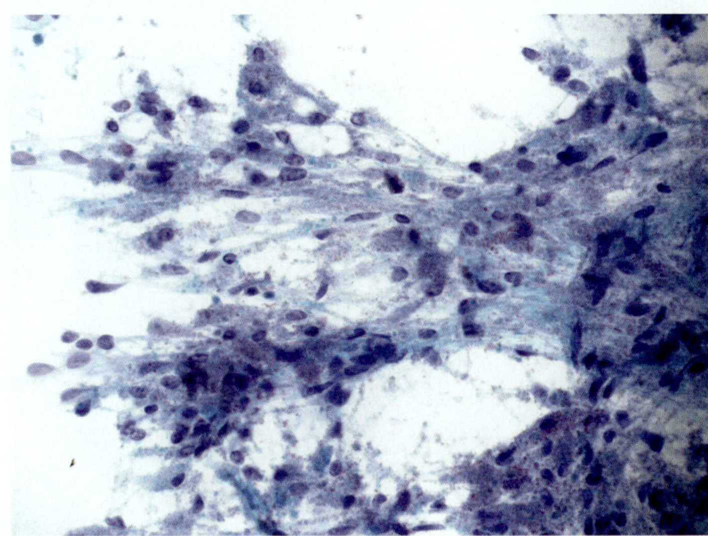

FIGURE 6.7 — Soft Tissue, Left Forearm, Granular Cell Tumor. The abundant granularity in the cytoplasm is quite apparent. Malignant melanoma could also be considered in the differential, though the nuclei here appear quite small and benign and lack nucleoli. (Papanicolaou stain, high power)

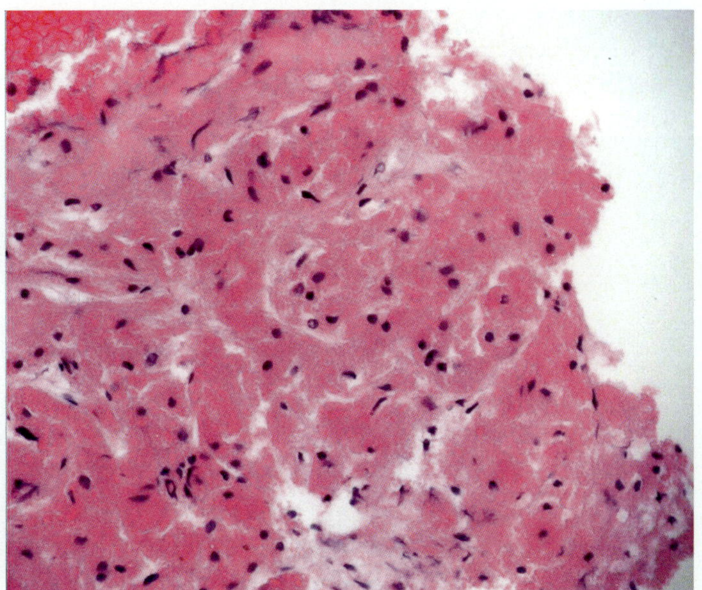

FIGURE 6.8 — Soft Tissue, Left Forearm, Granular Cell Tumor (Cell Block). On cell block preparation, the abundant eosinophilic granular cytoplasm is evident. Overlying pseudoepitheliomatous hyperplasia is characteristic, and can be misinterpreted as a squamous carcinoma. (Hematoxylin and eosin stain, high power)

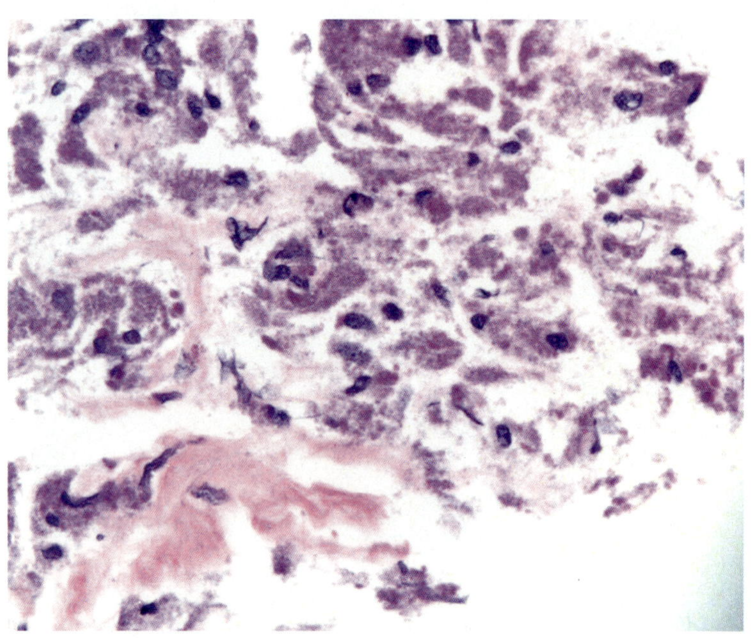

FIGURE 6.9 — Soft Tissue, Left Forearm, Granular Cell Tumor. PAS stain highlights the granules in the cytoplasm. These lesions are also positive for S-100 protein (not shown). (PAS stain, high power)

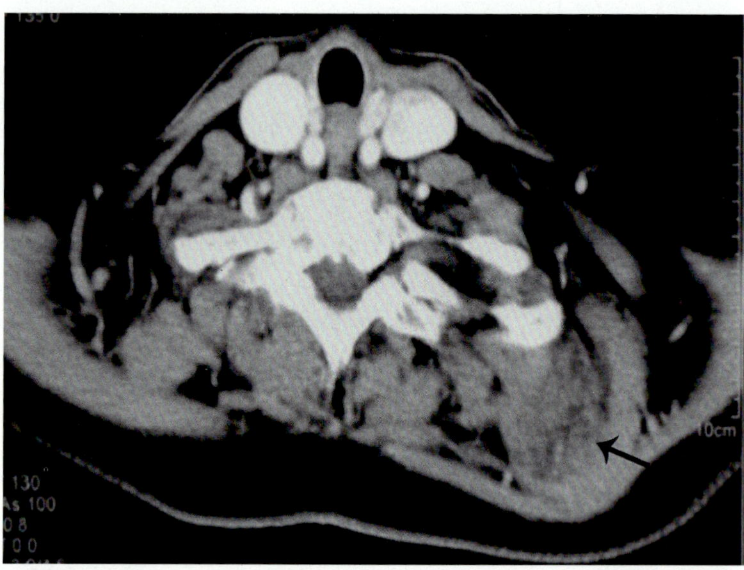

FIGURE 6.10 — Soft Tissue, Left Scapula, Elastofibroma. Axial contrast-enhanced CT demonstrates a mass in the left scapular region (arrow), which is similar in density to muscle and contains streaky areas of fat. Streaky areas of fat are often found in elastofibromas.

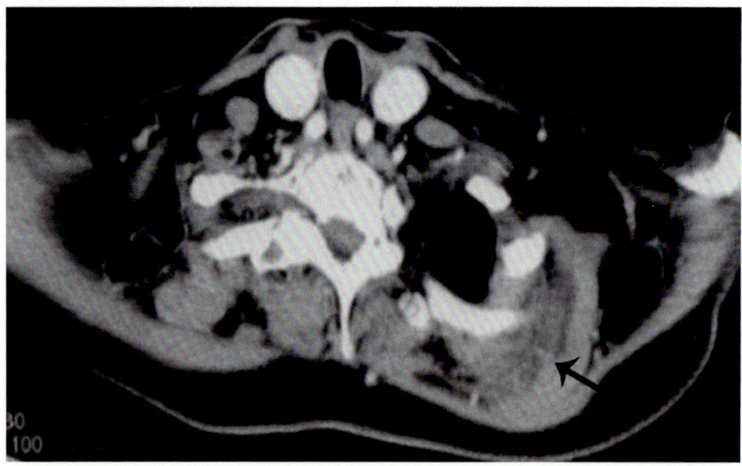

FIGURE 6.11 — Soft Tissue, Left Scapula, Elastofibroma. Axial contrast-enhanced CT more inferiorly shows further extent of mass (arrow). Elastofibromas are almost always seen in the scapular or infrascapular region and in older women. They may be multiple and bilateral.

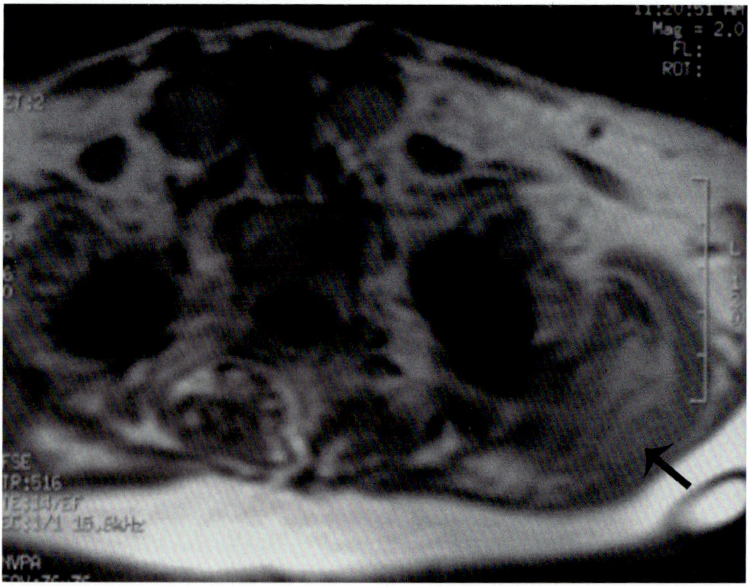

FIGURE 6.12 — Soft Tissue, Left Scapula, Elastofibroma. Axial T1-weighted MR image shows the left scapular mass (arrow), which is isointense to skeletal muscle and contains linear T1 hyperintense areas of fat.

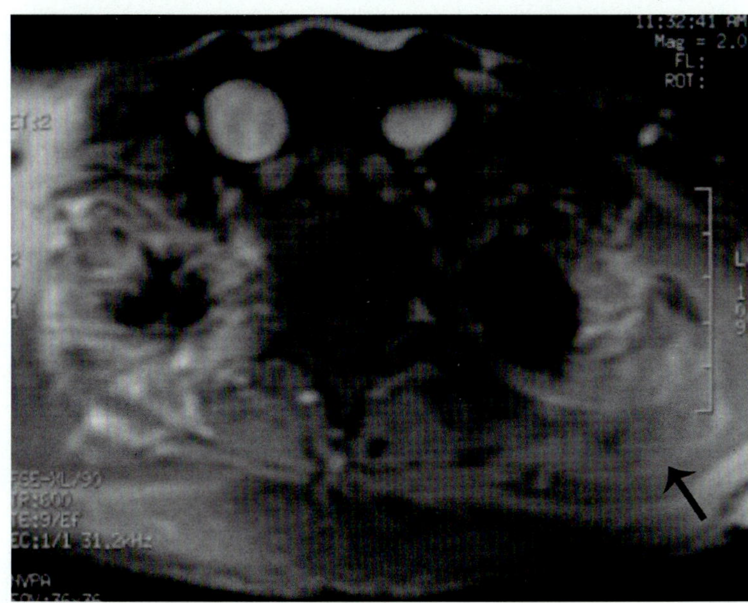

FIGURE 6.13 — Soft Tissue, Left Scapula, Elastofibroma. Axial T1-weighted MR with contrast. Mass shows mild enhancement postcontrast (arrow). Elastofibromas may be multiple and bilateral.

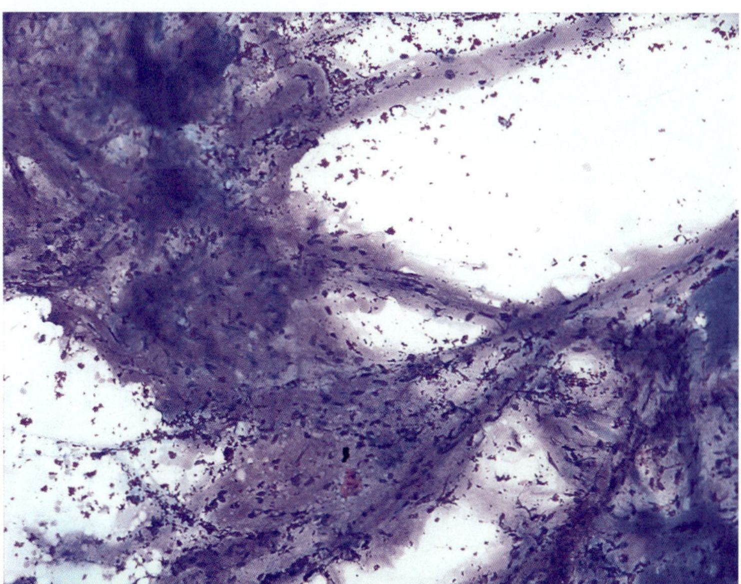

FIGURE 6.14 — Soft Tissue, Left Scapula, Elastofibroma. Elastofibromas consist of a collagenous background with thick bundles of elastic tissue, which often forms globular structures. Small, bland spindle cell nuclei are seen here embedded in a matrix of collagen. (Diff Quik stain, medium power)

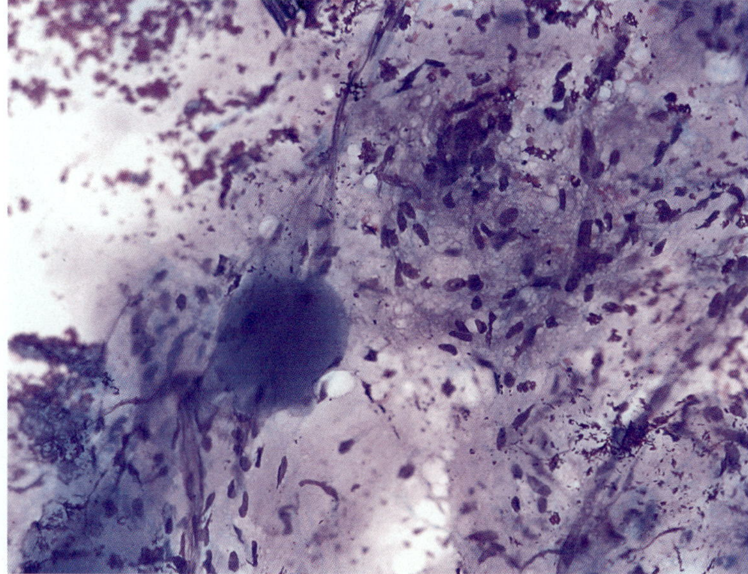

FIGURE 6.15 — Soft Tissue, Left Scapula, Elastofibroma. A globule of dense blue elastic tissue is present in a background of small, bland spindle cells. Aspirates from elastofibromas may be sparsely cellular due to the dense collagenous stroma. (Diff Quik stain, high power)

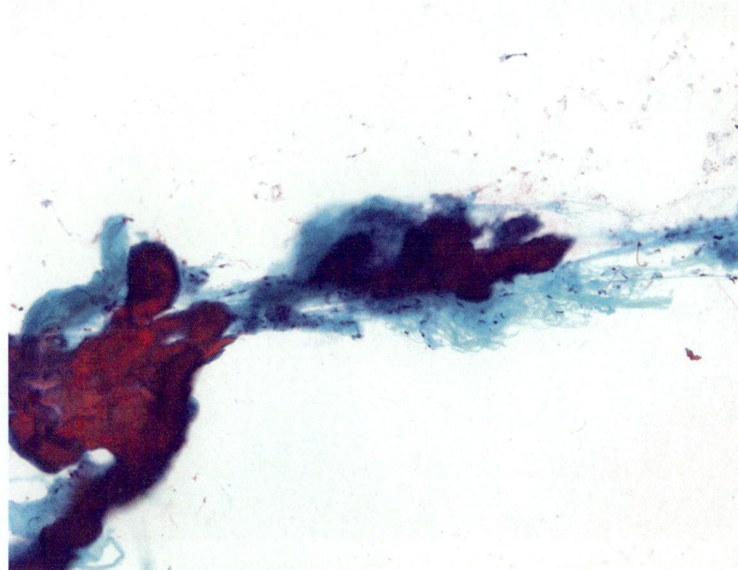

FIGURE 6.16 — Soft Tissue, Left Scapula, Elastofibroma. Large fragments of collagenized stroma are present (red-staining) in a background of small spindle cells with wispy cytoplasm. (Papanicolaou stain, low power)

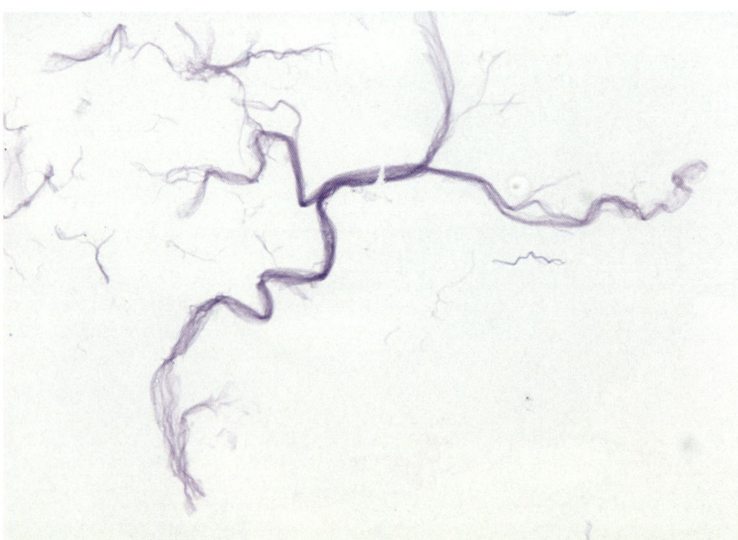

FIGURE 6.17 — Soft Tissue, Left Scapula, Elastofibroma. Aggregates of elastic tissue with a unique "braided" appearance are quite characteristic of elastofibroma. Differential diagnostic considerations such as fibromatosis and fibromas do not have such structures. (Papanicolaou stain, high power)

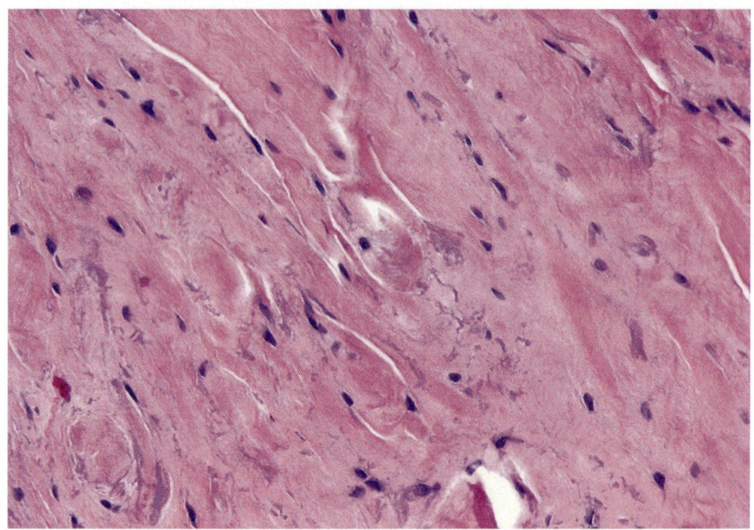

FIGURE 6.18 — Soft Tissue, Left Scapula, Elastofibroma (Histology). The predominant tissue present is collagen with scattered, small, spindled nuclei. Focal areas of dense tissue with deep eosinophilia represent the elastic component. (Hematoxylin and eosin stain, high power)

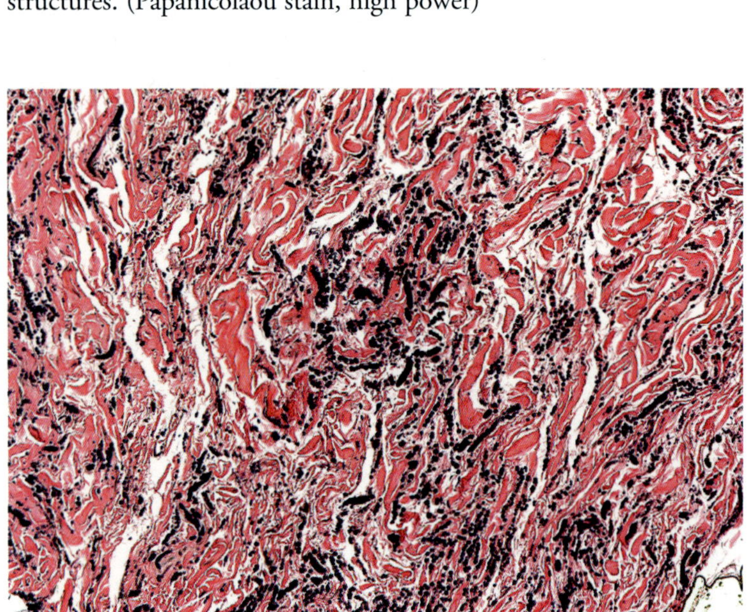

FIGURE 6.19 — Soft Tissue, Left Scapula, Elastofibroma (Histology). This elastic stain highlights the elastic fibers with dark black staining. Portions of the elastic tissue have a "beads on a string" appearance. The mixture of beaded and linear staining is characteristic of elastofibroma. (Elastic stain, high power)

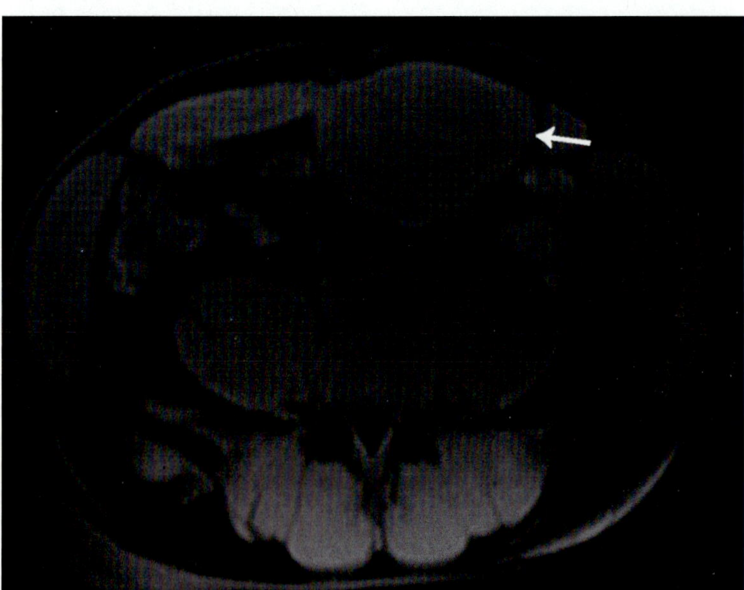

FIGURE 6.20 — Soft Tissue, Left Rectus Muscle, Fibromatosis. Axial T1-weighted MR image shows a well-defined, 7.5-cm mass in the left rectus muscle (arrow). The deep soft tissue type of fibromatosis is termed desmoid-type fibromatosis and is less common than the superficial types (palmar, plantar, and penile).

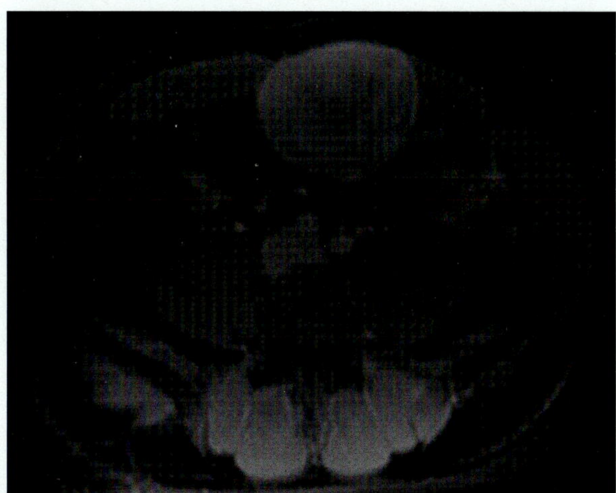

FIGURE 6.21 — Soft Tissue, Left Rectus Muscle, Fibromatosis. Axial T1-weighted MR with contrast shows the mass avidly enhances postcontrast. Fibromatosis can occur at areas of previous injury or surgery. It may occur intra-abdominally, related to surgery or in the setting of Gardner syndrome, or extra-abdominally, particularly in the area of the shoulder, chest, and back.

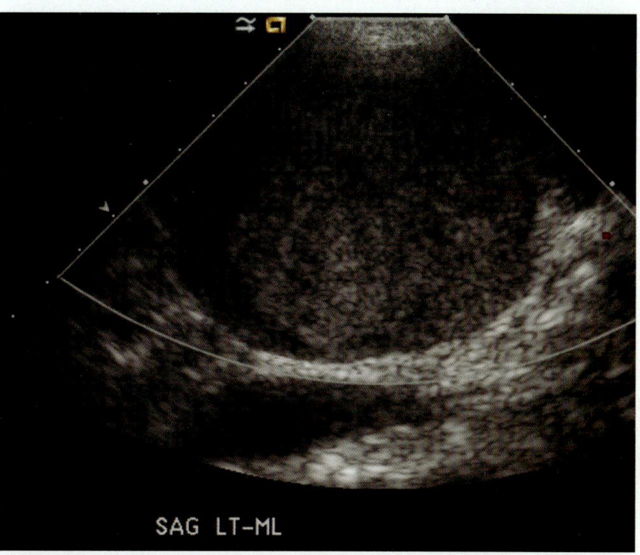

FIGURE 6.22 — Soft Tissue, Left Rectus Muscle, Fibromatosis. Sonographic image at the time of ultrasound-guided biopsy shows the large hypoechoic rectus muscle mass. Fibromatosis is benign but can be locally aggressive and often recurs despite negative resection margins.

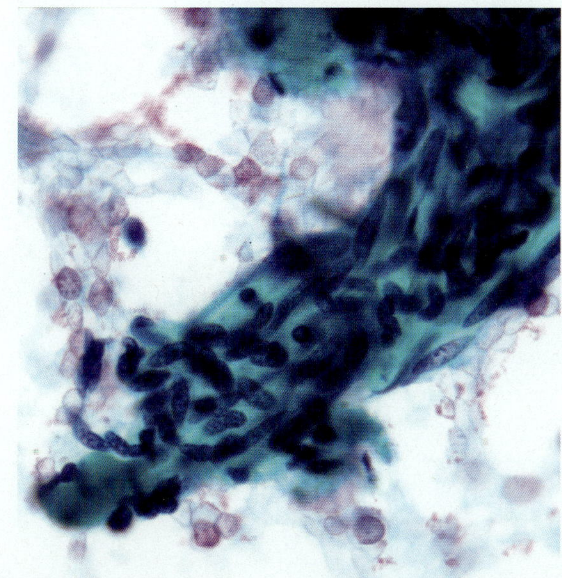

FIGURE 6.23 — Soft Tissue, Left Rectus Muscle, Fibromatosis. A single fragment of mesenchymal tissue is present with small, uniform, spindled nuclei. Aspirates from fibromatosis are commonly hypocellular due to the dense fibrous nature of the lesion. (Papanicolaou stain, high power)

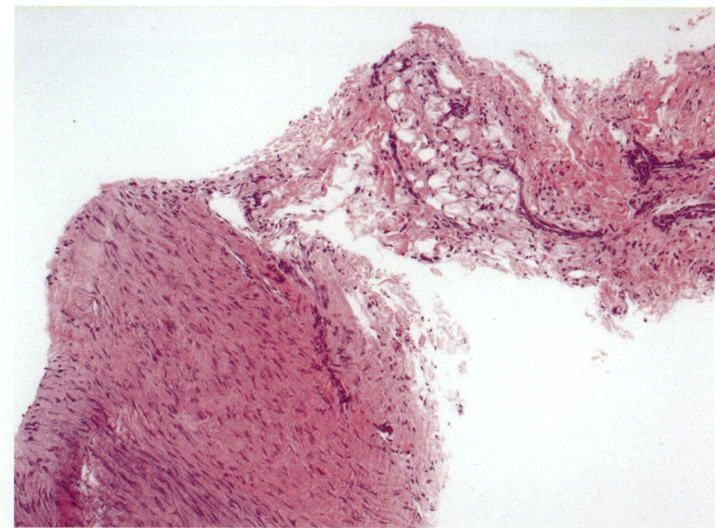

FIGURE 6.24 — Soft Tissue, Left Rectus Muscle, Fibromatosis (Core Biopsy). Dense fibrous tissue with small spindled nuclei is shown. Adipose tissue present in the top portion of the field is intimately admixed with the fibrous neoplastic tissue illustrating the infiltrative nature of the fibromatosis. (Hematoxylin and eosin stain, medium power)

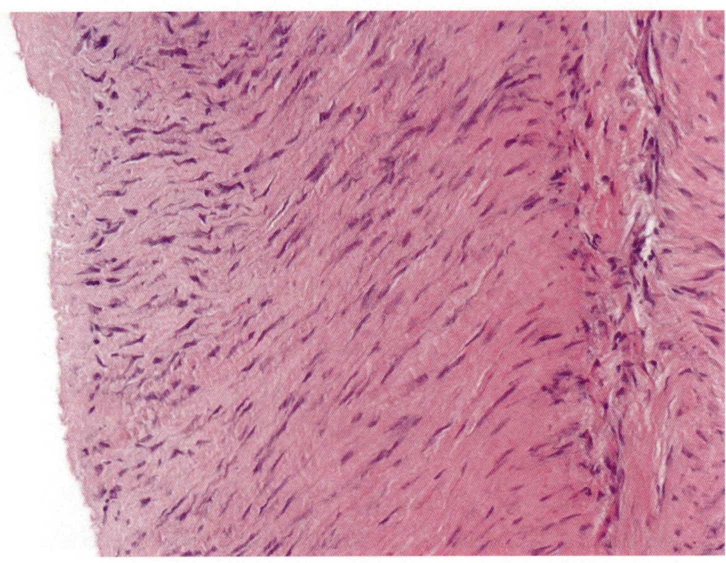

FIGURE 6.25 — Soft Tissue, Left Rectus Muscle, Fibromatosis (Core Biopsy). Fibrous tissue with bland nuclei is characteristic. Increased nuclear atypia may raise the possibility of fibrosarcoma. The cells show nuclear positivity for beta-catenin (not shown). (Hematoxylin and eosin stain, high power)

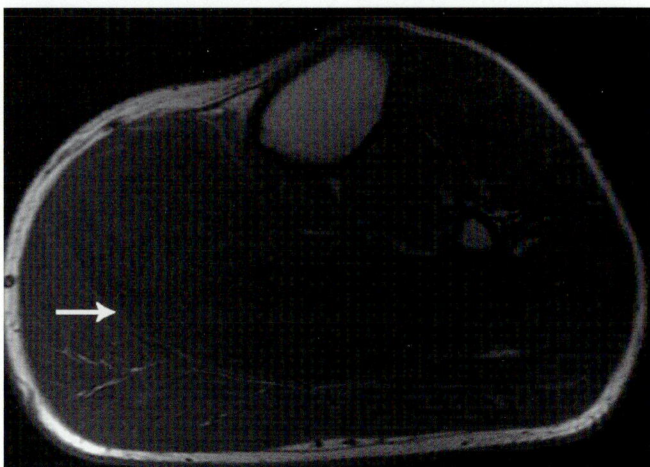

FIGURE 6.26 — Soft Tissue, Left Calf, Myxoid Liposarcoma. Axial T1-weighted MR image shows a well-defined 10.0 × 4.5-cm hypointense mass in the left calf (arrow). Myxoid liposarcomas are the second most common type of liposarcoma and are commonly T1 hypodense and T2 hyperintense due to lack of fat signal intensity.

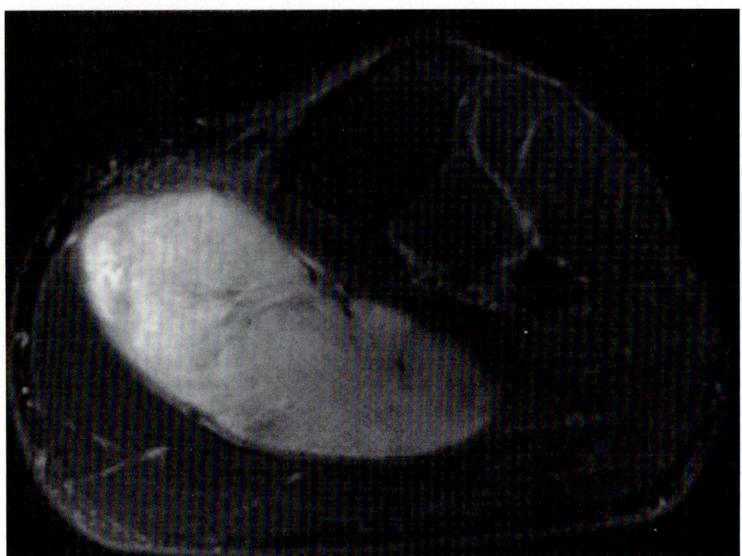

FIGURE 6.27 — Soft Tissue, Left Calf, Myxoid Liposarcoma. Axial T2-weighted MR image shows the mass is mostly T2 hyperintense with a few small linear hypointense areas. Myxoid liposarcoma typically occurs in the extremities.

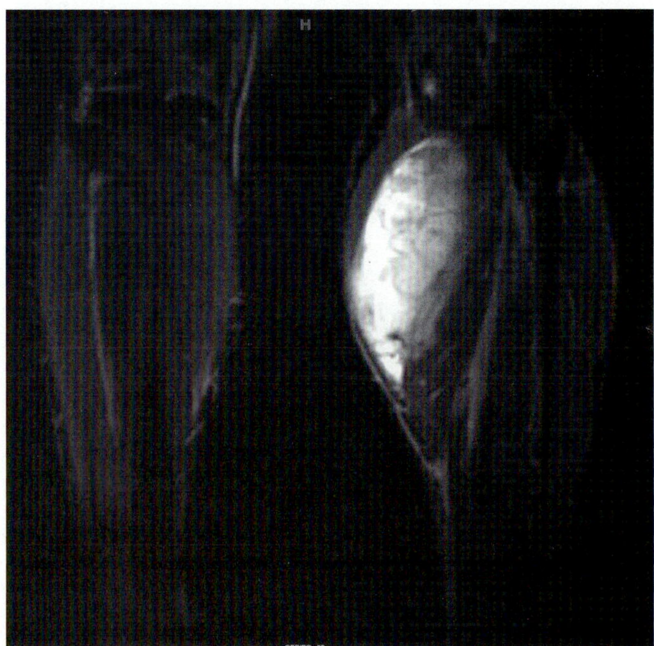

FIGURE 6.28 — Soft Tissue, Left Calf, Myxoid Liposarcoma. Coronal inversion recovery (IR) MR image shows the craniocaudal extent of the mass. These tumors are most often present in young to middle-aged adults and are rare in children.

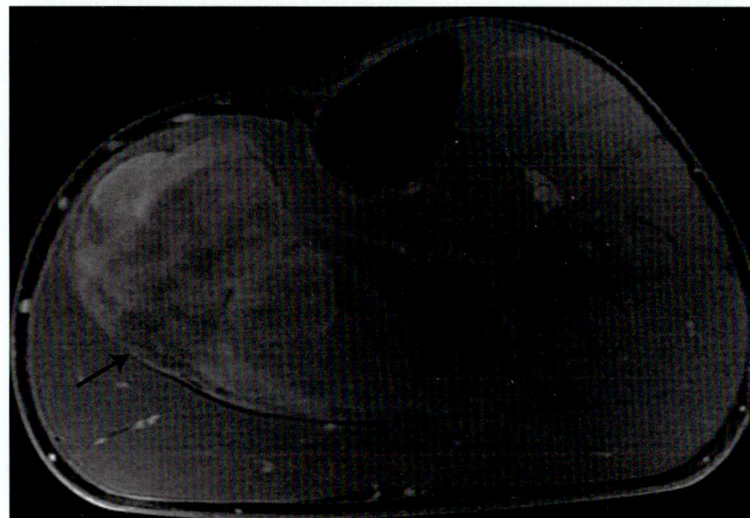

FIGURE 6.29 — Soft Tissue, Left Calf, Myxoid Liposarcoma. Axial T1-weighted MR image postcontrast demonstrates that the mass enhances mildly postcontrast (arrow).

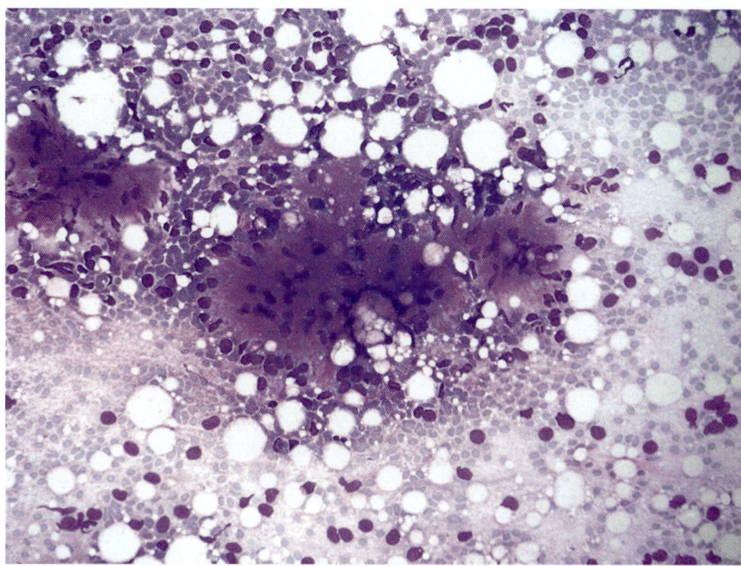

FIGURE 6.30 — Soft Tissue, Left Calf, Myxoid Liposarcoma. Spindle-shaped nuclei are embedded in a matrix of myxoid material, which appears bright purple on Diff Quik stain. (Diff Quik stain, medium power)

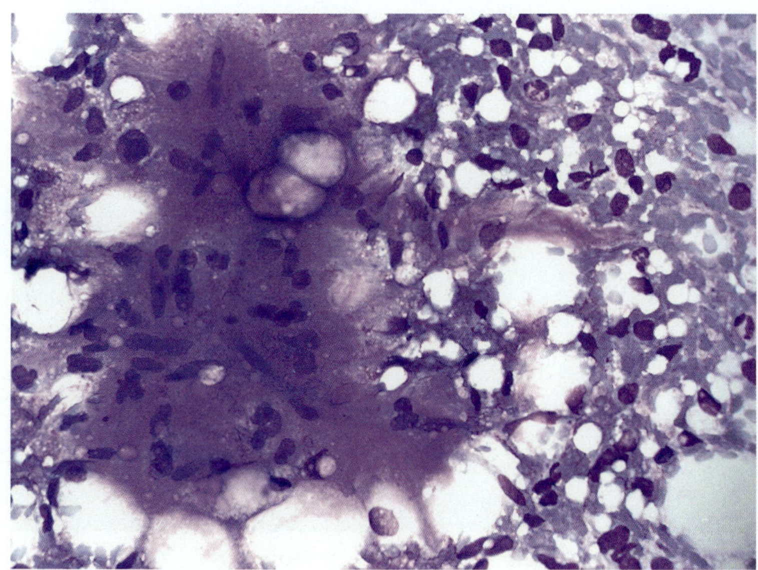

FIGURE 6.31 — Soft Tissue, Left Calf, Myxoid Liposarcoma. Bubbly or vacuolated areas within the myxoid matrix represent adipose tissue. Lipoblasts are positive for S-100 protein (not shown). (Diff Quik stain, high power)

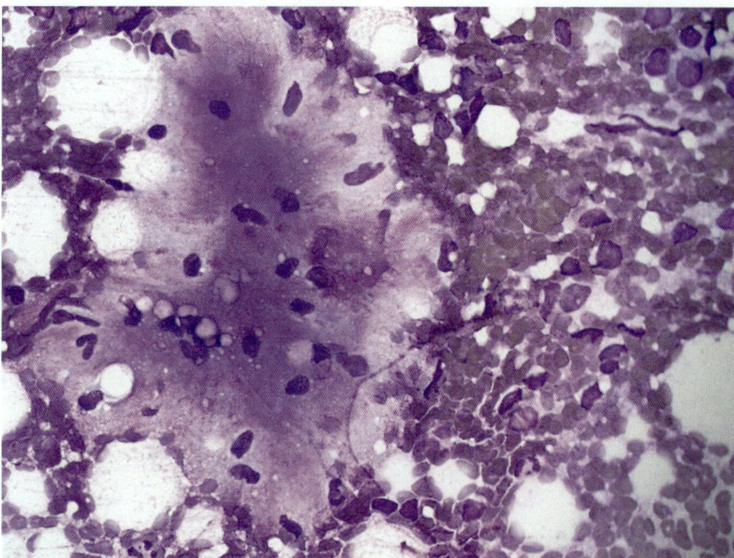

FIGURE 6.32 — Soft Tissue, Left Calf, Myxoid Liposarcoma. Wispy myxoid matrix contains spindle cells and vacuoles representing adipocytic differentiation. Myxoid liposarcoma is associated with a characteristic translocation t(12;16)(q13;p11), representing fusion of the TLS gene on 16p11 to the CHOP gene on 12q13. (Diff Quik stain, high power)

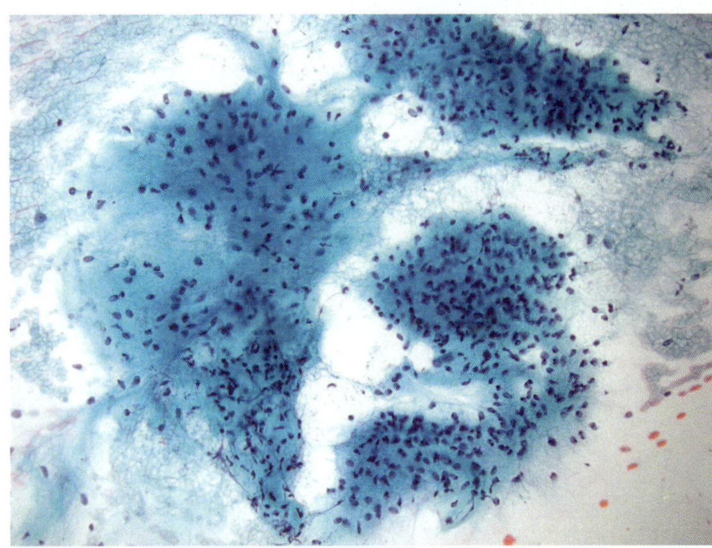

FIGURE 6.33 — – Soft Tissue, Left Calf, Myxoid Liposarcoma. Several cellular fragments show a myxoid stroma and small, bland spindle cells. The differential diagnosis includes a myxoma (less cellular) and myxofibrosarcoma (more nuclear atypia). (Papanicolaou stain, medium power)

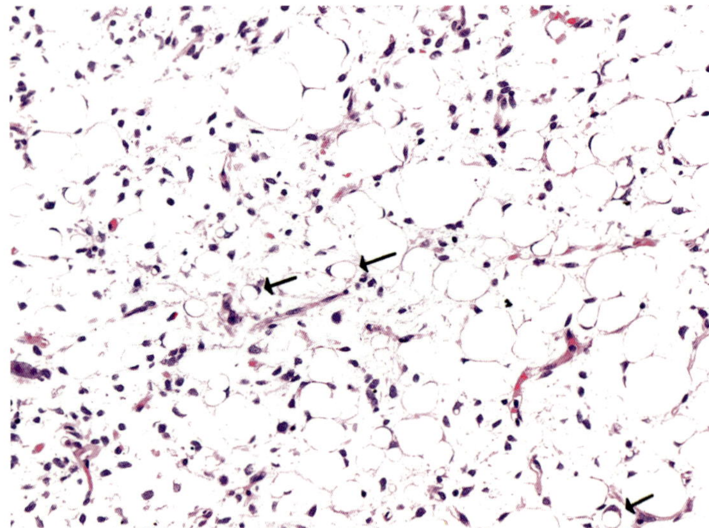

FIGURE 6.35 — Soft Tissue, Myxoid Liposarcoma (Histology). These lipoblasts show minimal nuclear atypia and mitotic figures are not seen. Occasional lipoblasts, commonly seen in well-differentiated myxoid liposarcoma, show a signet-ring cell morphology (arrows). Scattered small capillaries surround the lipoblasts. (Hematoxylin and eosin stain, medium power)

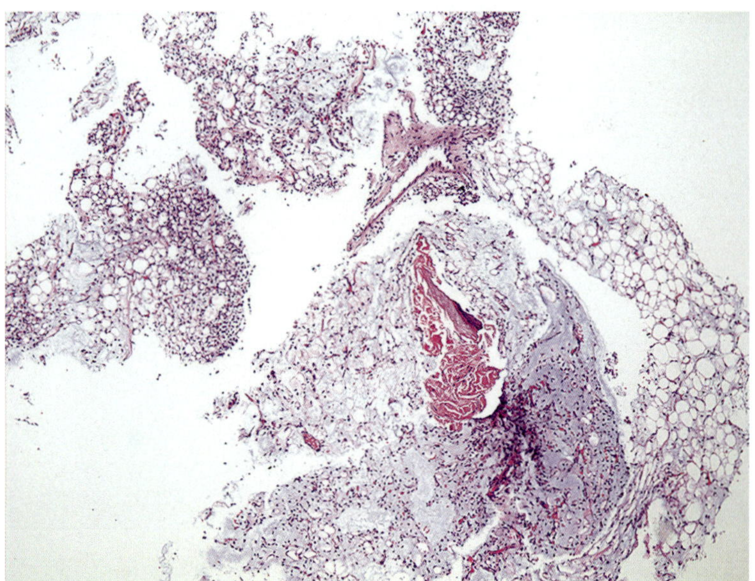

FIGURE 6.34 — Soft Tissue, Myxoid Liposarcoma (Core Biopsy). Myxoid liposarcoma is a common subtype of liposarcoma, accounting for one third to one half of cases. These core biopsies show blue-gray myxoid stroma (center of field) surrounded by neoplastic adipocytes. Delicate branching capillaries are scattered throughout the lesion. (Hematoxylin and eosin stain, low power)

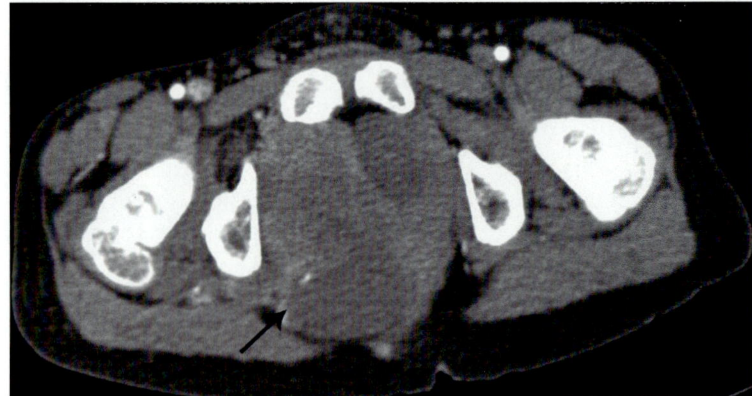

FIGURE 6.36 — Soft Tissue, Gluteal, Embryonal Rhabdomyosarcoma. Axial contrast-enhanced CT at the level of the pubic symphysis shows a heterogeneous mass in the right lower pelvis (arrow). Rhabdomyosarcoma is the most common soft tissue sarcoma of childhood and is rarely seen in adults.

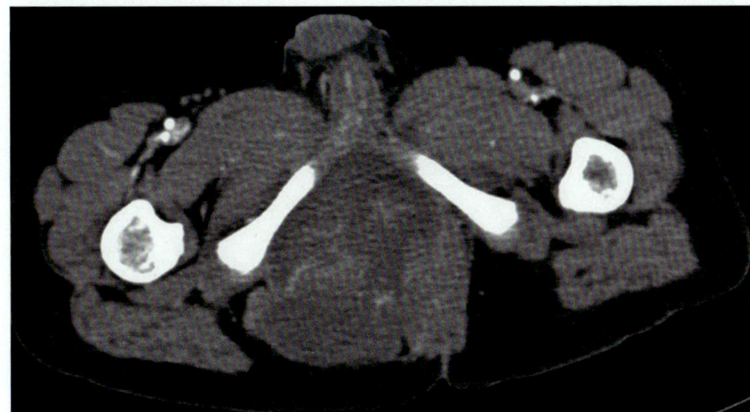

FIGURE 6.37 — Soft Tissue, Gluteal, Embryonal Rhabdomyosarcoma. Axial contrast-enhanced CT more inferiorly shows the mass extends into the right perineum and gluteal regions (arrow).

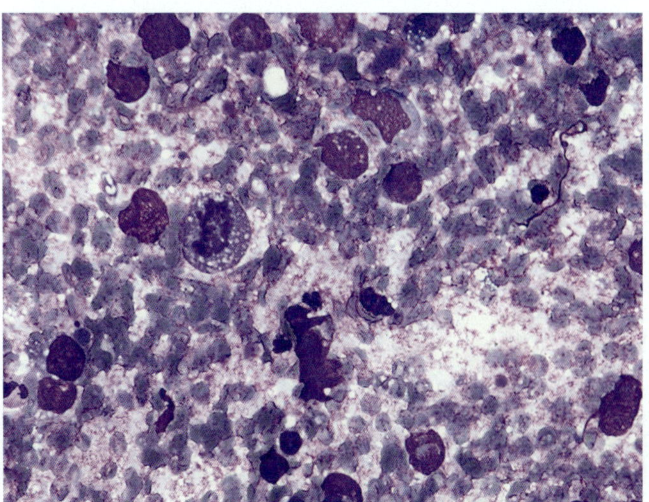

FIGURE 6.38 — Soft Tissue, Gluteal, Embryonal Rhabdomyosarcoma. A population of single cells with large, irregular nuclei is shown. Many of the cells have scant cytoplasm or are bare nuclei. A mitotic figure is present. (Diff Quik stain, high power)

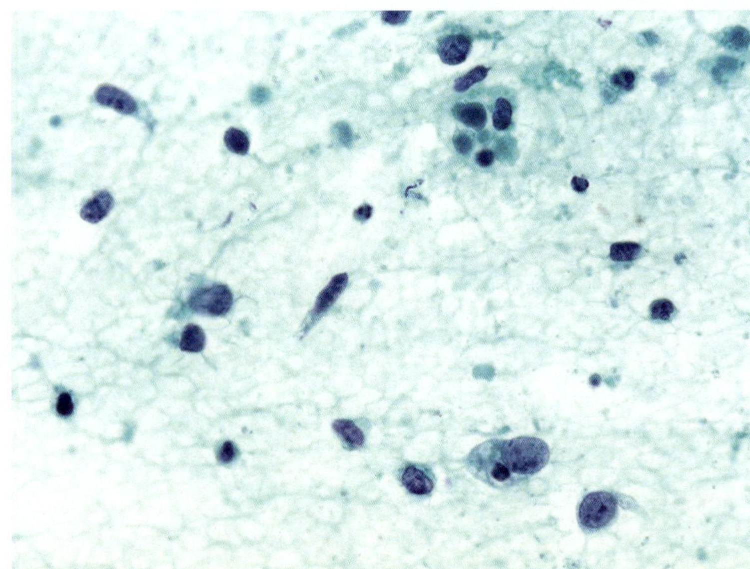

FIGURE 6.39 — Soft Tissue, Gluteal, Embryonal Rhabdomyosarcoma. The cells here show marked pleomorphism with irregular nuclei. Spindle-shaped skeletal muscle cells with cross-striations are quite specific, but are rarely seen on smears. (Papanicolaou stain, high power)

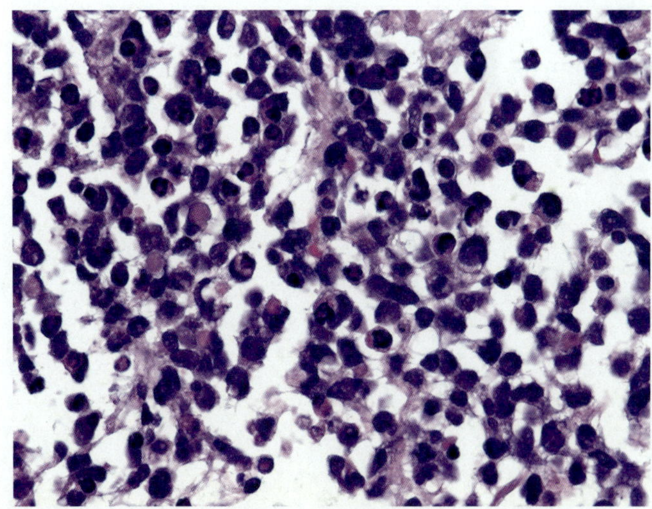

FIGURE 6.40 — Soft Tissue, Gluteal, Embryonal Rhabdomyosarcoma (Core Biopsy). Core biopsy material shows a population of predominantly single cells with irregular, hyperchromatic nuclei. While most cells have scant cytoplasm, occasional cells are seen with dense eosinophilic cytoplasm suggestive of skeletal muscle differentiation. (Hematoxylin and eosin stain, high power)

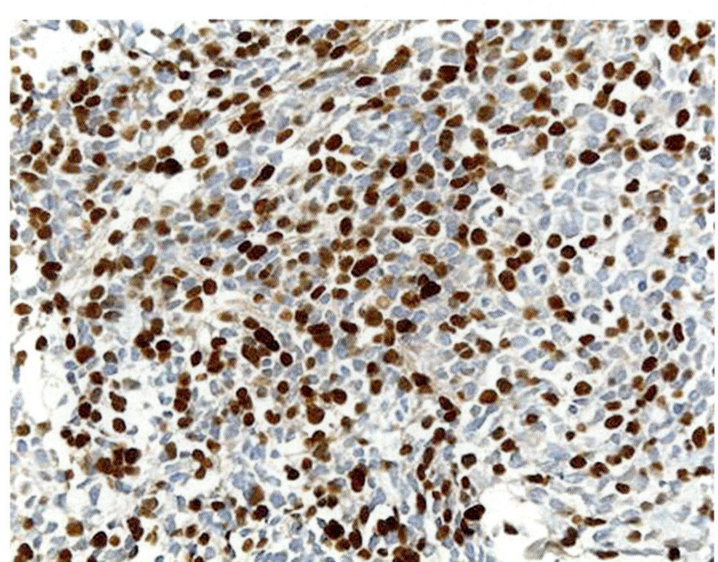

FIGURE 6.41 — Soft Tissue, Gluteal, Embryonal Rhabdomyosarcoma (Core Biopsy). Myogenin immunostain shows strong nuclear positivity consistent with muscular origin. Embryonal is the most common subtype of rhabdomyosarcoma. (Myogenin immunostain, high power)

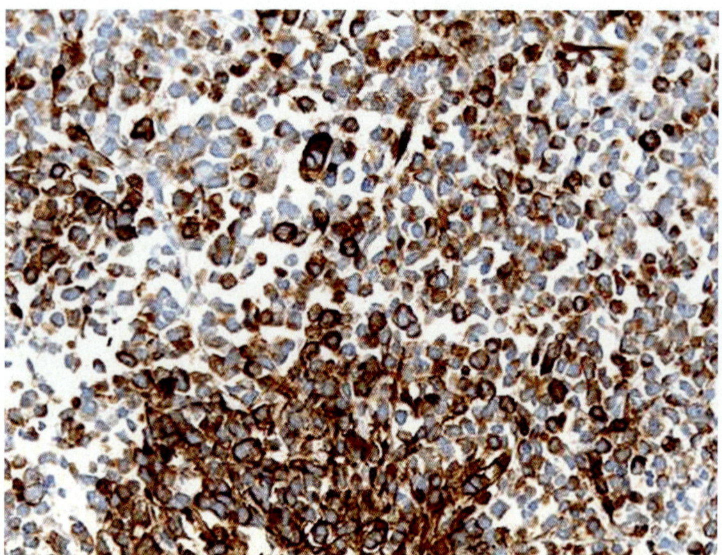

FIGURE 6.42 — Soft Tissue, Gluteal, Embryonal Rhabdomyosarcoma (Core Biopsy). A desmin immunostain is positive in most of the tumor cells, supporting the diagnosis. Desmoplastic small round cell tumor may also be included in the differential and is also desmin positive, but keratin immunostains can distinguish the two. (Desmin immunostain, high power)

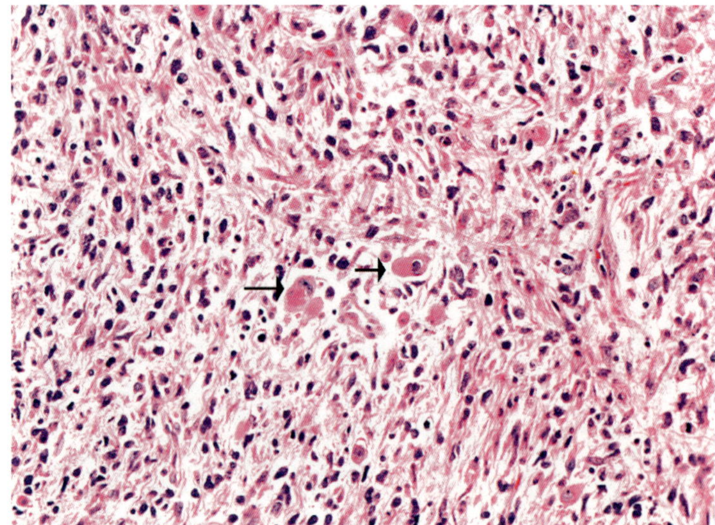

FIGURE 6.43 — Soft Tissue, Embryonal Rhabdomyosarcoma (Histology). This case of embryonal rhabdomyosarcoma demonstrates focal cells with rhabdoid morphology (arrows). These cells have abundant dense eosinophilic cytoplasm and eccentrically placed nuclei. The background is composed of spindled cells. (Hematoxylin and eosin stain, medium power)

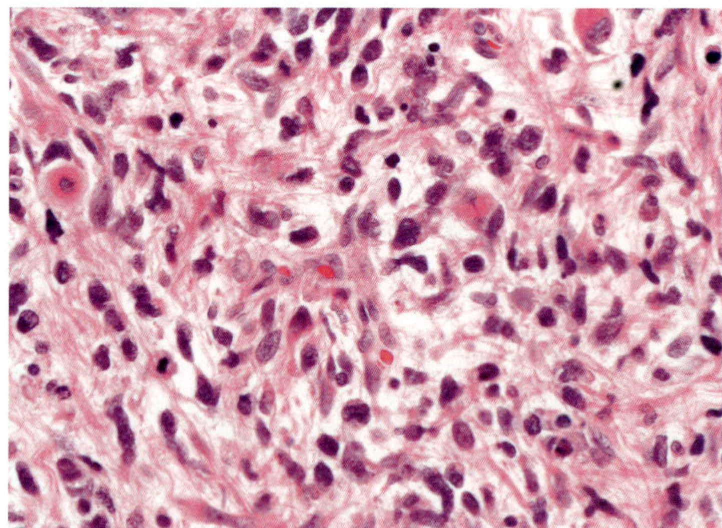

FIGURE 6.44 — Soft Tissue, Embryonal Rhabdomyosarcoma (Histology). On high power, rare rhabdoid cells are seen admixed with small malignant cells with irregularly shaped nuclei and scant cytoplasm. Apoptotic bodies and mitotic figures are readily identified. (Hematoxylin and eosin stain, high power)

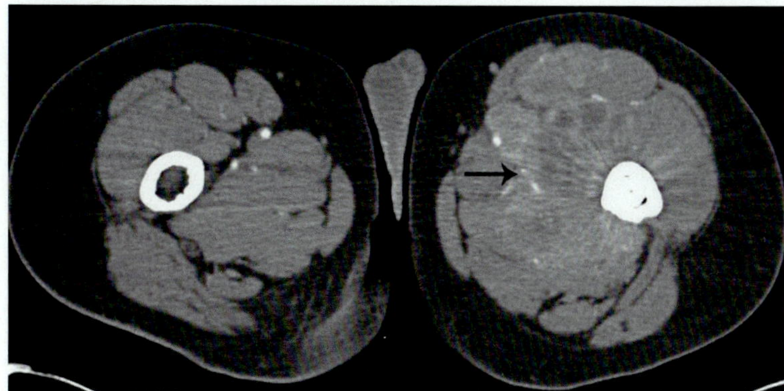

FIGURE 6.45 — Soft Tissue, Left Thigh, Diffuse Large B-Cell Lymphoma. Axial contrast-enhanced CT shows a lobulated enhancing mass in the medial left thigh (arrow). The patient has a history of lymphoma as well as a prior left femur fracture with an intramedullary rod.

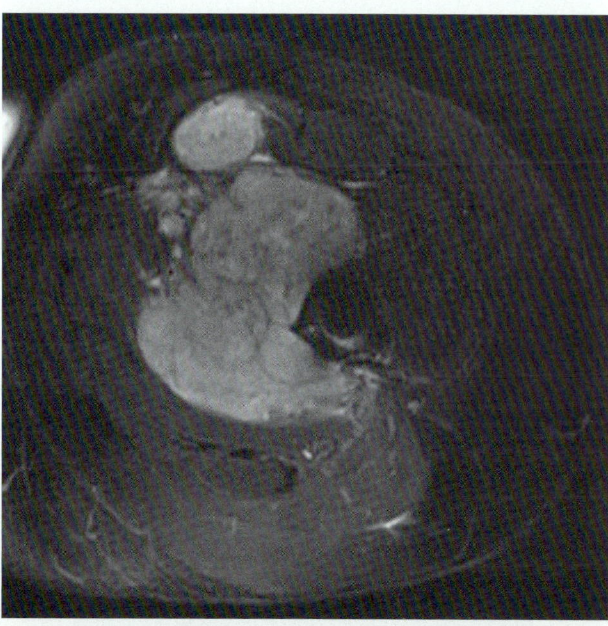

FIGURE 6.46 — Soft Tissue, Left Thigh, Diffuse Large B-Cell Lymphoma. Axial T2-weighted MR image shows the mass in the medial left thigh is T2 hyperintense.

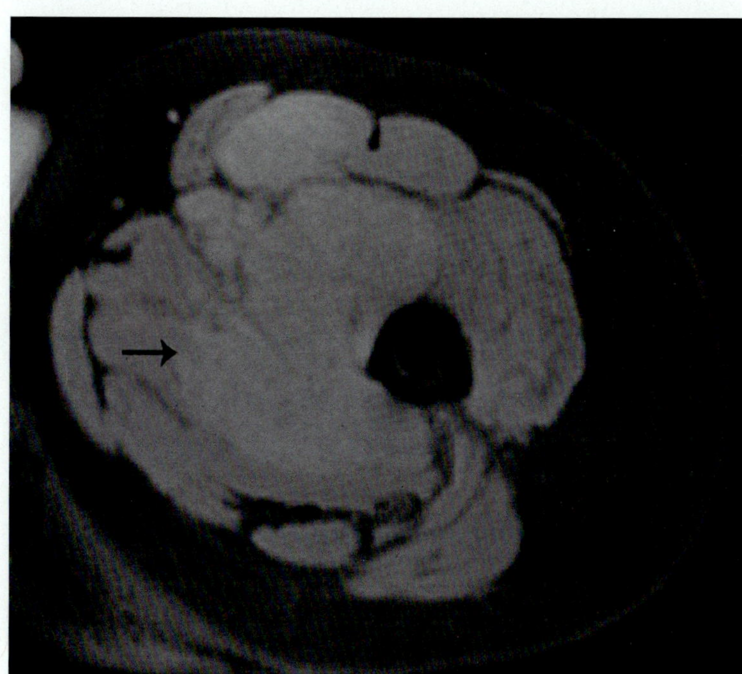

FIGURE 6.47 — Soft Tissue, Left Thigh, Diffuse Large B-Cell Lymphoma. On axial T1-weighted MR image, the mass (arrow) is similar in intensity to muscle.

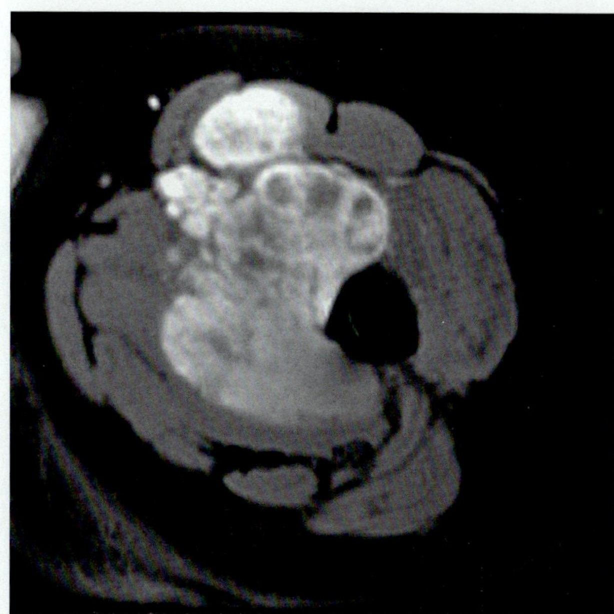

FIGURE 6.48 — Soft Tissue, Left Thigh, Diffuse Large B-Cell Lymphoma. Axial T1-weighted MR image postcontrast is shown. The mass avidly enhances postcontrast.

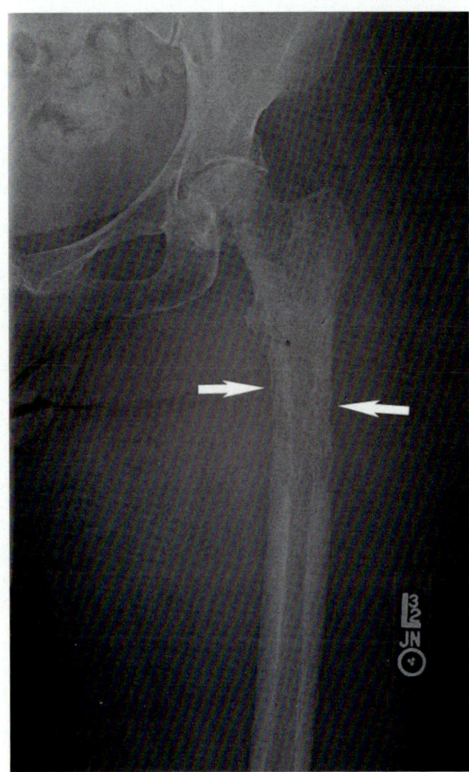

FIGURE 6.49 — Soft Tissue, Left Thigh, Diffuse Large B-Cell Lymphoma. X-ray in a different patient shows a permeative lytic lesion in the left femoral head and proximal left femoral shaft, which involves the cortex (arrows). Lymphoma, myeloma, and metastatic disease are included in the differential diagnosis.

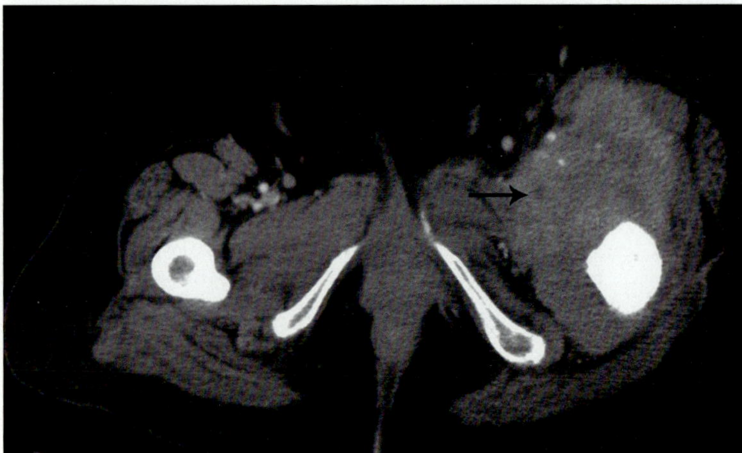

FIGURE 6.50 — Soft Tissue, Left Thigh, Diffuse Large B-Cell Lymphoma. Corresponding axial contrast-enhanced CT shows an associated enhancing soft tissue mass in the adjacent proximal left thigh (arrow). Biopsy was consistent with lymphoma.

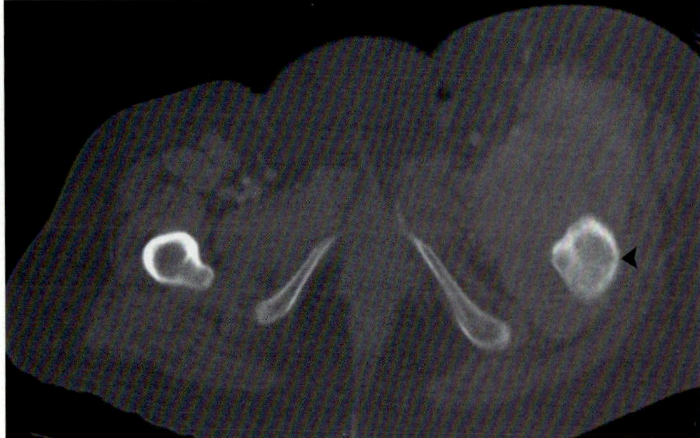

FIGURE 6.51 — Soft Tissue, Left Thigh, Diffuse Large B-Cell Lymphoma. Associated lytic changes in the bone are also noted on bone windows (arrowhead).

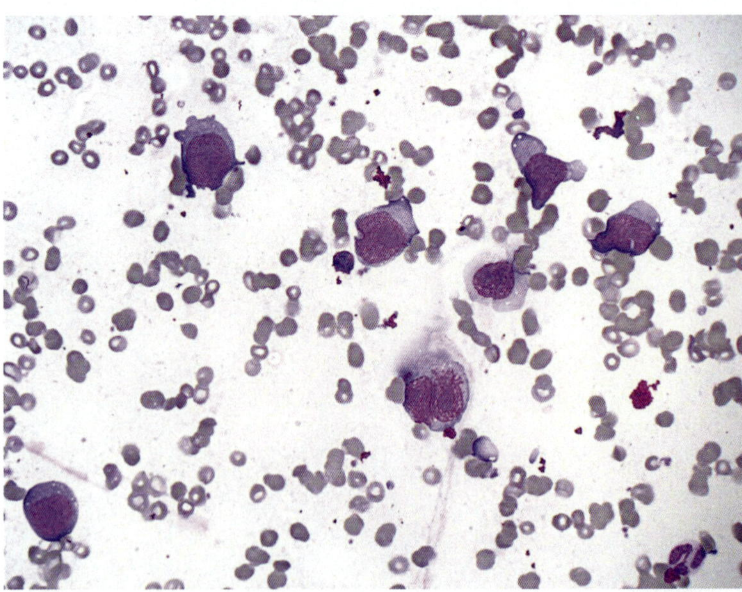

FIGURE 6.52 — Soft Tissue, Left Thigh, Diffuse Large B-Cell Lymphoma. A population of dispersed cells with large, irregular nuclei and deep blue cytoplasm is present. The differential diagnosis includes lymphoma and malignant melanoma. (Diff Quik stain, high power)

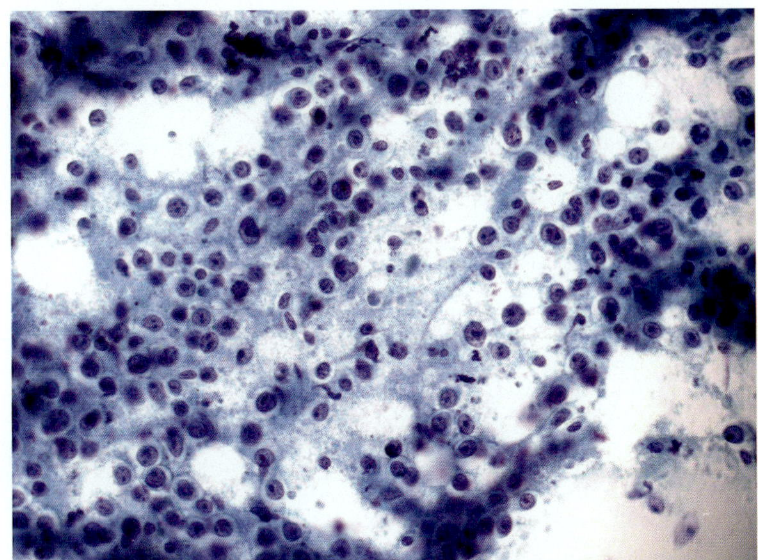

FIGURE 6.53 — Soft Tissue, Left Thigh, Diffuse Large B-Cell Lymphoma. The malignant cells have scant cytoplasm and show frequent prominent nucleoli. Single, prominent nucleoli are often seen in cells of large B-cell lymphoma, but are uncommon in low-grade lymphoma cells. (Papanicolaou stain, high power)

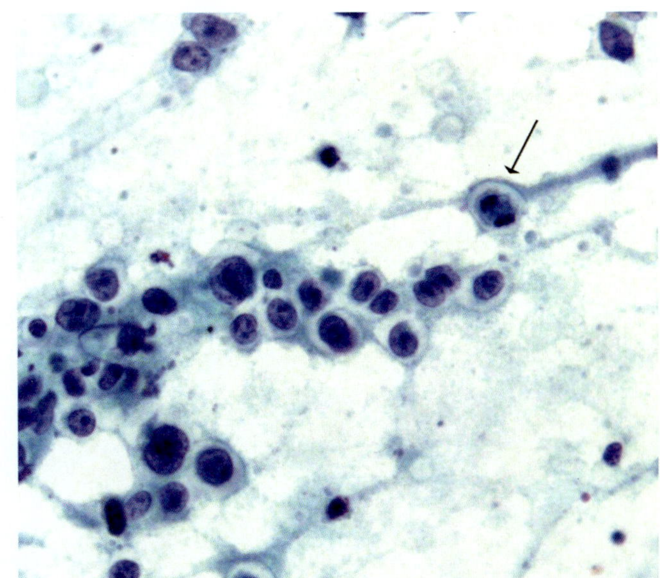

FIGURE 6.54 — Soft Tissue, Left Thigh, Diffuse Large B-Cell Lymphoma. Tumor cells show scant to absent cytoplasm and prominent nucleoli. A mitotic figure is present (arrow), an indication that this tumor is of a high grade. (Papanicolaou stain, high power)

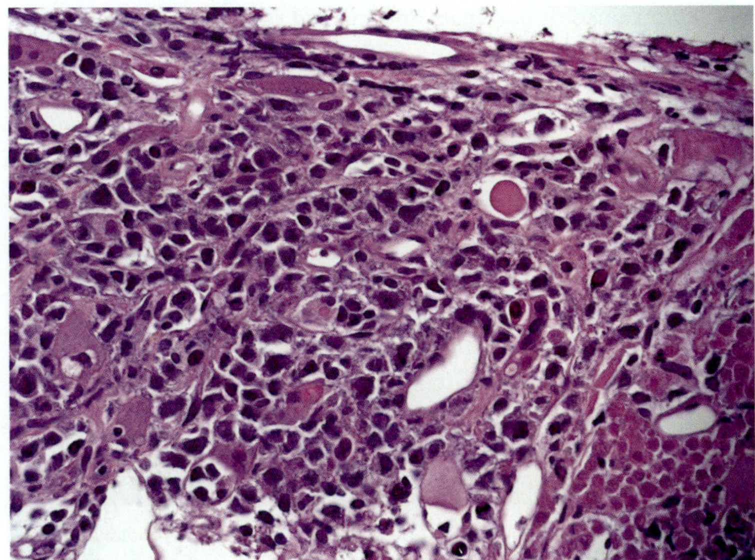

FIGURE 6.55 — Soft Tissue, Left Thigh, Diffuse Large B-Cell Lymphoma (Core Biopsy). Variably sized tumor cells are present in a sheet. An area of tumor necrosis is shown in the bottom right portion of the field. (Hematoxylin and eosin stain, high power)

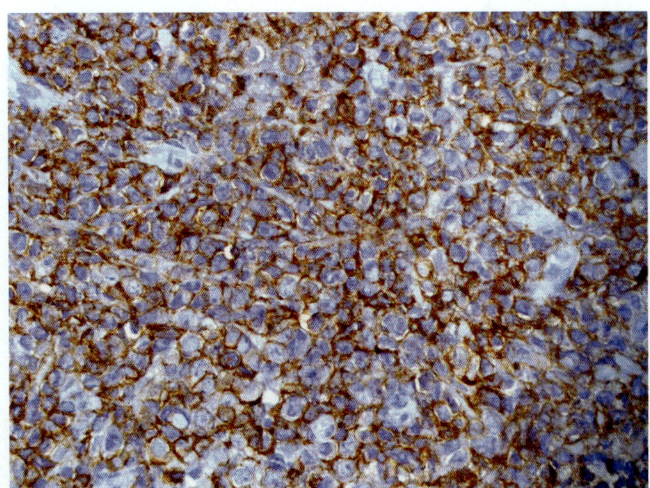

FIGURE 6.56 — Soft Tissue, Left Thigh, Diffuse Large B-Cell Lymphoma (Core Biopsy). A CD20 immunostain, a marker of B-lymphocytes, is diffusely positive. Lymphomas treated with anti-CD20 therapy may develop clones of CD20 negative B-cells. (CD20 immunostain, high power)

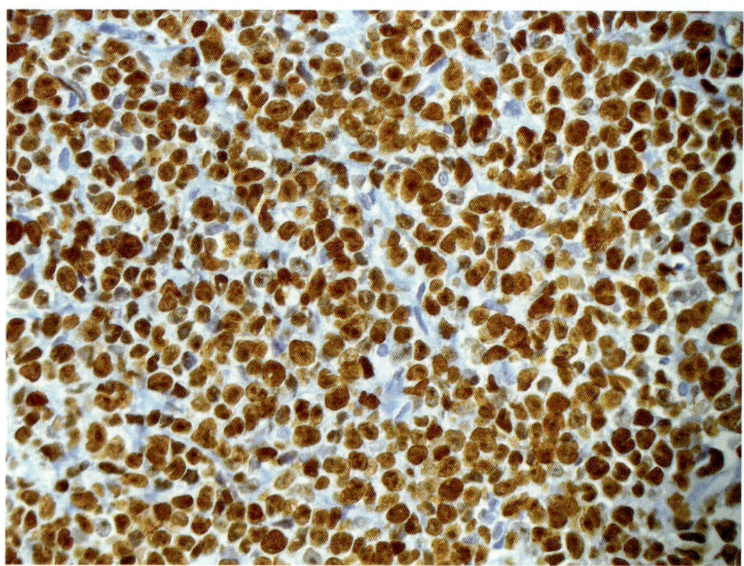

FIGURE 6.57 — Soft Tissue, Left Thigh, Diffuse Large B-Cell Lymphoma (Core Biopsy). This Ki67 immunostain is positive in almost every tumor cell nucleus, indicating a very high proliferative rate. These tumors often respond well to aggressive chemotherapy regimens. (Ki67 immunostain, high power)

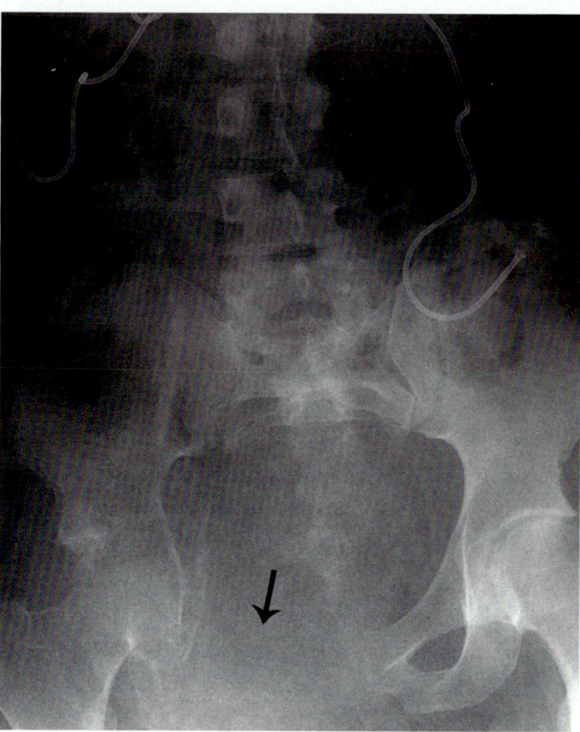

FIGURE 6.58 — Bone, Acetabulum, and Pubic Rami, Ewing Sarcoma (Peripheral Neuroectodermal Tumor). This 29-year-old man complained of back pain and marked right sciatica symptoms. X-ray of the pelvis shows lytic destruction of the right acetabulum and right superior and inferior pubic rami (arrow).

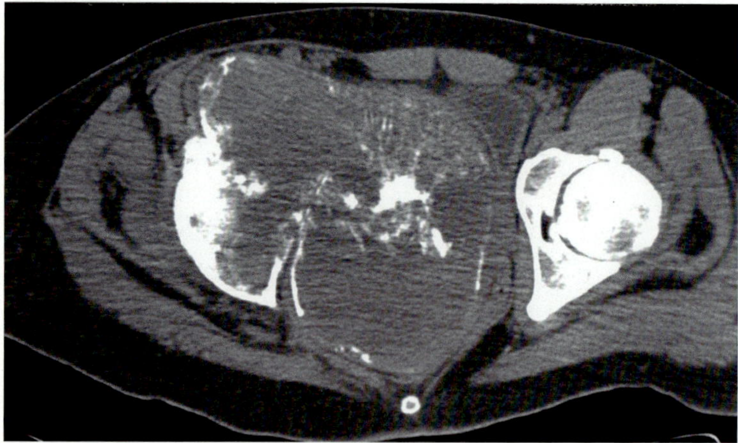

FIGURE 6.59 — Bone, Acetabulum, and Pubic Rami, Ewing Sarcoma (Peripheral Neuroectodermal Tumor). Axial CT demonstrates an expansile lytic lesion involving the right acetabulum and right superior and inferior pubic rami. There is a large associated soft tissue mass with calcifications.

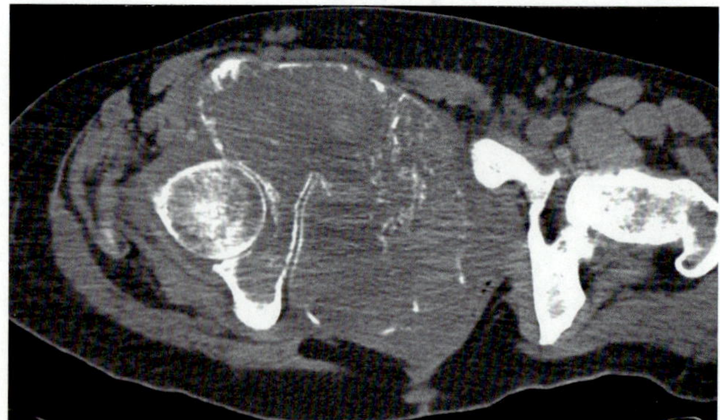

FIGURE 6.60 — Bone, Acetabulum, and Pubic Rami, Ewing Sarcoma (Peripheral Neuroectodermal Tumor). Axial CT image slightly more inferiorly shows further extent of lytic lesion and associated soft tissue mass. Ewing sarcoma commonly presents as a lytic or permeative lesion with an associated soft tissue mass and periosteal reaction.

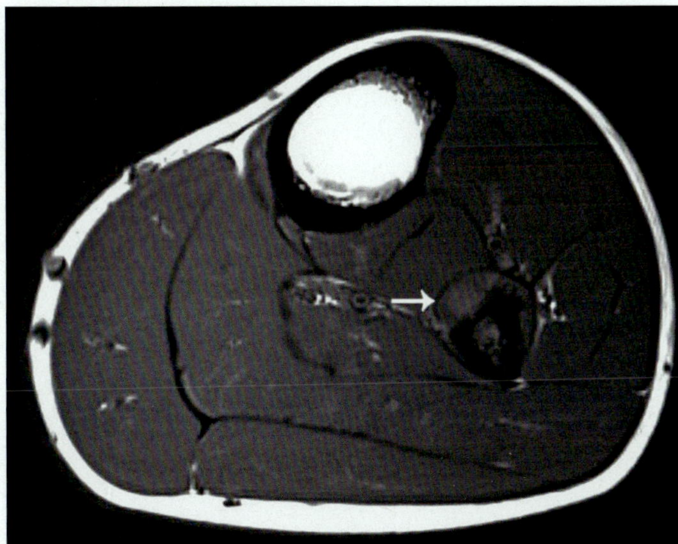

FIGURE 6.61 — Soft Tissue, Left Lower Leg, Ewing Sarcoma (Peripheral Neuroectodermal Tumor). Axial T1-weighted MR image of the left lower leg demonstrates abnormal T1 hypointense signal in the marrow (arrowhead) and a T1 hypointense mass (arrow) surrounding the fibular diaphysis in this region.

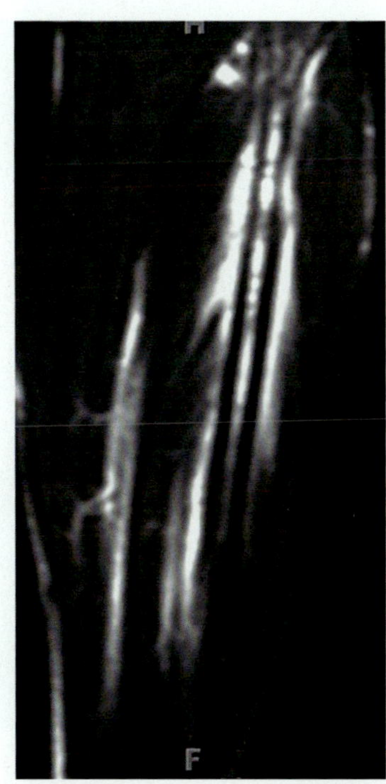

FIGURE 6.62 — Soft Tissue, Left Lower Leg, Ewing Sarcoma (Peripheral Neuroectodermal Tumor). Coronal T2 fat-saturated MR image shows extent of abnormal T2 hyperintense signal in the marrow and T2 hyperintense mass surrounding the fibular diaphysis.

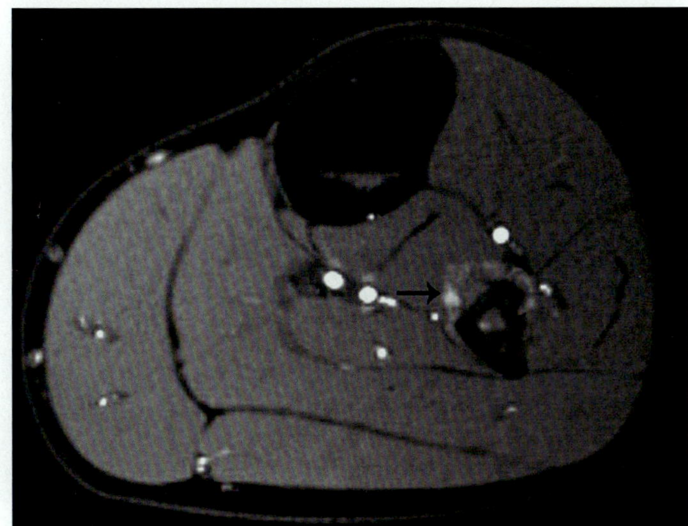

FIGURE 6.63 — Soft Tissue, Left Lower Leg, Ewing Sarcoma (Peripheral Neuroectodermal Tumor). Axial T1 fat-saturated MR image demonstrate enhancement of the marrow (arrowhead) and mass (arrow) postcontrast.

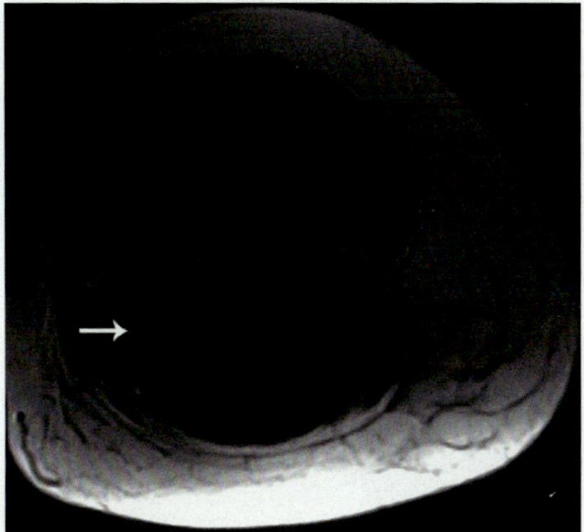

FIGURE 6.64 — Soft Tissue, Left Thigh, Ewing Sarcoma (Peripheral Neuroectodermal Tumor). This 17-year-old girl complained of left lower extremity pain for the past 3 years. Axial T1-weighted MR image demonstrates a large, heterogeneous T1 hypointense mass (arrow) in the muscles posterior to the left femoral shaft.

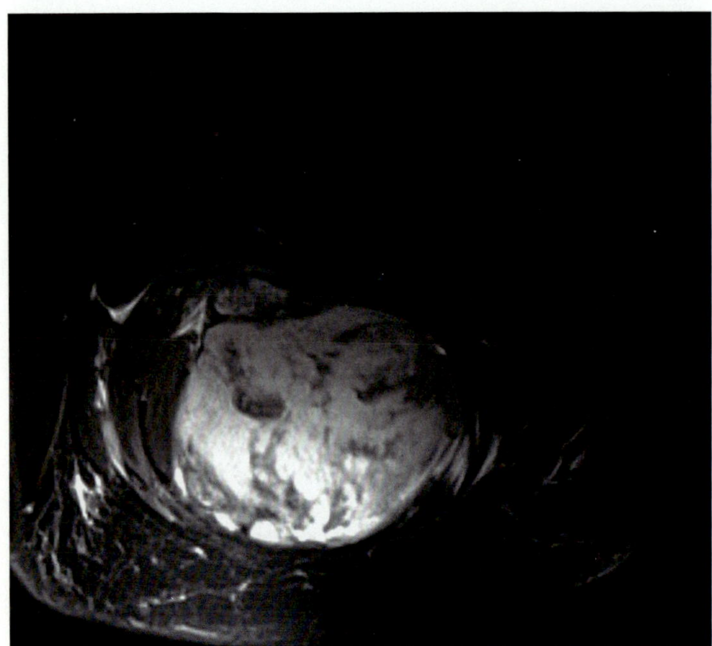

FIGURE 6.65 — Soft Tissue, Left Thigh, Ewing Sarcoma (Peripheral Neuroectodermal Tumor). Axial T2-weighted MR shows the mass is markedly T2 hyperintense. There is no evidence of bone invasion.

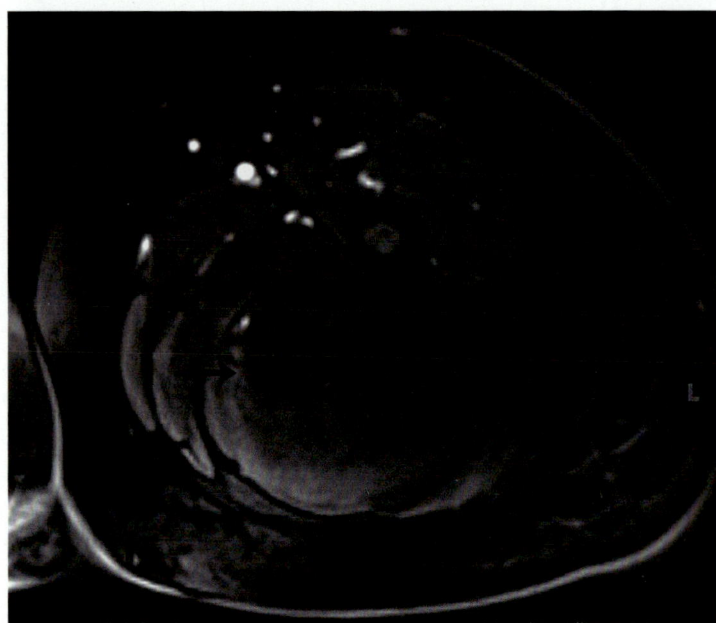

FIGURE 6.66 — Soft Tissue, Left Thigh, Ewing Sarcoma (Peripheral Neuroectodermal Tumor). Axial T1-weighted MR image with fat saturation postcontrast demonstrates minimal enhancement of the mass (arrow).

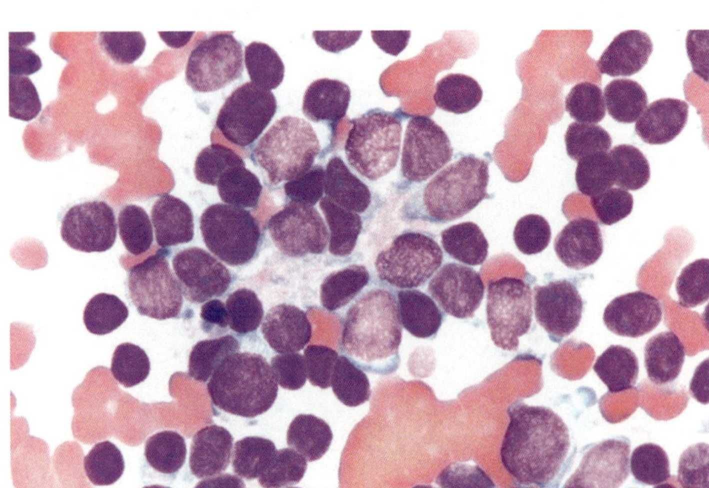

FIGURE 6.67 — Soft Tissue, Left Thigh, Ewing Sarcoma (Peripheral Neuroectodermal Tumor). A population of predominantly dispersed cells with round to oval nuclei and scant cytoplasm prompts consideration of the "small round blue cell" tumors, including Ewing sarcoma, rhabdomyosarcoma, and lymphoma. (Diff Quik stain, high power)

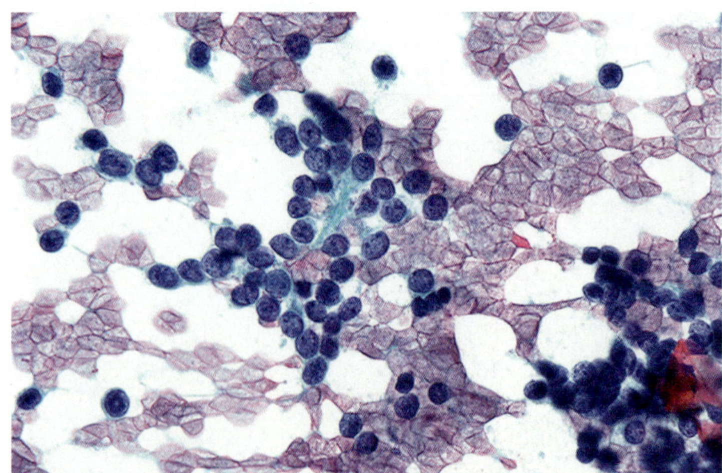

FIGURE 6.68 — Soft Tissue, Left Thigh, Ewing Sarcoma (Peripheral Neuroectodermal Tumor). The neoplastic cells show uniform nuclei and evenly dispersed chromatin. A rosette formation is seen in the center of the field, consistent with a Ewing sarcoma. (Papanicolaou stain, high power)

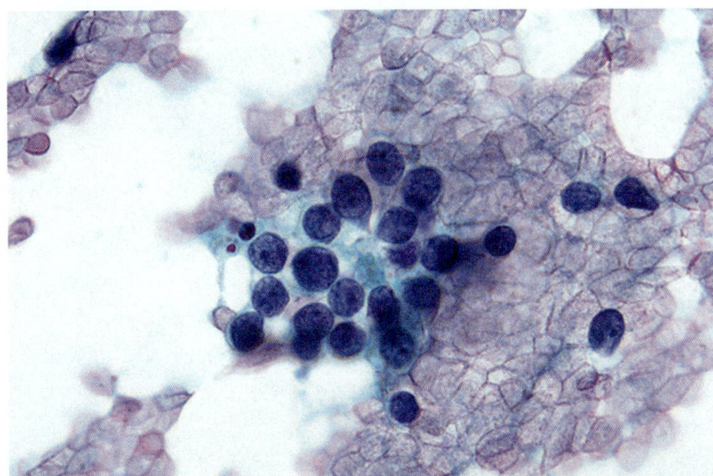

FIGURE 6.69 — Soft Tissue, Left Thigh, Ewing Sarcoma (Primitive Neuroectodermal Tumor). A Homer Wright-type rosette is present with tumor cells surround a central core of fibrillary material. Ewing sarcoma most often shows a translocation t(11;22), involving the EWS gene at 22q12. (Papanicolaou stain, high power)

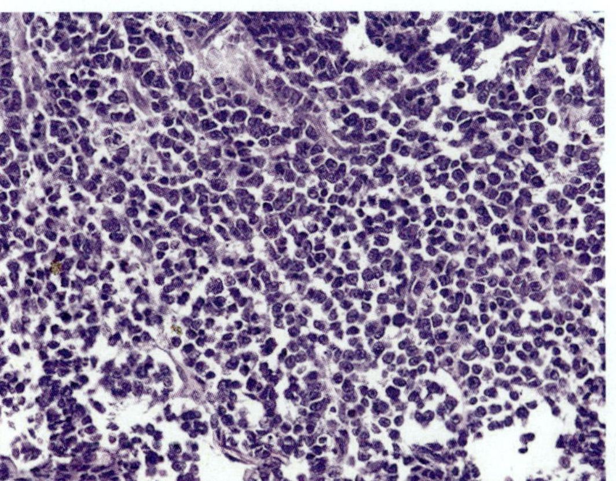

FIGURE 6.70 — Bone, Acetabulum, and Pubic Rami, Ewing Sarcoma (Primitive Neuroectodermal Tumor) (Histology). The neoplasm is composed of a monotonous population of small cells with hyperchromatic nuclei and scant cytoplasm. A diagnosis of Ewing sarcoma cannot be made exclusively on morphologic grounds. (Hematoxylin and eosin stain, high power)

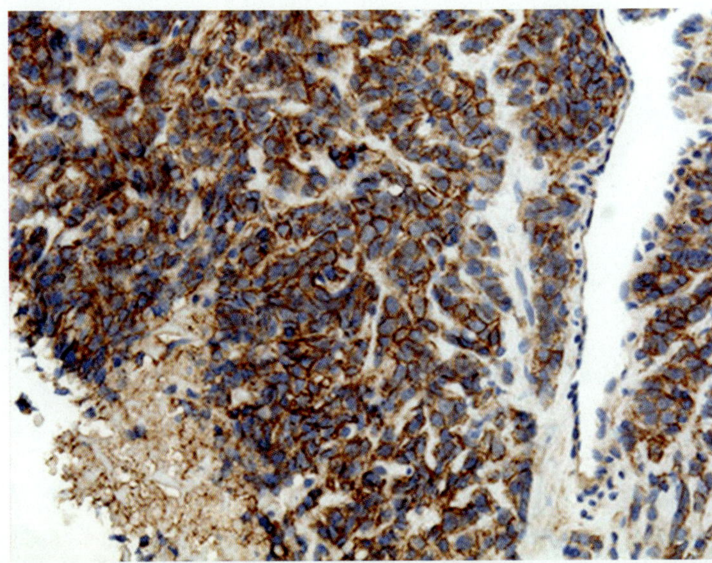

FIGURE 6.71 — Bone, Acetabulum, and Pubic Rami, Ewing Sarcoma (Primitive Neuroectodermal Tumor) (Histology). This CD99 (O13) immunostain shows the distinct membranous staining pattern of Ewing sarcoma. CD99 is positive, but typically in a cytoplasmic pattern, in many other neoplasms, including synovial sarcoma and some rhabdomyosarcomas. (CD99 immunostain, high power)

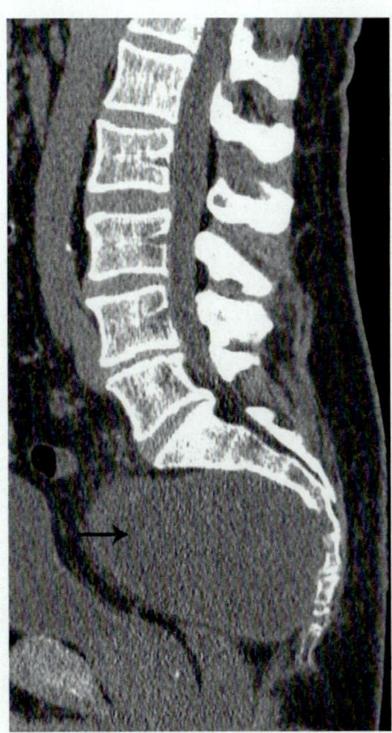

FIGURE 6.72 — Bone and Soft Tissue, Presacral, Chordoma. A 56-year-old man presented with a long history of progressive back pain and right lower extremity discomfort following trauma. The patient had a remote history of lumbar laminectomy and facet injections. There was no history of bladder or bowel dysfunction. Sagittal CT without contrast shows a large presacral soft tissue mass (arrow) with anterior sacral bone erosion.

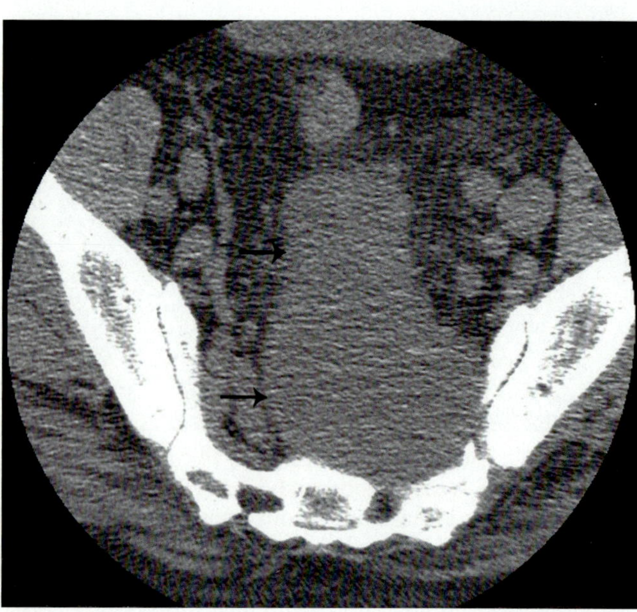

FIGURE 6.73 — Bone and Soft Tissue, Presacral, Chordoma. Axial CT without IV contrast confirms presacral soft tissue mass (arrows) in the midline. Chordomas are most common in the midline in the sacrococcygeal region followed by the clivus. A giant cell tumor, chondrosarcoma, and metastasis are included in the differential diagnosis.

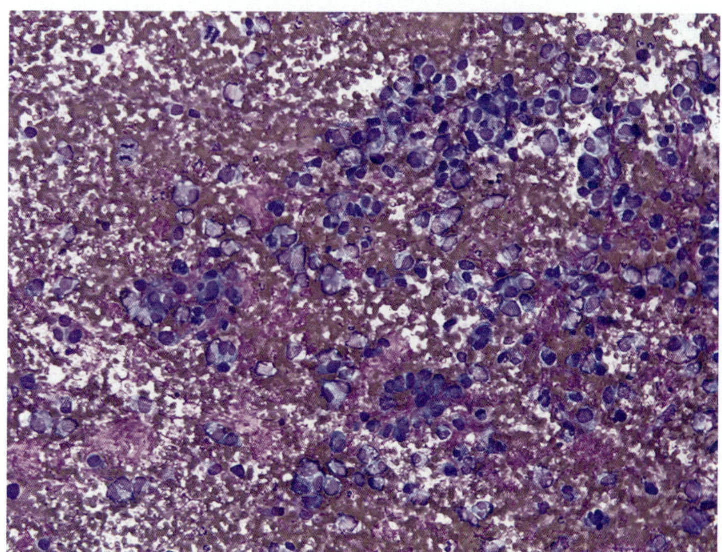

FIGURE 6.74 — Bone and Soft Tissue, Presacral, Chordoma. Numerous, dispersed, single tumor cells are present showing low nuclear-to-cytoplasmic ratios and fairly abundant cytoplasm. An eosinophilic matrix material is seen in the background and admixed with the neoplastic cells. (Diff Quik stain, medium power)

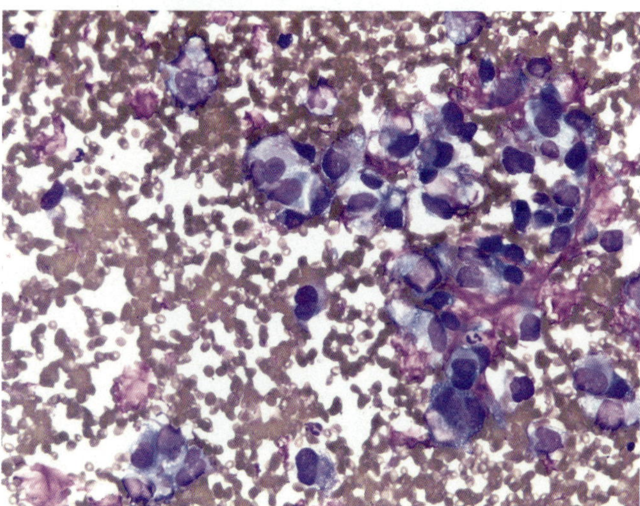

FIGURE 6.75 — Bone and Soft Tissue, Presacral, Chordoma. On higher power, the neoplastic cells show abundant vacuolated cytoplasm, characteristic of the physaliferous cells of chordoma. There is a brightly eosinophilic, myxoid-appearing matrix present in the background. (Diff Quik stain, high power)

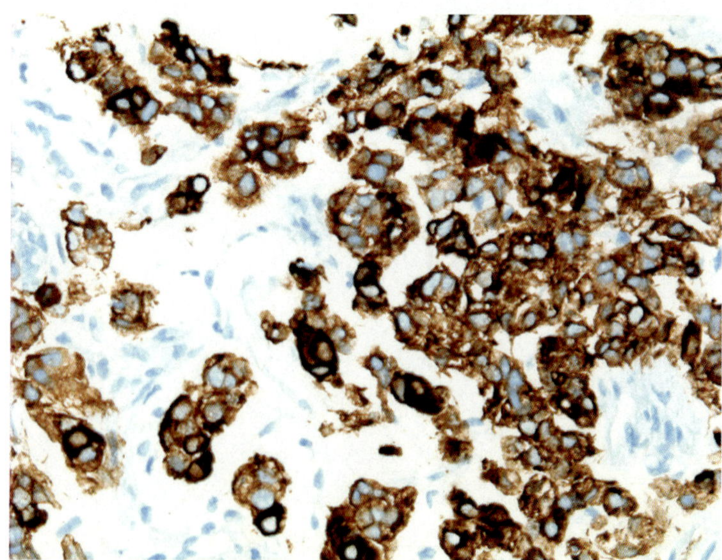

FIGURE 6.76 — Bone and Soft Tissue, Presacral, Chordoma (Cell Block). A cell block was available for confirmatory immunostains. A cytokeratin AE1/3 shows strong and diffuse positivity. These tumors are also positive for S-100 protein and EMA (not shown). (Cytokeratin AE1/3 immunostain, high power)

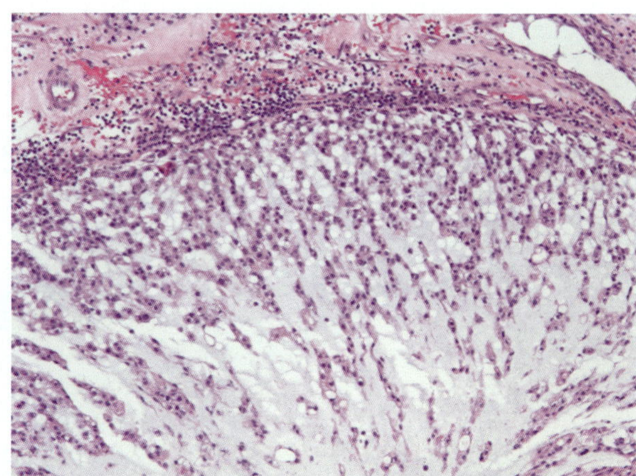

FIGURE 6.77 — Bone and Soft Tissue, Presacral, Chordoma (Histology). Chordoma is a primary bone tumor arising from notochordal rests. About 80% of the tumors arise in the sacrum. The neoplasm consists of chords or nests of rounded cells in a myxoid matrix. The characteristic cells often have prominent vacuolated cytoplasm and are termed "physaliferous" cells from the Greek meaning "having vacuoles." (Hematoxylin and eosin stain, low power)

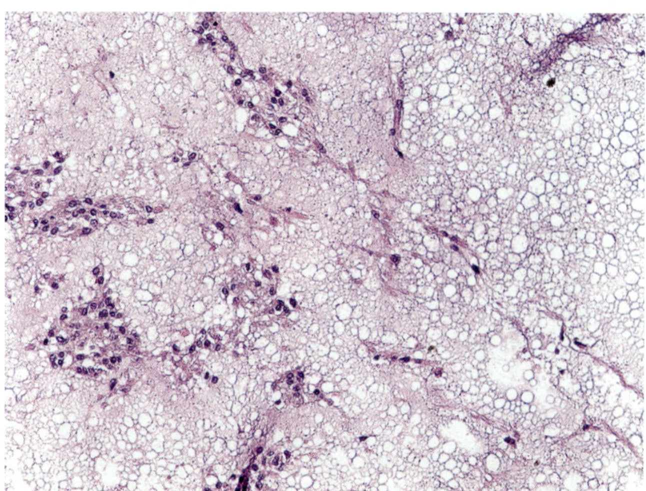

FIGURE 6.78 — Bone and Soft Tissue, Presacral, Chordoma (Histology). Neoplastic cells with vacuolated cytoplasm are seen in a myxoid matrix. The differential diagnosis includes a myxoid chondrosarcoma. Chordomas are positive for keratins and epithelial membrane antigen whereas chondrosarcomas are negative for both. (Hematoxylin and eosin stain, high power)

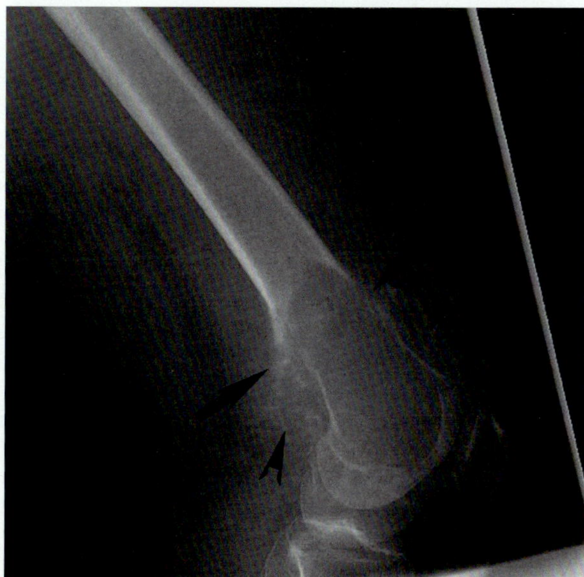

FIGURE 6.79 — Bone, Distal Femur, Giant Cell Tumor of Bone. Lateral radiograph of the left knee demonstrates an expansile lytic lesion in the distal femur involving the metaphysis and epiphysis and abutting the articular surface (arrows). There is associated periosteal reaction (arrowheads).

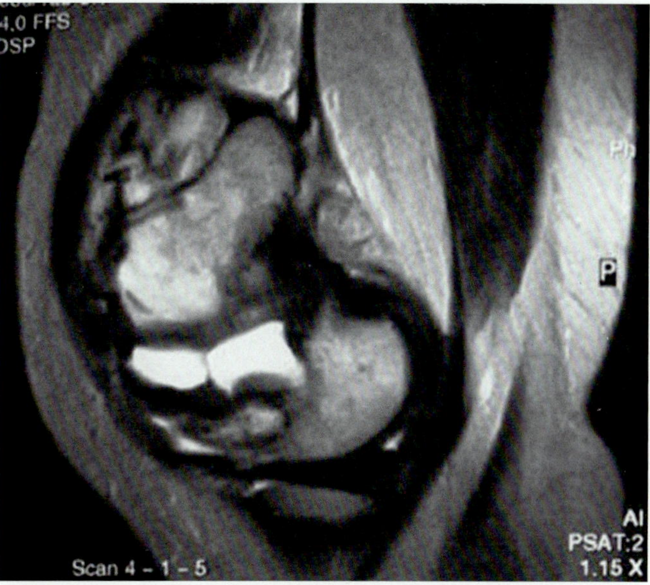

FIGURE 6.80 — Bone, Distal Femur, Giant Cell Tumor of Bone. This patient was a 39-year-old woman with a 1-month history of rapidly enlarging left lower thigh mass, difficulty walking, and leg pain awakening her from sleep. Sagittal MR image demonstrates fluid levels and associated soft tissue mass.

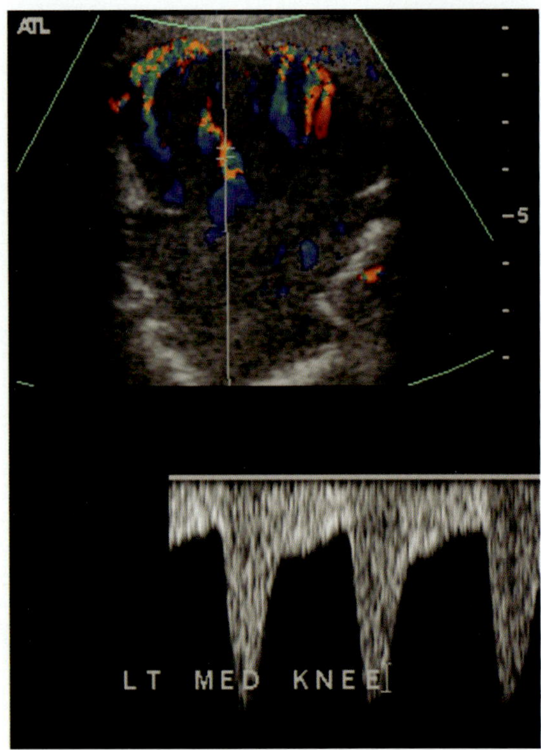

FIGURE 6.81 — Bone, Distal Femur, Giant Cell Tumor of Bone. Sonographic image confirms large associated soft tissue mass with internal vascularity, which was targeted for biopsy.

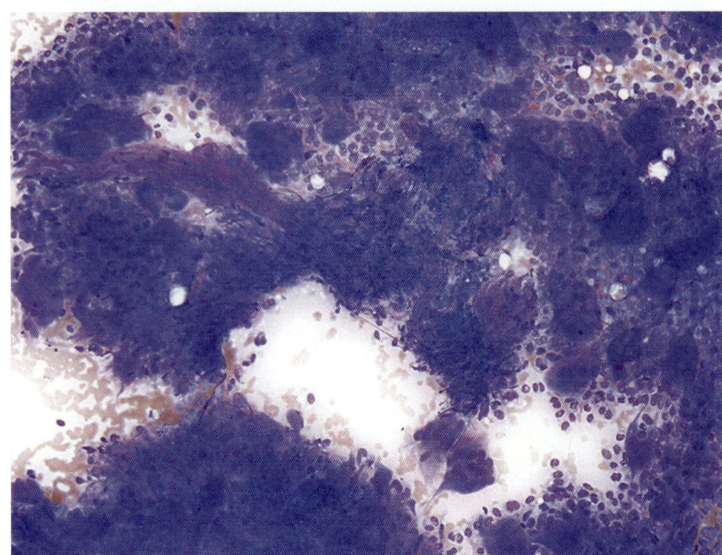

FIGURE 6.82 — Bone, Distal Femur, Giant Cell Tumor of Bone. This densely cellular aspirate smear shows numerous multinucleated cells and a fibrous background. Giant cells are present in many bone lesions, both benign and malignant. (Diff Quik stain, medium power)

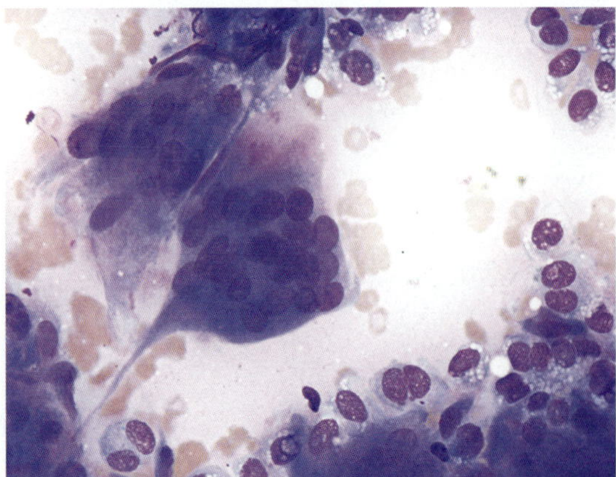

FIGURE 6.83 — Bone, Distal Femur, Giant Cell Tumor of Bone. Two multinucleated giant cells are present in the center of the field. Surrounding single cells show nuclei similar to those of the giant cells, a characteristic of giant cell tumor. (Diff Quik stain, high power)

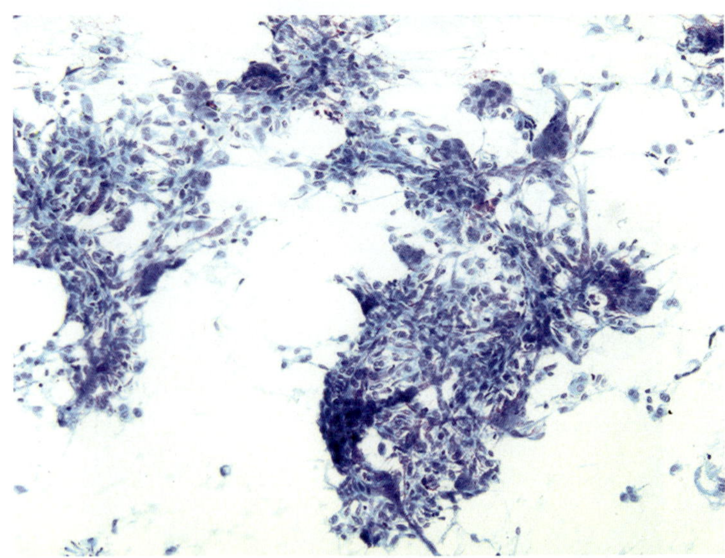

FIGURE 6.84 — Bone, Distal Femur, Giant Cell Tumor of Bone. Cohesive fragments of stromal cells are admixed with scattered giant cells. Giant cell tumors are benign, but may be locally aggressive. Necrosis and hemorrhage may be encountered. (Papanicolaou stain, medium power)

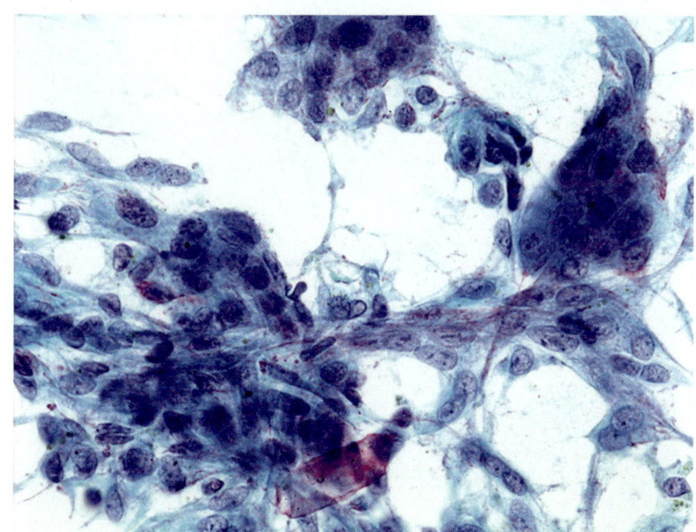

FIGURE 6.85 — Bone, Distal Femur, Giant Cell Tumor of Bone. Stroma and giant cells are present. The differential diagnosis includes "brown tumor" of hyperparathyroidism, pigmented villonodular synovitis, aneurysmal bone cyst, and chondroblastoma. (Papanicolaou stain, high power)

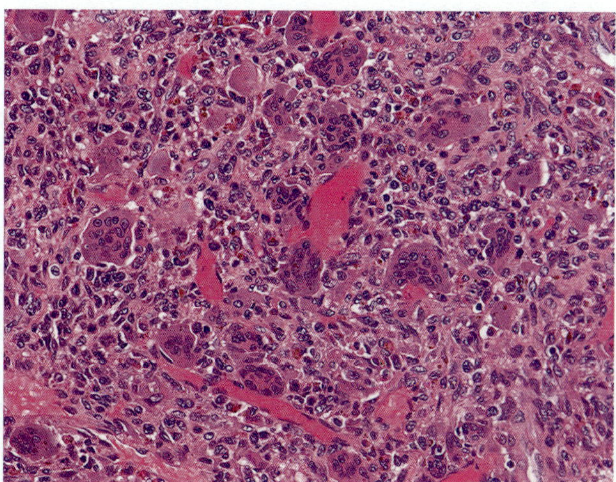

FIGURE 6.86 — Bone, Distal Femur, Giant Cell Tumor of Bone (Histology). The lesion consists of multinucleated giant cells admixed with mononuclear cells admixed with plump spindle to epithelioid mononuclear cells. There is some hemosiderin (brown pigment) in the background. (Hematoxylin and eosin stain, medium power)

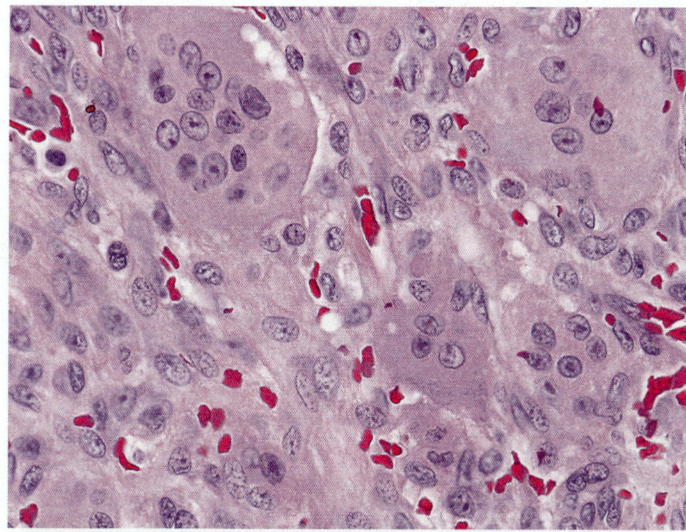

FIGURE 6.87 — Bone, Distal Femur, Giant Cell Tumor of Bone (Histology). Multinucleated giant cells are admixed with stromal cells. Note that the nuclei of the giant cells are cytologically very similar to the background mononuclear cells. Occasional small nuclei are seen but nuclear atypia is minimal. (Hematoxylin and eosin stain, low power)

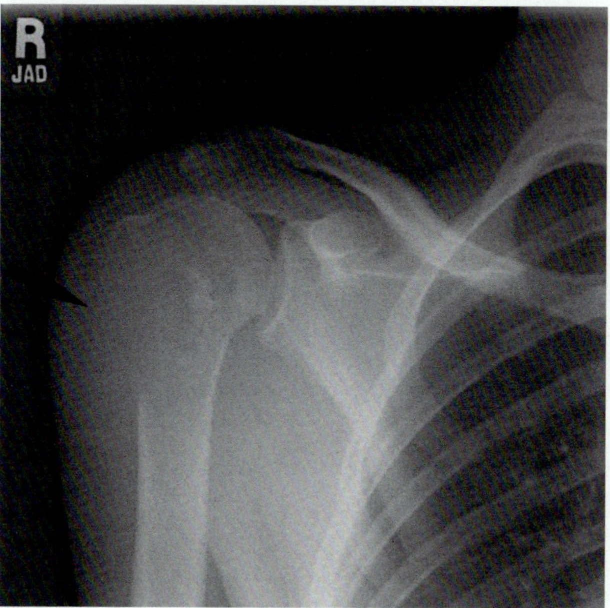

FIGURE 6.88 — Bone, Right Humerus, Osteosarcoma. X-ray of the right shoulder shows a large lytic lesion with ill-defined borders centered in the proximal right humeral metaphysis (arrow). There is expansion of the lateral cortex. Osteosarcomas involve cortical and medullary bone destruction.

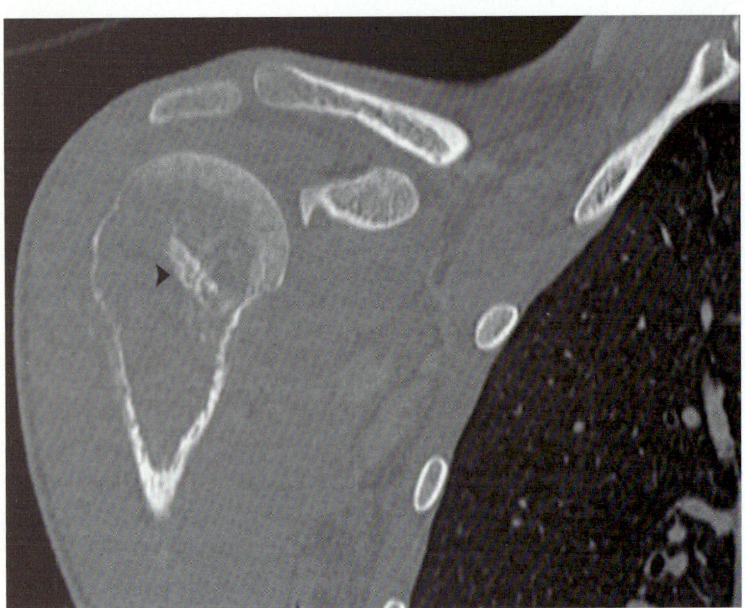

FIGURE 6.89 — Bone, Right Humerus, Osteosarcoma. Coronal CT in bone windows shows the permeative lesion involving the cortex. Osteoid-type matrix is seen within this lesion (arrowhead) suggestive of an osteosarcoma.

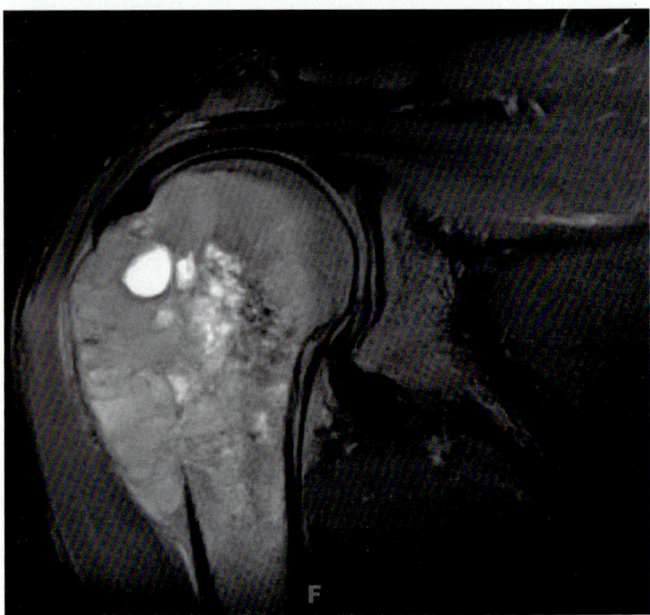

FIGURE 6.90 — Bone, Right Humerus, Osteosarcoma. Coronal fat-saturated proton density MR image shows a large associated soft tissue mass, which is heterogeneous in signal intensity. An associated soft tissue mass is often seen with osteosarcomas.

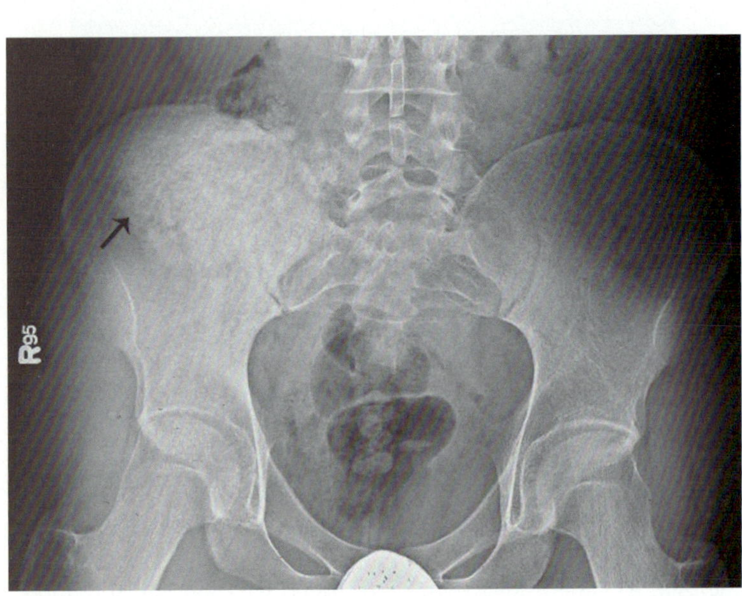

FIGURE 6.91 — Bone, Right Iliac Wing, Osteosarcoma. Frontal x-ray of the pelvis shows a large area of tumor bone formation in the right iliac wing (arrow).

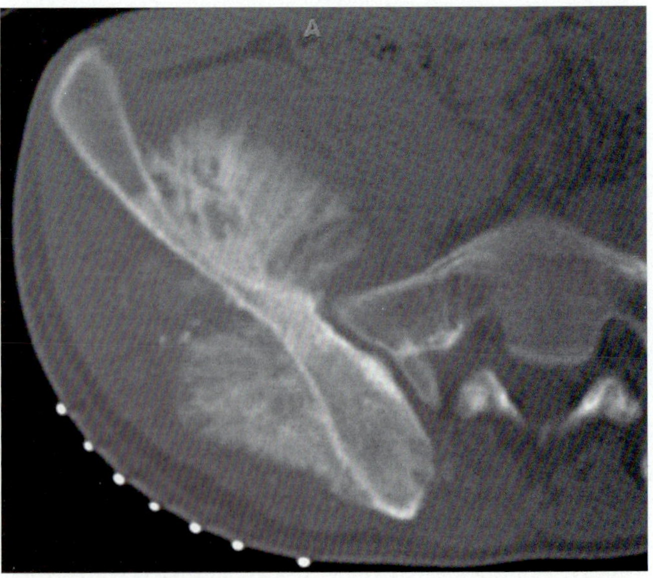

FIGURE 6.92 — Bone, Right Iliac Wing, Osteosarcoma. Axial CT of the pelvis in bone windows shows the corresponding aggressive sunburst periosteal reaction and the extent of anterior and posterior bone formation.

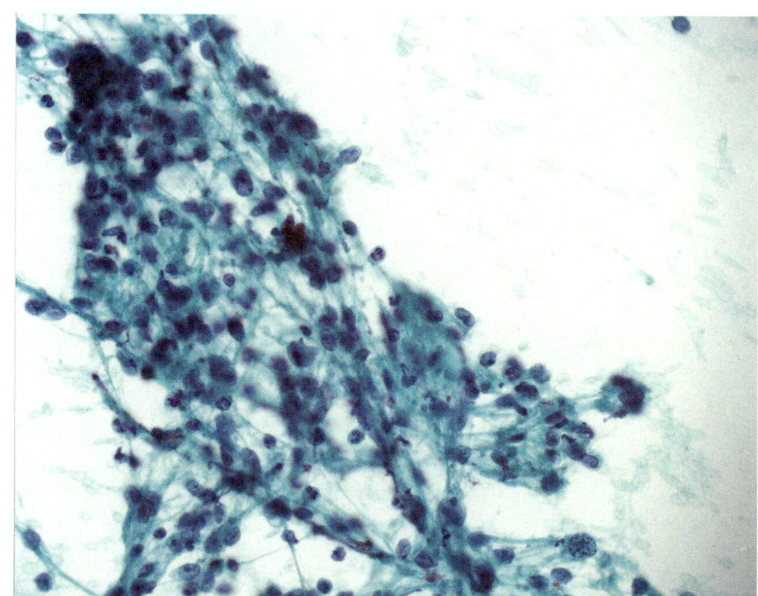

FIGURE 6.93 — Bone, Right Iliac Wing, Osteosarcoma. A loose fibrous meshwork contains numerous small- to medium-sized cells with slightly hyperchromatic cells. Aspirates from osteosarcoma may be variably cellular, and core biopsy may be required for definitive diagnosis. (Papanicolaou stain, high power)

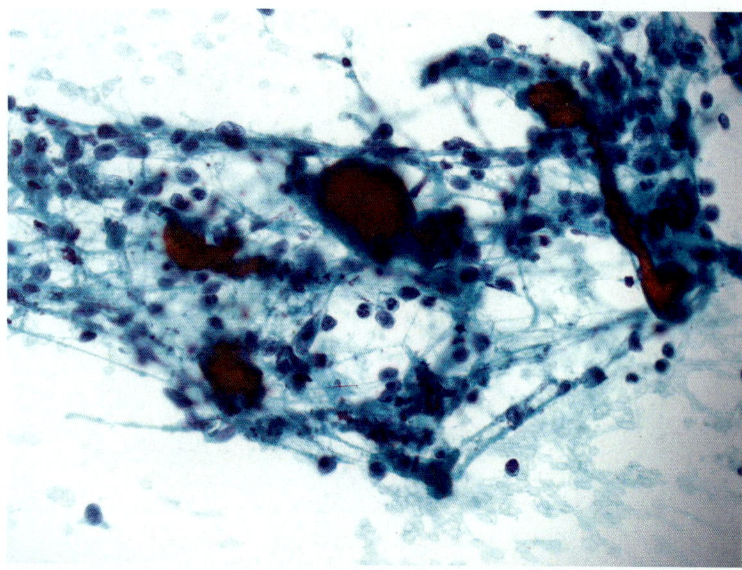

FIGURE 6.94 — Bone, Right Iliac Wing, Osteosarcoma. Dense, glassy acellular material is consistent with osteoid. Osteoid should be distinguished from benign bone fragments, which may be admixed with any tumor aspirate. (Papanicolaou stain, high power)

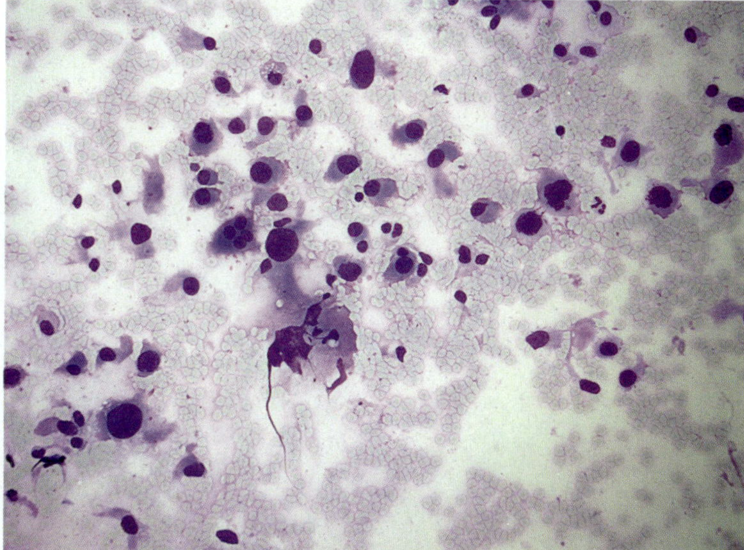

FIGURE 6.95 — Bone, Right Iliac Wing, Osteosarcoma. A dispersed population of markedly atypical cells is shown. A small giant cell is present, which may be seen in osteosarcoma. (Diff Quik stain, high power)

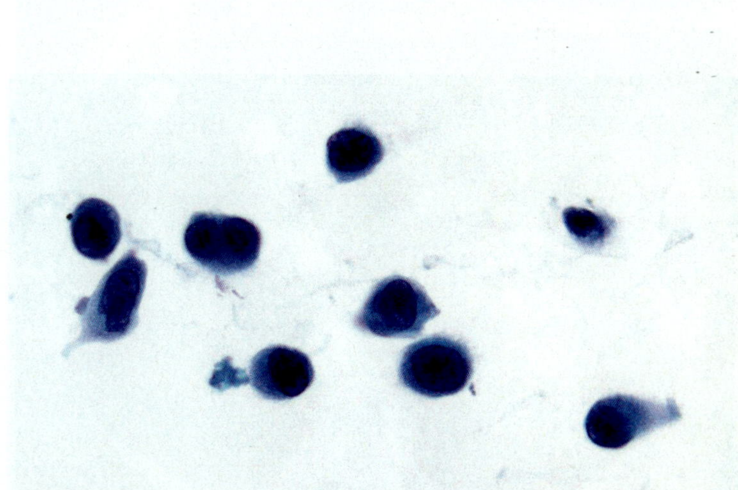

FIGURE 6.96 — Bone, Right Iliac Wing, Osteosarcoma. These malignant cells show very high nuclear-to-cytoplasmic ratio and irregular, hyperchromatic nuclei. There is no evidence of differentiation here, and the differential diagnosis includes mesenchymal, lymphoid, and epithelial neoplasms. (Papanicolaou stain, high power)

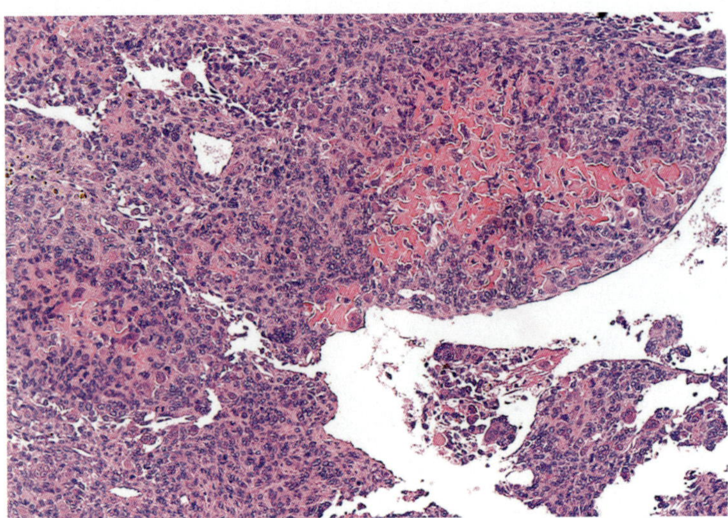

FIGURE 6.97 — Bone, Right Humerus, Osteosarcoma (Histology). This neoplasm shows a densely cellular proliferation of small- to medium-sized cells with moderate nuclear atypia. Osteoid (dense, eosinophilic, acellular material) production is evident in the right portion of the field. (Hematoxylin and eosin stain, medium power)

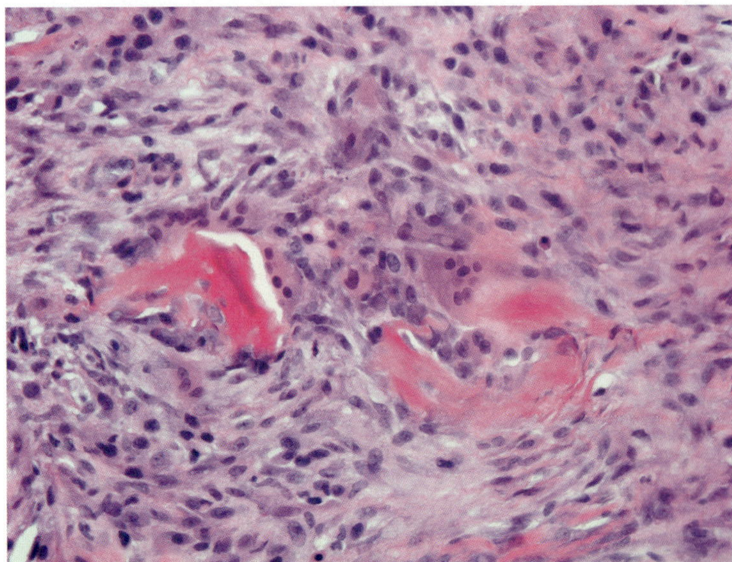

FIGURE 6.98 — Bone, Right Humerus, Osteosarcoma (Histology). Glassy, eosinophilic material consistent with osteoid is seen surrounded by a densely cellular proliferation of spindle cells. Osteoblasts are seen rimming the neoplastic bone. (Hematoxylin and eosin stain, high power)

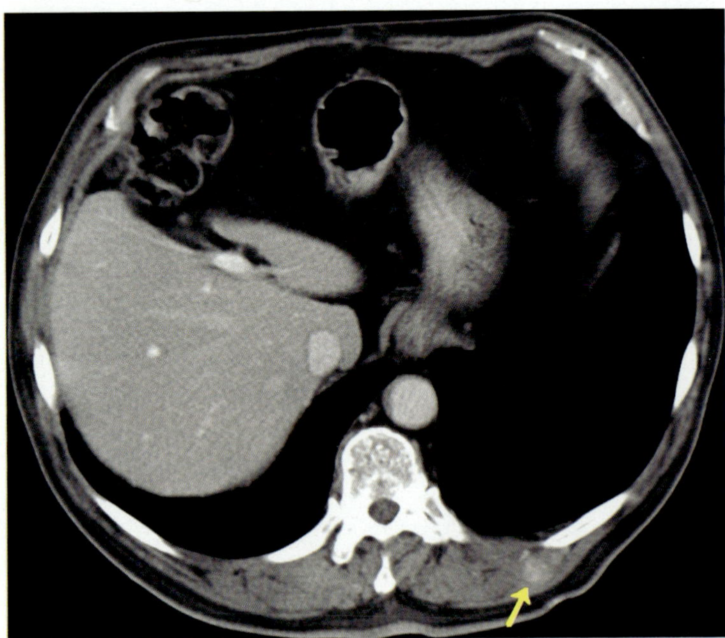

FIGURE 6.99 — Soft Tissue, Paraspinal, Metastatic Renal Cell Carcinoma. Axial contrast-enhanced CT shows a small, enhancing mass in the left paraspinal muscles (arrow).

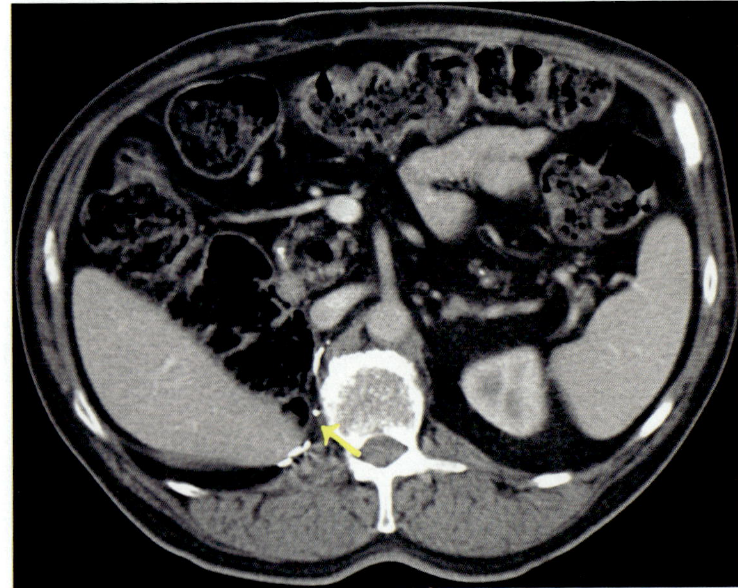

FIGURE 6.100 — Soft Tissue, Paraspinal, Metastatic Renal Cell Carcinoma. The patient has a history of right nephrectomy for renal cell carcinoma. Note the surgical clips in the right renal fossa (arrow).

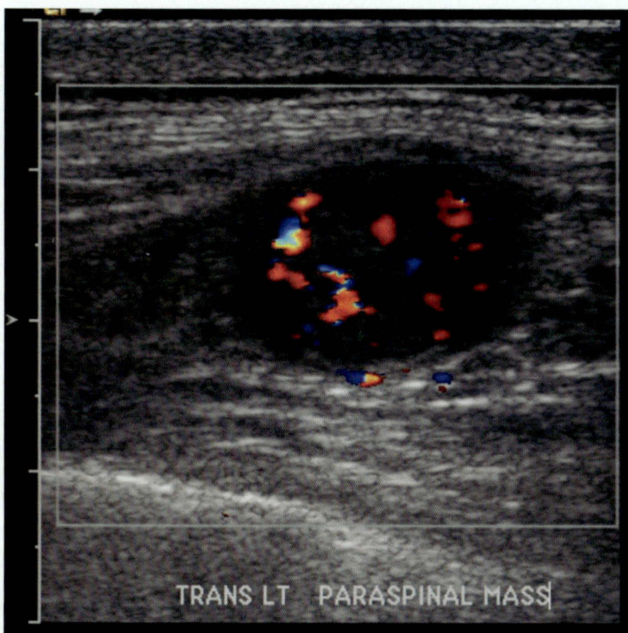

FIGURE 6.101 — Soft Tissue, Paraspinal, Metastatic Renal Cell Carcinoma. Sonographic image confirms hypoechoic left paraspinal mass with marked internal vascularity. Metastases from renal cell carcinoma are commonly hypervascular.

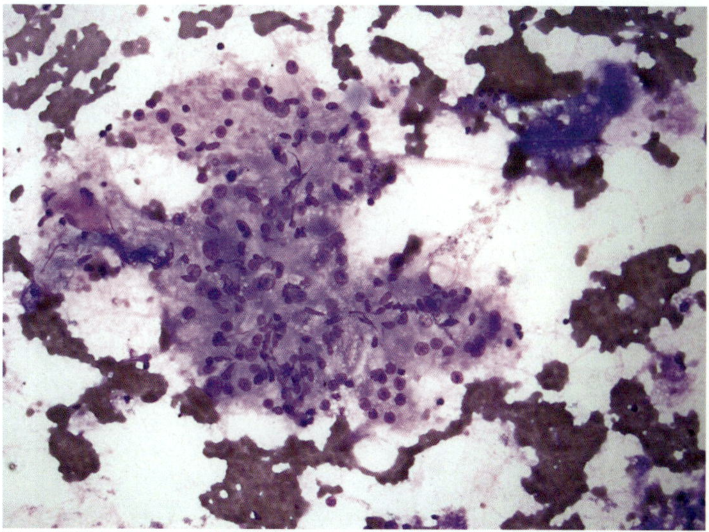

FIGURE 6.102 — Soft Tissue, Paraspinal, Metastatic Renal Cell Carcinoma. This cohesive fragment of cells shows abundant vacuolated cytoplasm and round, uniform nuclei. The nuclei show prominent nucleoli. (Diff Quik stain, medium power)

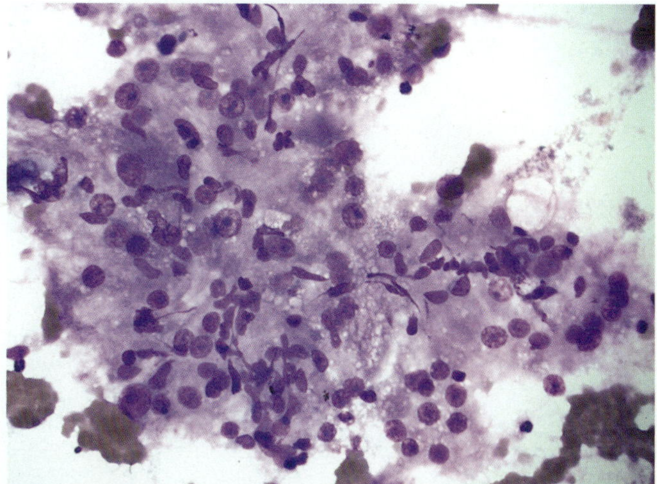

FIGURE 6.103 — Soft Tissue, Paraspinal, Metastatic Renal Cell Carcinoma. Vacuolated cytoplasm and round nuclei with prominent nucleoli are characteristic of clear cell renal cell carcinoma. Renal cell carcinoma may present as a metastasis as the primary tumors are often undetected due to lack of clinical symptoms. (Diff Quik stain, high power)

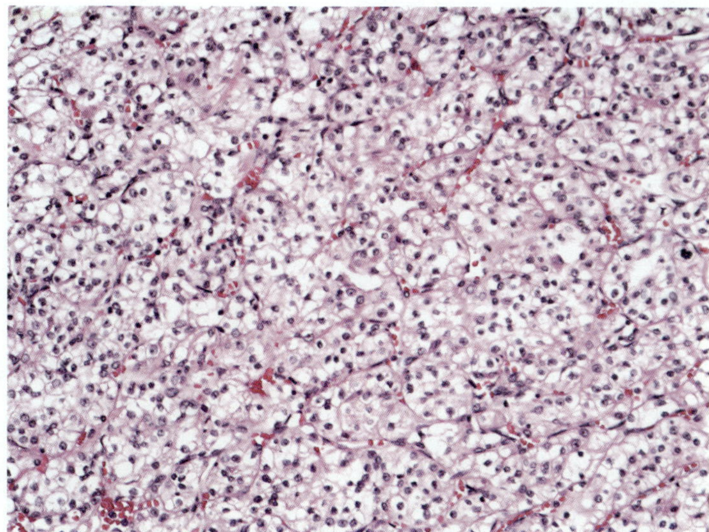

FIGURE 6.104 — Soft Tissue, Paraspinal, Metastatic Renal Cell Carcinoma (Histology). Nests of clear cells are seen surrounded by a rich network of small capillaries. The nuclei are round and have inconspicuous nucleoli. By immunohistochemistry, these cells were positive for carbonic anhydrase 9 and CD10. (Hematoxylin and eosin stain, medium power)

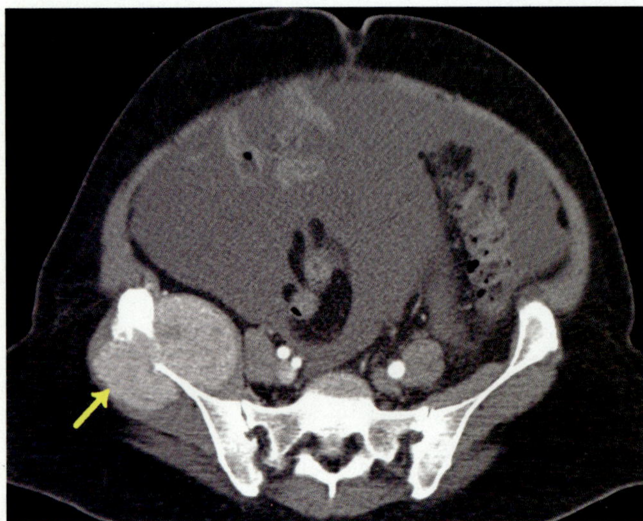

FIGURE 6.105 — Bone, Right Iliac Wing, Metastatic Adenocarcinoma. Axial contrast-enhanced CT image demonstrates an enhancing mass in the right iliac wing (arrow). There is associated destruction of the right iliac bone.

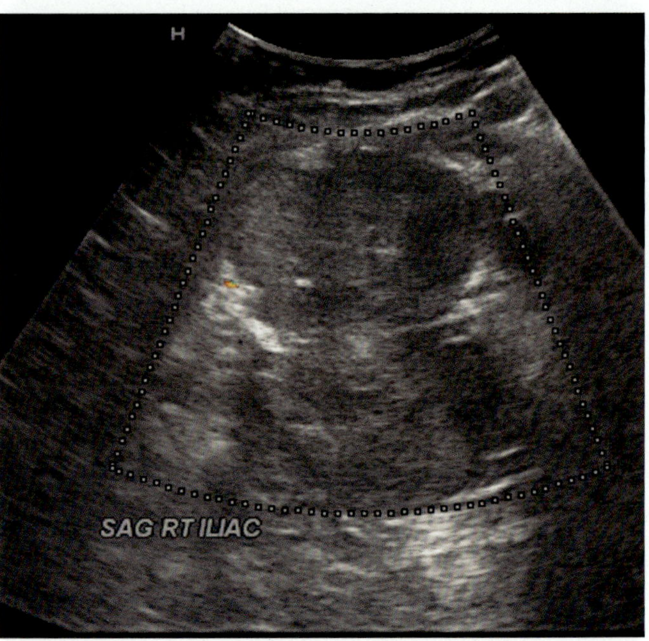

FIGURE 6.106 — Bone, Right Iliac Wing, Metastatic Adenocarcinoma. Sonographic image at the time of ultrasound-guided biopsy with color Doppler confirms heterogeneous right iliac wing mass with minimal vascularity.

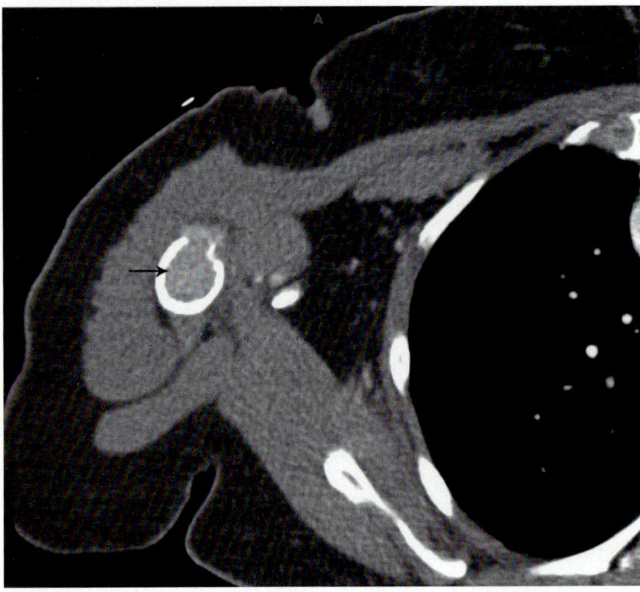

FIGURE 6.107 — Bone, Right Iliac Wing, Metastatic Adenocarcinoma. Patient has an additional soft tissue mass in the right humerus (arrow) with cortical destruction anteriorly. This represented another metastasis.

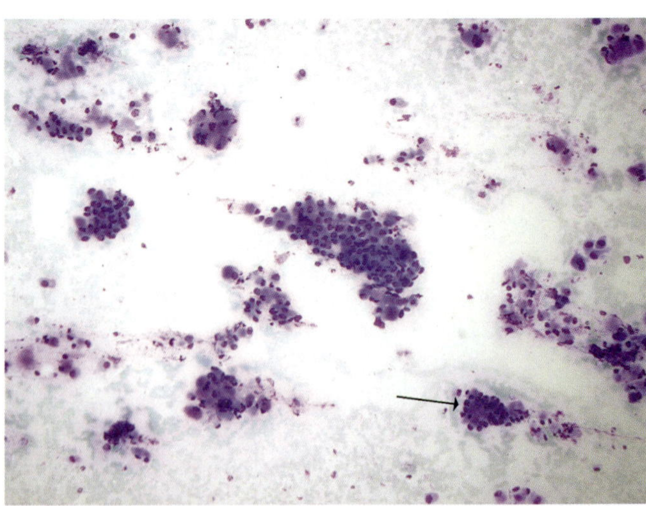

FIGURE 6.108 — Bone, Right Iliac Wing, Metastatic Adenocarcinoma. A cellular aspirate is shown with predominantly cohesive fragments of cells consistent with epithelial differentiation. A glandular structure is present (arrow) in addition to sheets of tumor cells. (Diff Quik stain, medium power).

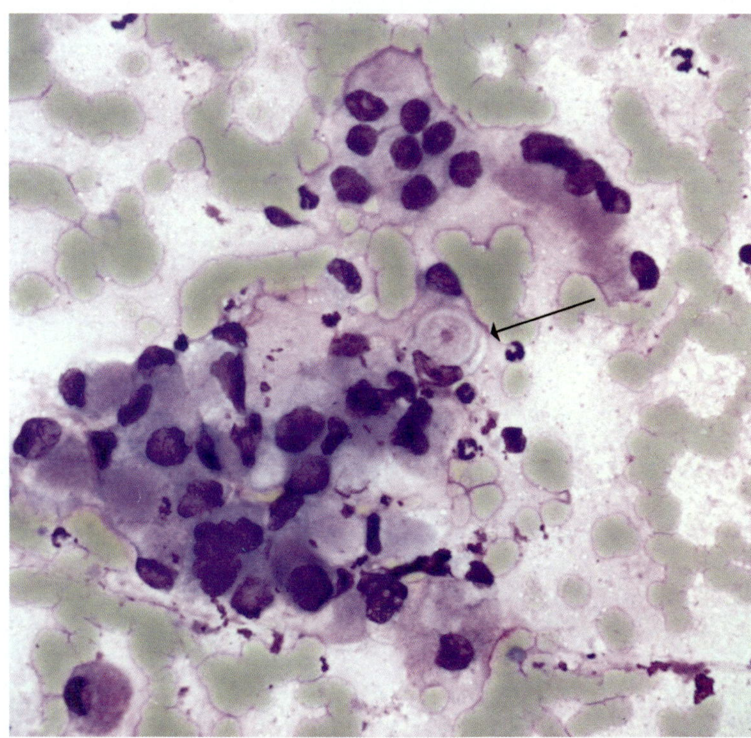

FIGURE 6.109 — Bone, Right Iliac Wing, Metastatic Adenocarcinoma. This fragment of cells shows a haphazard architectural arrangement. A single cell shows a cytoplasmic vacuole representing a mucin droplet (arrow). This patient had a history of lung adenocarcinoma. (Diff Quik stain, high power)

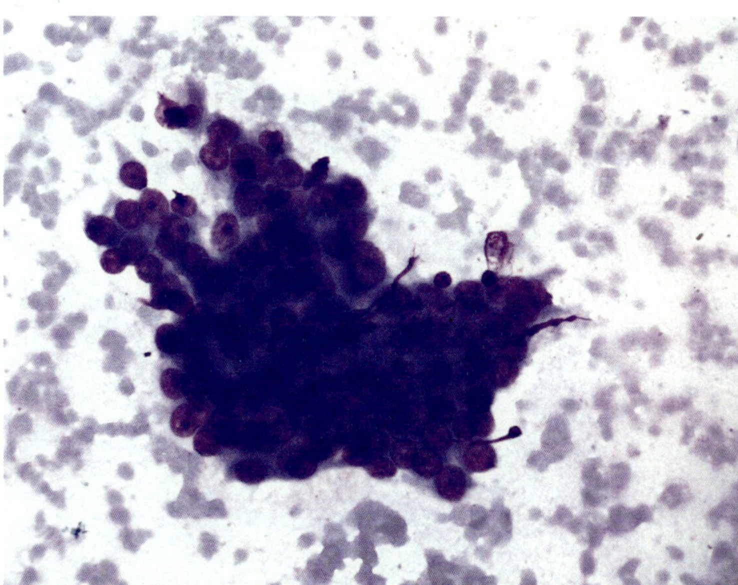

FIGURE 6.110 — Bone, Right Iliac Wing, Metastatic Adenocarcinoma. A sheet of epithelial cells shows a high nuclear-to-cytoplasmic ratio and occasional prominent nucleoli. Tumors that commonly metastasize to bone include lung, thyroid, kidney, prostate, and breast. (Diff Quik stain, high power)

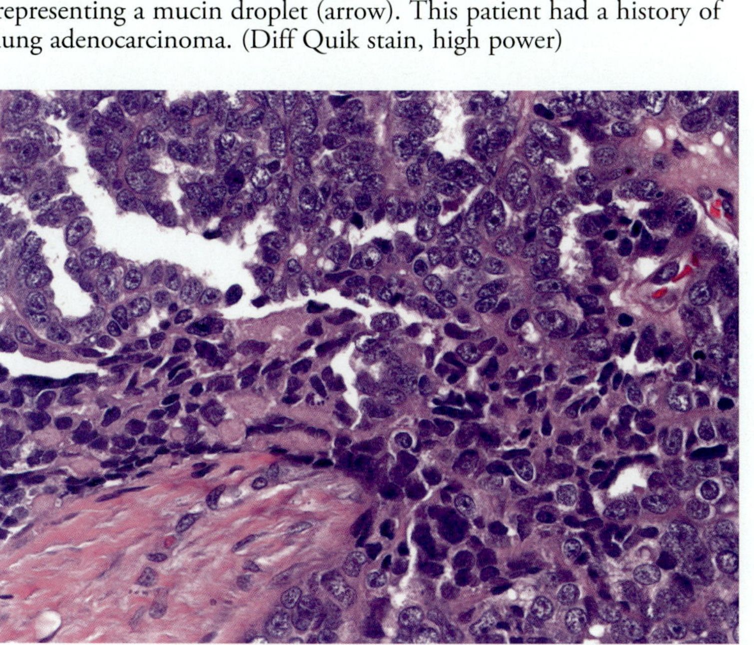

FIGURE 6.111 — Bone, Right Iliac Wing, Metastatic Adenocarcinoma (Histology). Malignant glandular formations are present. The nuclei are hyperchromatic and show prominent nucleoli. Immunohistochemistry was positive for CK7 and TTF-1, supporting a lung origin of the lesion. (Hematoxylin and eosin stain, high power)

Index